S0-BQI-348

Methods of Cell Separation

Volume 2

BIOLOGICAL SEPARATIONS

Series Editor: **Nicholas Catsimpoolas**
Massachusetts Institute of Technology
Cambridge, Massachusetts

Methods of Protein Separation, Volume 1
Edited by Nicholas Catsimpoolas

Methods of Protein Separation, Volume 2
Edited by Nicholas Catsimpoolas

Biological and Biomedical Applications of Isoelectric Focusing
Edited by Nicholas Catsimpoolas and James Drysdale

Methods of Cell Separation, Volume 1
Edited by Nicholas Catsimpoolas

Methods of Cell Separation, Volume 2
Edited by Nicholas Catsimpoolas

A Continuation Order Plan is available for this series. A continuation order will bring delivery of each new volume immediately upon publication. Volumes are billed only upon actual shipment. For further information please contact the publisher.

Methods of Cell Separation

Volume 2

Edited by
Nicholas Catsimpoolas
Massachusetts Institute of Technology

Plenum Press · New York and London

Library of Congress Cataloging in Publication Data

Main entry under title:

Methods of cell separation.

(Biological separations)
Includes bibliographies and index.
1. Cell separation. I. Catsimpoolas, Nicholas. II. Series. [DNLM: 1. Cell separation–Methods. WH25 M592]
QH585.M49 574.8'7'0724 77-11018
ISBN 0-306-40094-4 (vol. 2)

A Division of Plenum Publishing Corporation
227 West 17th Street, New York, N.Y. 10011

Printed in the United States of America

Contributors

Nicholas Catsimpoolas, *Biophysics Laboratory, Department of Nutrition and Food Science, Massachusetts Institute of Technology, Cambridge, Massachusetts*

Ann L. Griffith, *Biophysics Laboratory, Department of Nutrition and Food Science, Massachusetts Institute of Technology, Cambridge, Massachusetts*

Jack Y. Josefowicz, *Xerox Research Centre of Canada, Mississauga, Ontario, Canada*

Alexander Kolin, *Molecular Biology Institute, University of California, Los Angeles, California*

Robert C. Leif, *Papanicolaou Cancer Research Institute, Miami, Florida*

Howard C. Mel, *Institut de Pathologie Cellulaire, Hôpital Bicètre, Le Kremlin Bicètre, France, and Division of Medical Physics and Donner Laboratory, Lawrence Berkeley Laboratory, University of California, Berkeley, California*

Narla Mohandas, *Institut de Pathologie Cellulaire, Hôpital Bicètre, Le Kremlin Bicètre, France, and Departments of Laboratory Medicine and Medicine, Cancer Research Institute, University of California, San Francisco, California*

Preface

Presently, the need for methods involving separation, identification, and characterization of different kinds of cells is amply realized among immunologists, hematologists, cell biologists, clinical pathologists, and cancer researchers. Unless cells exhibiting different functions and stages of differentiation are separated from one another, it will be exceedingly difficult to study some of the molecular mechanisms involved in cell recognition, specialization, interactions, cytotoxicity, and transformation. Clinical diagnosis of diseased states and use of isolated cells for therapeutic (e.g., immunotherapy) or survival (e.g., transfusion) purposes are some of the pressing areas where immediate practical benefits can be obtained by applying cell separation techniques. However, the development of such useful methods is still in its infancy. A number of good techniques exist based either on the physical or biological properties of the cells, and these have produced some valuable results. Still others are to be discovered. Therefore, the purpose of this open-end treatise is to acquaint the reader with some of the basic principles, instrumentation, and procedures presently in practice at various laboratories around the world and to present some typical applications of each technique to particular biological problems. To this end, I was fortunate to obtain the contribution of certain leading scientists in the field of cell separation, people who in their pioneering work have struggled with the particular problems involved in separating living cells and in some way have won. It is hoped that new workers with fresh ideas will join us in the near future to achieve further and much needed progress in this important area of biological research.

Nicholas Catsimpoolas

Cambridge, Massachusetts

Contents

Chapter 1

1

Transient Electrophoretic and Sedimentation Analysis of Cells in Density Gradients

NICHOLAS CATSIMPOOLAS AND
ANN L. GRIFFITH

I. INTRODUCTION

Separation, identification, and characterization of mammalian cells represents one of the great challenges of present-day biological research. The elucidation of some of the most intricate problems in immunology, cell and molecular biology, and cancer research depends on new developments in the cell separations field. However, the diversity of mammalian cell properties can act both as a deterrent and as an enhancer of progress in this area. Therefore the coordinated utilization of physical, morphological, biological, and immunological characteristics of cells and their surfaces is necessary to accomplish the task of separation and analysis.

Recently, a new instrumentation system has been described (Catsimpoolas, 1974; Catsimpoolas *et al.*, 1975; Catsimpoolas and Griffith, 1977a,b) for the separation and characterization of cells by transient state electrophoresis (TRANS-EL), isoelectric focusing (TRANS-IF), and velocity sedimentation at 1*g* (TRANS-VELS) in isosmolar density gradients. These instruments are based on earlier prototypes (Catsimpoolas, 1971a,b) designed for the electrophoretic study of proteins. Monitoring of the cell

NICHOLAS CATSIMPOOLAS AND ANN L. GRIFFITH • Biophysics Laboratory, Department of Nutrition and Food Science, Massachusetts Institute of Technology, Cambridge, Massachusetts 02139.

migration in the electrical and 1*g* gravitational fields is performed *in situ* repetitively by "absorbance" (light extinction) and scattering measurements. Data acquisition, processing, and display is performed by a computer. Kinetic analysis of the cell distribution provides precise information on the electrophoretic mobility and sedimentation velocity of mammalian cells under standardized conditions. Selective applications of these methods to biological samples involving mammalian erythrocytes and lymphocytes have been reported (Catsimpoolas *et al.*, 1975, 1975; Catsimpoolas and Griffith, 1977a; Agathos *et al.*, 1977).

The availability of these techniques provides a new approach to biophysical studies concerning the surface charge and hydrodynamic properties of sedimenting cells. These parameters may be used as criteria of physical homogeneity and as a means in assessing alterations induced by experimental conditions (e.g., method of preparation, radiation, cryopreservation, etc.) or by events of immunological significance such as antigen and mitogen activation, cytotoxicity, interaction with surface probes, mixed culturing, and others. Additionally, diseased states may alter in some way the physical characteristics of cells, which if measured precisely may provide supplementary information for diagnosis and the monitoring of therapeutic progress.

II. INSTRUMENTATION

A. General Considerations

Cell surface charge density has been traditionally measured indirectly by the technique of microscope chamber electrophoresis (Ambrose, 1965) and recently by laser Doppler spectroscopy (Uzgiris and Kaplan, 1974; Smith *et al.*, 1976) and endless fluid belt electrophoresis (Sturgeon *et al.*, 1972). These instrumental techniques provide valuable information regarding the electrophoretic mobility of cells in free solution; although actual physical separation of cells is not achieved by the first two methods. With the advent of isosmolar preparative density gradient electrophoresis (Boltz *et al.*, 1973; Griffith *et al.*, 1975), the need was realized for measuring the mobility of cells in gradients of supporting media rather than in free solution and under conditions of actual physical separation. In addition, there was a need to explore other types of electrophoresis (e.g., isoelectric focusing and isotachophoresis) which cannot be investigated by the above-mentioned instruments and procedures. Furthermore, the sedimentation behavior of cells at 1*g* cannot be measured precisely by the available preparative techniques.

For the aforementioned reasons, a single-column prototype instrument was constructed which allowed electrophoretic analysis of cells in density gradients (Catsimpoolas, 1974; Catsimpoolas *et al.*, 1975). The small-diameter (i.e., 6 mm i.d.) column of the instrument required careful coating of the walls to avoid electroosmosis. Also light-scattering measurements could not be performed. Consequently, a multicolumn (bearing large-diameter, 16 mm i.d. tubes) instrument called TRANS-Analyzer was designed and constructed (Catsimpoolas and Griffith, 1977b) which permitted simultaneous measurement of absorbance and scattering or fluorescence. In parallel and in consultation with one of the authors (N.C.), a commercial instrument (TRANSANALYZER™) was developed by Bascom–Turner Instruments, Inc., Newton, Massachusetts, employing a novel optical scanning system. All three instruments are briefly described below, as their design varies.

B. The Single-Column Instrument

A schematic diagram of the single-column instrument is shown in Fig. 1 and a photograph in Fig. 2. A 200-W xenon–mercury arc lamp and associated power supply (Schoeffel) are used in conjunction with a tandem grating monochromator (Schoeffel GM100D) to produce monochromatic energy in the 200- to 700-nm-wavelength range of very low stray light characteristics (e.g., $1{:}10^4$ at 220 nm) (Fig. 3). The monochromatic light beam is subsequently collimated by a quartz lens, shaped by a variable horizontal slit (50 to 100 μm), passes through the electrophoresis cells, and is thereafter directed to the sample and reference photomultipliers. The light beam is divided to simultaneously illuminate the sample and reference cells. Each beam is detected separately by its photomultiplier and the log of the ratio of both signals, i.e., the linear absorbance, is provided electronically (Schoeffel Model SD 3000 Spectrodensitometer). The ratioing of the signals eliminates errors due to possible fluctuations of light intensity and photomultiplier high voltage. A knob balance control and zero meter (provided on the panel) permit matching spectral sensitivity levels of the photomultipliers in any desired spectral range. This adjustment makes the electrical outputs equal (signal ratio of 1:1) which is equivalent to zero optical density (O.D.) at the beginning of the scan, with the sample beam in a "neutral" area of the media to be measured. A panel meter (0.0–3.0 O.D. units) is also provided with a "zero" control knob. Seven O.D. full-scale ranges (0.1, 0.2, 0.4, 1.0, 2.0, 4.0, and 10.0) can be selected on the front panel. The photometer supplies an electrical output of 1 V per 1 O.D. unit for computer processing and 100 mV full scale (at any O.D. range) for operating a recorder. Single (sample photomultiplier only) or ratio recording of absorbance and scattering is available in the instrument.

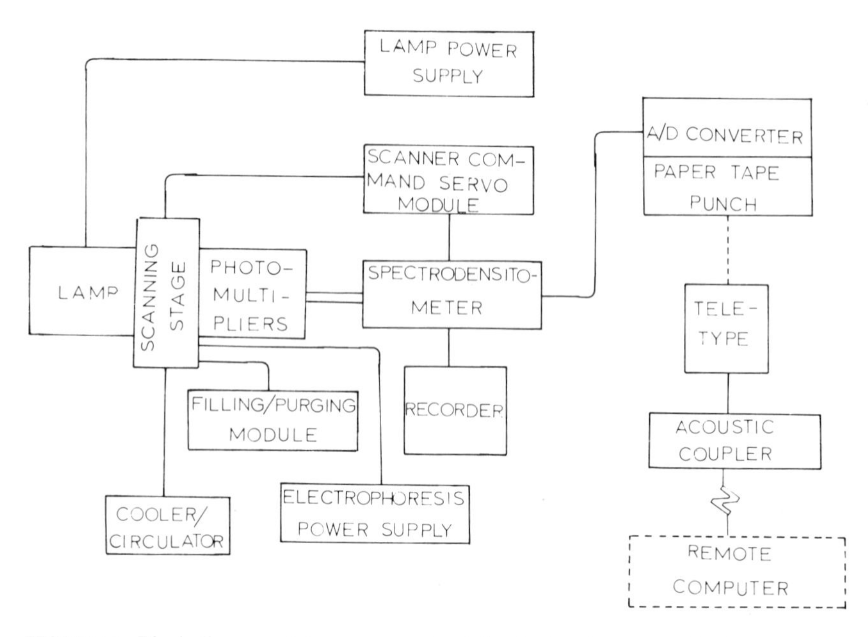

FIGURE 1. Block diagram of the components of the single-column scanning instrument.

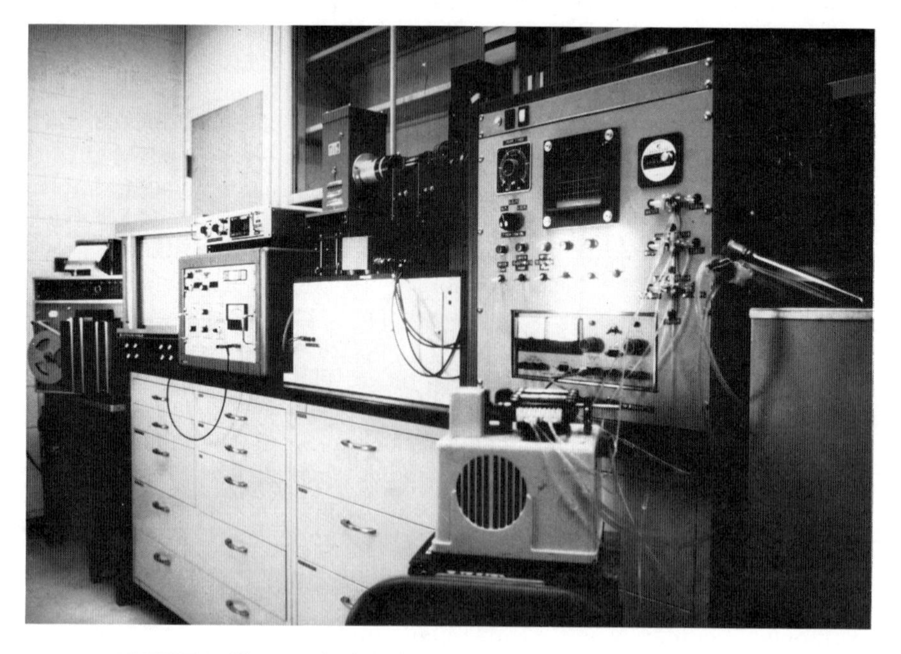

FIGURE 2. Photograph of the instrumentation system shown in Fig. 1.

The scanning-stage module provides dark housing for the removable electrophoresis cassette, and vertical (linear) transport stage by means of a reversible stepping motor attached to a leadscrew (Fig. 3). The stepping motor and adjustable frequency generator provide six reversible scanning speeds of 5, 10, 20, 40, 80, and 160 s/cm. Upper and lower microswitch stops make possible manual actuation and automatic stopping of the scanner at predetermined column intervals.

The linear transport stage and associated instrumentation are automatically controlled by the "scanner control servo unit." This is accomplished as follows. A 2.5K "scanner pickoff" linear displacement potentiometer is mechanically fixed to the moving stage. The potentiometer is driven from an appropriately scaled voltage source; this results in the potentiometer output voltage being numerically equivalent to the position of the scanner in centimeters to 0.05% accuracy. This potential is impedance transformed and fed to a digital panel meter (Newport 2000) which provides a digital readout of the scanner position in centimeters. The signal is also supplied to two amplifiers which are in a double limit comparator configuration. Two 10K ten-turn potentiometers serve to allow setting up "high" and "low" scanner-travel-limit positions and are calibrated directly in centimeters to

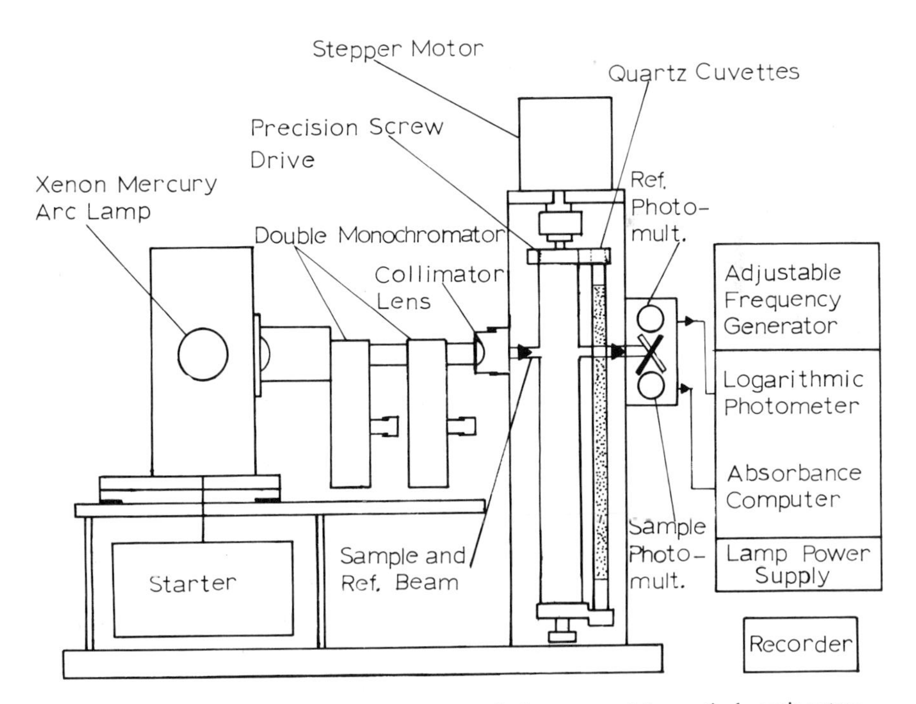

FIGURE 3. Schematic diagram of the electrooptical system and the vertical scaning stage.

three places. The comparator continuously compares the limit potentiometer settings with the pickoff signal and issues motor-reversing commands to the memory/switching element accordingly. The memory/switching element is essentially equivalent to a set–reset flip flop, but features versatile switching capability and high noise immunity. One set of relay contacts function as a latch and provide the "memory" function. A second set of contacts sources the reversing information to the motor. Another set of contacts automatically operates the "sweep" and "reset" functions of an X-Y recorder and also commands the paper tape punch to issue a leader (blank) space on the tape. A final set of contacts provides for the motor to run at a higher speed in the "down" scan mode. All the functions of the scanner command servo may be overridden (and performed manually) through panel switches.

The practical implications of the scanner control servo unit are several. The scanning interval (in centimeters) can be selected digitally and be set at any part in the column by means of two control knobs (high and low position). A digital display of column position with respect to the light beam is available at all times during scanning. The recorder and paper tape punch are actuated automatically during the entire electrophoretic experiment. Finally the scanner can be commanded to run automatically at different speeds in the "up" or "down" mode of travel. This allows collecting data either in both directions of travel, or preferentially at normal speed in the "up" mode accompanied by fast reversal in the "down" mode without data collection.

The column cassette is removable and accommodates two quartz columns (Amersil, Suprasil T-20) (Fig. 4). The dimensions of the columns are: 6.0 mm i.d., 8.0 mm o.d., and 142 mm long. Only one column carries the sample for analysis, the other acts as reference background in balancing the photometer output. In density gradient experiments the bottom of the column is covered either with a semipermeable membrane, or with a polyacrylamide gel plug. The cassette also accommodates the upper and lower flow-through electrolyte reservoirs with removable platinum electrodes and a flow-through cooler block for circulating cooling liquid. An additional outlet is provided at the top of the lower reservoir to allow escape of air bubbles during loading. The total cassette can be easily disassembled for cleaning.

The filling/purging/cooling module consists of a multichannel Technicon Autoanalyzer proportioning pump, a vacuum pump, Hamilton chemically inert valves, a thermostatted cooler–circulator, and associated tubing (Fig. 5). The function of the assembly is to recirculate the buffers into the upper and lower electrolyte reservoirs during the electrophoretic run, purge and wash the flow system at the end of the run, and circulate fluid through

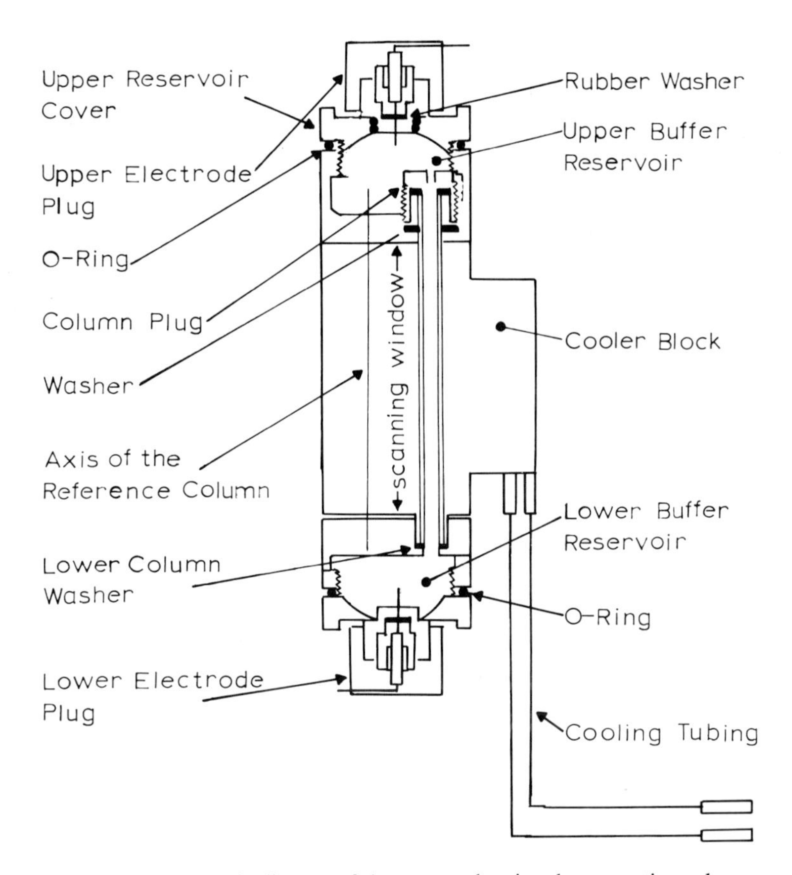

FIGURE 4. Schematic diagram of the cassette bearing the separation column.

the cooling block. The buffer glass reservoirs are kept in the bath of the cooler for temperature equilibration.

A regulated DC power supply providing both constant voltage and constant current operation is used for electrophoresis and isoelectric focusing experiments. The photometer output is recorded with an Esterline–Angus Model 2417 TB X-Y and Y-t recorder automatically controlled by the scanner control servo unit.

The digital data acquisition module consists of an analog-to-digital converter with visual display, two-channel analog multiplexer, variable-speed sampler, a paper tape punch, a teletype, and an acoustic coupler. Data can be punched at a switch-selectable rate of one to twenty readings per second. Other provisions include choice of three gain settings, single- or double-channel operation, and single or continuous sampling of the data.

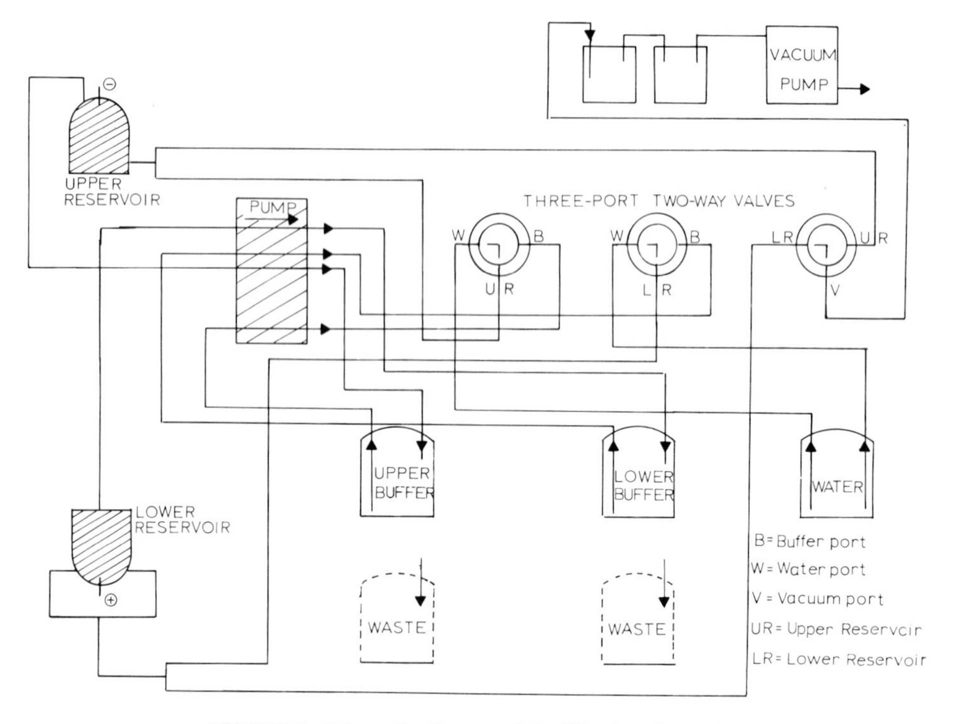

FIGURE 5. Schematic diagram of the filling/purging unit.

The acquired data punched on the paper tape are processed by a remote computer via the teletype acoustic coupler module. In addition a digital multiplexer–logger provides readout of temperature, voltage, current, and power on a teletype.

Operation of the instrument is performed as follows. The upper and lower buffer in glass containers are placed in the constant temperature bath for thermal equilibration. Cooling fluid also is allowed to flow through the cooling block of the cassette. The quartz column, covered at the lower end with a dialysis membrane sheet premoistened with the lower buffer, is placed in the cassette, and the density gradient is prepared *in situ*. Concurrent with the above operation, the buffer is pumped into the lower electrolyte reservoir. The sample solution is then applied on top of the gradient and carefully layered with the upper buffer; thus filling the remainder of the column. Subsequently, the buffer is pumped into the upper reservoir with the upper chamber cover in position. The upper electrode plug is then inserted carefully to avoid pressure in the column. The electrophoresis power supply is turned on for a few seconds to establish the passage of current. The electrophoresis cassette is placed in the scanning-stage module and the lid is closed. The photometer is adjusted to zero at a "neutral" area of the column and a preliminary scan is obtained to establish the baseline before the current is turned on for the experiment. During electrophoresis the buffers are circulating through the upper and lower electrode reservoirs thus removing undesirable products and air bubbles generated by the platinum electrodes. The column is scanned continuously during the experiment, providing both an analog signal recorded on the recorder chart and digital data punched on the paper tape. At the conclusion of the experiment, the pump is stopped and the buffer in the reservoirs and tubing is removed by vacuum suction. The column is removed, appropriate plugs are inserted, and the total buffer circulation system is washed with water and purged repetitively by means of the filling/purging module.

Because of its small diameter, the quartz column is coated before use with density gradients to prevent electroendosmosis by a modification of the procedure described by Hjertén (1967). Methylcellulose (Methocel, visc. 8000 centipoise, Dow Chemical Company) (0.4*g*) is dispersed in 30 ml hot (boiling) water and stirred until a lumpfree dispersion is formed. An additional 70 ml of cold (4°C) water is added and stirring is resumed in the cold room until the solution appears clear. Formic acid (7 ml) and then formaldehyde (35 ml) are added, with stirring. The final solution is clarified by filtration and can be stored in the refrigerator for at least 6 months. The quartz tube is washed thoroughly with a detergent solution, hot and cold tap water, distilled water, and dried. The methylcellulose solution is drawn into the tube by suction and after 5 min is allowed to run out slowly. Subsequently, the tube is dried in a 120°C oven for 40 min. The coating and drying procedures are repeated once more. Care should be exercised to avoid air bubble adherence to the tube wall and to keep the tube in the vertical position during coating.

C. The TRANS-Analyzer Prototype System

A block diagram of the TRANS-Analyzer is shown in Fig. 6. Cell separation takes place in jacketed quartz tubes (16 mm i.d., 18 mm o.d., and 150 mm length) made of Suprasil T20 (Amersil, Inc., Hillside, N.J.) which bear upper and lower Pt electrode reservoirs with provisions for continuous buffer circulation (Fig. 7). The inlet and outlet ports are machined to accept Cheminert (Laboratory Data Control, Riviera Beach, Fla.) tubing connectors to facilitate cleaning and sterilization. Up to ten interconnected columns can be accommodated on the scanner. Alterna-

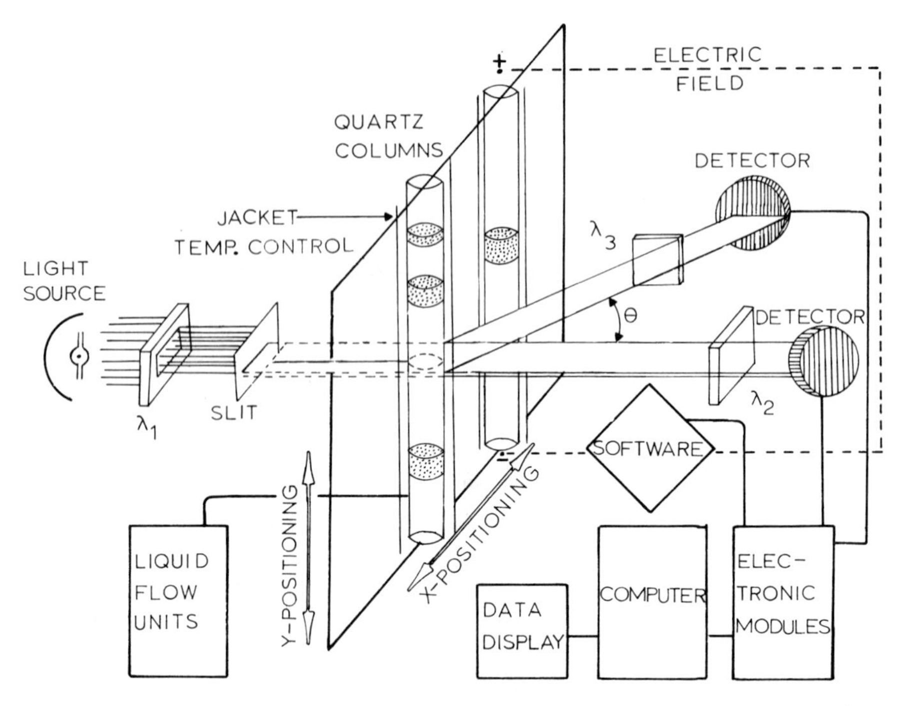

FIGURE 6. Schematic diagram of the prototype TRANS-Analyzer multicolumn scanning instrument.

tively, a six-column cassette (see below) designed for the commercial instrument TRANSANALYZER™ can be employed.

A Lauda K-4/R cooler–circulator (Brinkmann Instruments) provides temperature control for the column(s). An ISCO Model 570 gradient former (Instrumentation Specialties, Lincoln, Neb.) is used to prepare the stabilization gradient. An ISCO Model 1330 syringe pump and a SAGE Model 375A peristaltic pump are used for chase-solution infusion and buffer recirculation, respectively. Distribution of fluids is carried out by the use of Cheminert (Laboratory Data Control) and Hamilton (Hamilton Co., Reno, Nev.) valves.

The X and Y movement of the scanner is controlled by two stepping motors (Fig. 8). The vertical (Y) scanning rate can be varied from 0.01 to 1.00 mm/s and it is used to move each column up and down in front of a stationary slit (100 μm) of light. The horizontal (X) movement of the scanner positions each column sequentially in the path of the light beam which is generated by 200-W xenon–mercury compact arc lamp (Hanovia

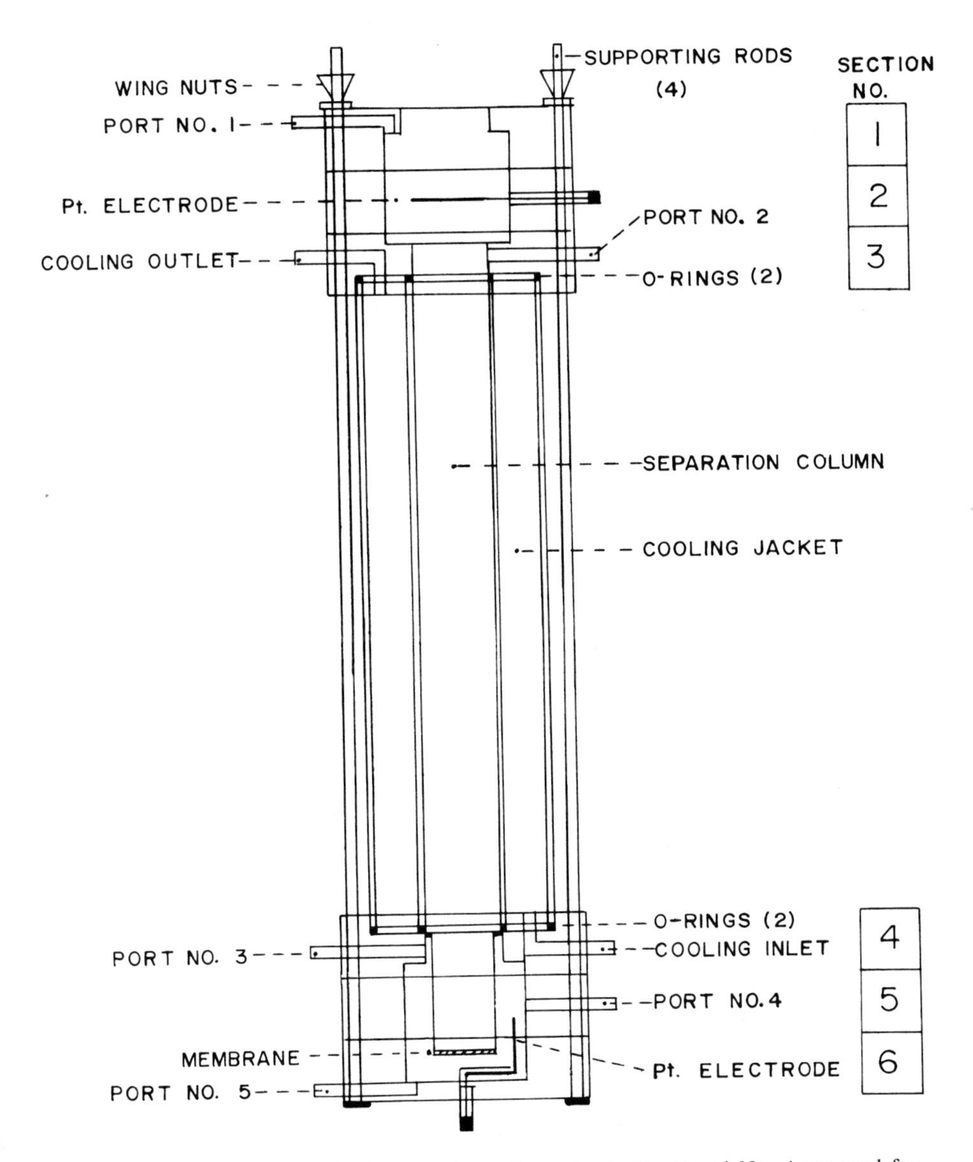

FIGURE 7. Diagram of a single separation column. Ports No. 5 and No. 4 are used for circulating the lower buffer and ports No. 2 and No. 1 for the upper buffer. The column consists of six sections and two concentric cylindrical tubes which can be easily disassembled for cleaning.

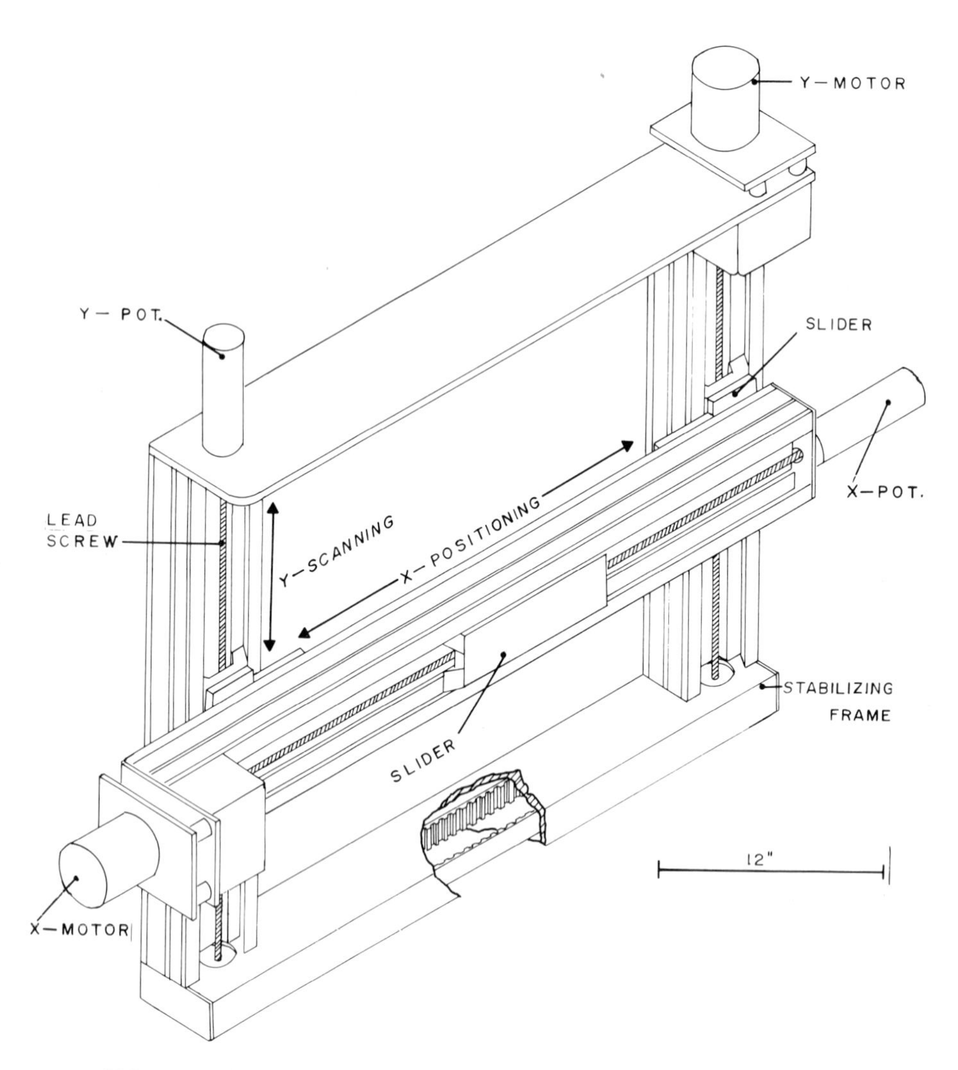

FIGURE 8. Diagram of the X-Y scanning-stage module of the TRANS-Analyzer.

901B-1) housed in a Schoeffel (Westwood, N.J.) Model LH 150 unit (Fig. 9). The lamp housing features a fused silica lens (f/1.5) in a focusing sleeve and forced air cooling. The lamp is started and operated by a Schoeffel Model LPS 251 current-regulated DC power source. The collimated beam is UV-filtered and is refocused as a horizontal slit of light in the cross-sectional center of the column. At the exit, the beam is detected at 0° and 15° angles by two side-on photomultipliers (Hamamatsu R777) after refocusing and passage through a second set of filters of selective wavelength. The "absorbance" light is filtered (λ_2) through an ORIEL (Stamford, Conn.) No. G522-6200 filter peaking at 6192 Å. The "scattering" light is filtered (λ_3) through ORIEL No. G522-5200 filter peaking at 5206 Å with half-band width of 92 Å. An aus JENA (Fairfield, N.J.) No. 304758:131.008 frosted glass is used as UV-absorbing filter and diffuser (λ_1).

The "absorbance" (light extinction) and "scattering" of the cells in the column are recorded by two Schoeffel M460 photometers coupled to a dual-channel strip-chart recorder (Model 2802, Laboratory Data Control) (Fig. 10). In addition, the photometer output is digitized (DATOS 308, EH Research Laboratories, Oakland, Cal.) and punched by a Roytron 500 unit (Litton ABS, Pine Brook, N.J.) on paper tape for off-line computer data processing and display. Additional electronic units (homemade) instruct the recorder, A/D multiplexer, and paper tape punch to record data at the initiation of a scan and also to issue leader tape at its termination. An auxiliary data logger/multiplexer is interfaced to the X-Y scanner control unit and provides a teletype output identifying the column being scanned, the elapsed time, column temperature, and electric output of the electrophoresis power supply (Williams and Catsimpoolas, 1976).

A block diagram of the data processing and display system is shown in Fig. 11. It consists of a PDP-11/10 computer (Digital Equipment Corpora-

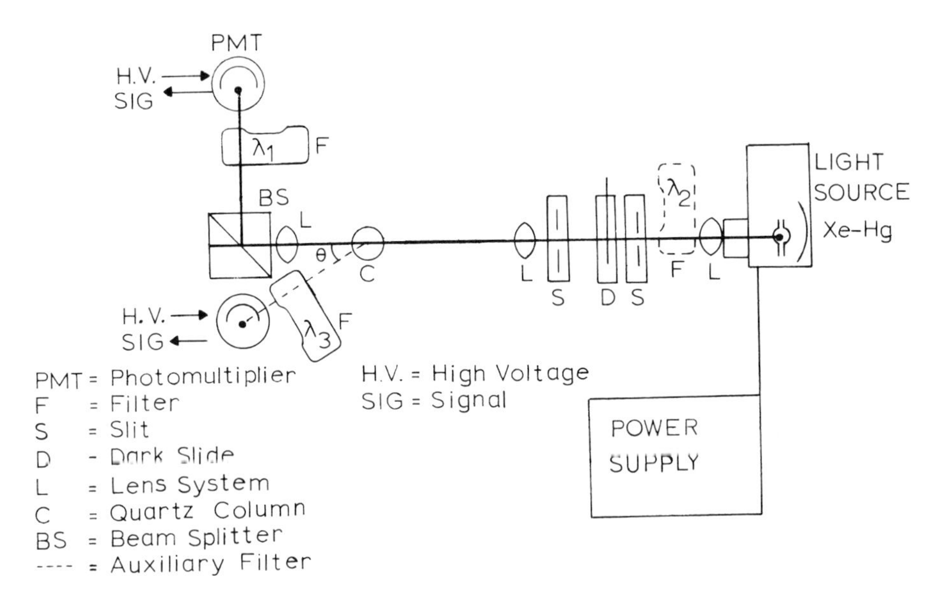

FIGURE 9. The optical system of the TRANS-Analyzer.

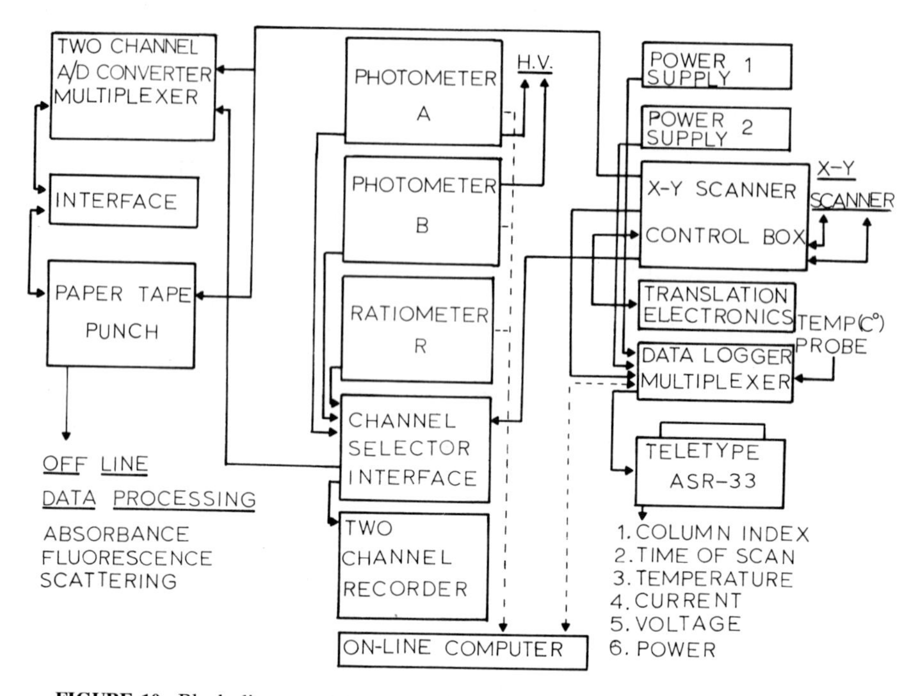

FIGURE 10. Block diagram of the electronic control units and data-acquisition modules.

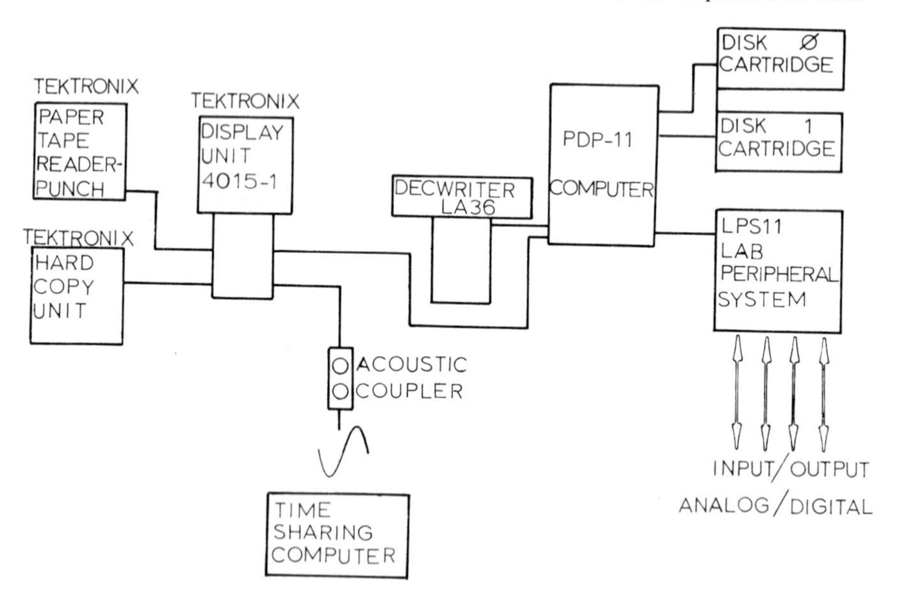

FIGURE 11. Block diagram of the data processing and display system.

tion, Maynard, Mass.) with 16K memory, dual RK05 disk cartridge, LA36 DECKWRITER II, and LPS11 lab peripheral system. The latter includes programmable real-time clock with dual Schmitt triggers, selectable differential input for 4 A/D channels, program-transfer 12-bit A/D with dual sample hold, 8-channel expansion multiplexer, and 16-bit buffered digital I/O with TTI capabilities. The PDP-11 computer is coupled to a Tektronix 4015-1 computer display terminal (Tektronix, Beaverton, Ore.) via a KL11-S interface (DEC). The Tektronix display is equipped with a Model 4911 high-speed tape reader/perforator unit (Tektronix) and a Model 4631 hard-copy unit (Tektronix). In addition the display terminal is interfaced via an acoustic coupler to a large digital computer (time sharing). This arrangement allows for fast acquisition, processing, storage, and display of data from the TRANS-Analyzer instrument.

D. The TRANSANALYZER™

1. The Optical System

Bascom–Turner Instruments (Newton, Mass.) produces a commercial version of the scanning apparatus called the TRANSANALYZER™ which is based on prototype designs by Catsimpoolas.

The optical system employs a series of scanning and stationary mirrors to move the light beam from a fixed source vertically along a single separation column (Y scanning). X-positioning of a series of columns in the light path is carried out by a mechanically moving stage. In more detail the system works as follows. The light source is a General Electric GE 1974, 6-V, 20-W tungsten–halogen lamp regulated by a power supply. As shown in Fig. 12, the horizontal slit S1(100–150 μm) shapes the beam which is reflected by mirror M1 and passes through filter F1. F1 is a narrow-band filter used to select the desired part of the spectral output. Mirror M2 reflects the beam onto mirror M3. Mirror M3 and its twin M3′ are mounted at the opposite ends of a shaft and perform the vertical (Y) scanning function. The movement of the shaft is regulated through the cam to produce a uniform scanning velocity along the separation column. The shaft and the cam are mechanically actuated by a stepper motor. As the scanning mirror M3 oscillates between the limits of a fixed angle, the beam travels vertically on the flat mirror M4, is reflected on the curved mirror M5, and scans the length of the column. A mirror-strip M6 mounted on the rear optical plate of the cassette redirects the beam between two columns and through mirrors M5′, M4′, M3′, and M7, and a diffuser D1 onto the photomultiplier window. The optical system is designed to produce an approximately perpendicular beam at all positions of the column.

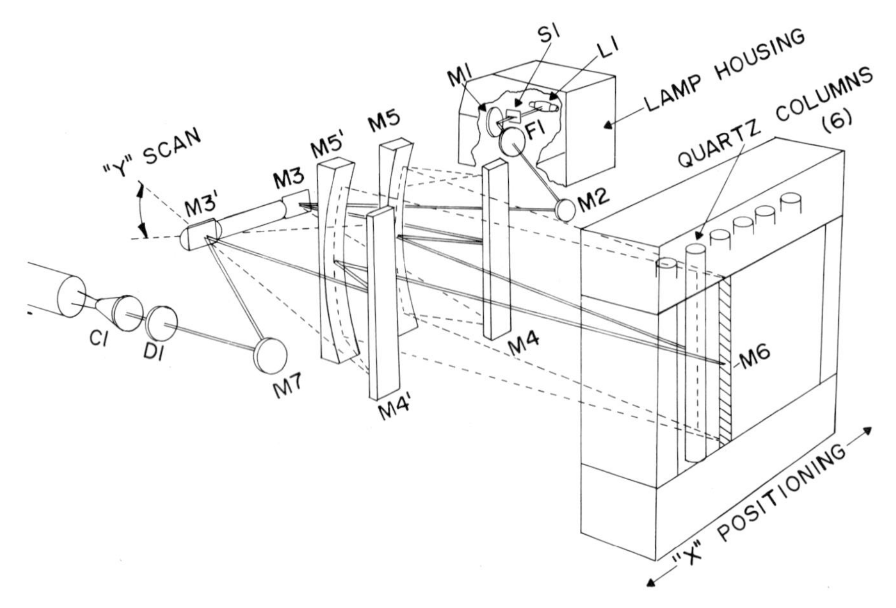

FIGURE 12. Diagram of the optical system of the TRANSANALYZER™ (courtesy Bascom–Turner Instruments).

2. *The Cassette Module*

The electrophoresis cassette shown in Fig. 13 consists of two buffer chambers (upper and lower), a central cooling compartment, and six removable columns (18 mm o.d., 16 mm i.d., 21.6 cm length). Platinum wire electrodes and parts for buffer circulation are provided in the upper and lower chambers. The cassette surfaces exposed to the light beam are made of special optical glass. The rear plate (facing the operator) bears the mirror-strips for beam reflection. The individual columns and the main cassette can be entirely disassembled for cleaning.

A reversible roller pump with individual pumping heads and control valves is used for filling, purging, and washing the buffer chambers. The coolant is supplied by an external cooler/circulator bath. However, coolant flow rate is adjusted by means of a panel flow meter and a bypass valve in order to avoid undue pressure to the plates of the cassette.

The horizontal (X) movement of the cassette is done by a stepper motor through a leadscrew mounted on the front side of cabinet B. Sensing switches limit the cassette travel distance on both sides of the leadscrew. The X movement positions either sequentially or selectively the six columns in the path of the Y-scanning beam.

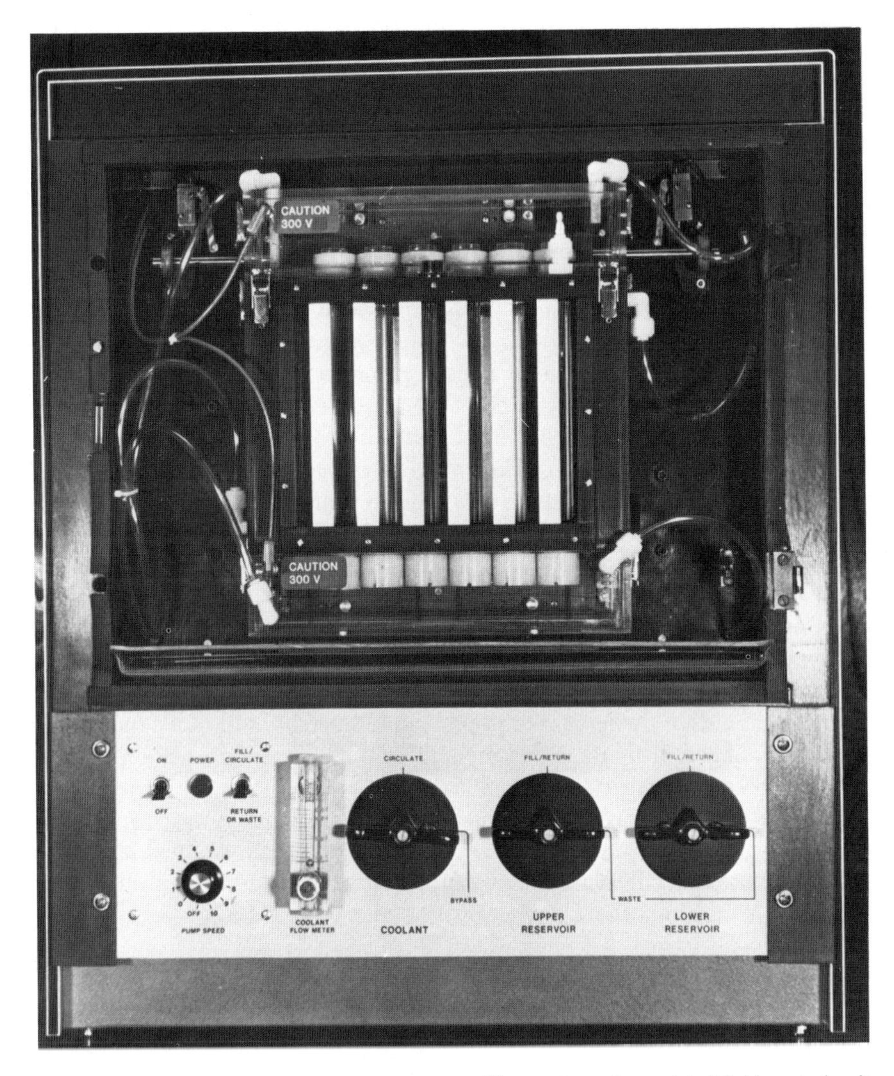

FIGURE 13. Photograph of the TRANSANALYZER™ cassette and associated fluid control unit (courtesy Bascom–Turner Instruments).

3. *The Electronic Modules*

A digital photometer capable of measuring optical density or percent transmittance is an integral part of the instrument. This unit permits selection of gain and dark current and full scale adjustments for optical performance when different stabilization media are used in the column (Fig. 14). A stepwise adjustment of high voltage (400, 600, 800, 1000, and 1200 V) is provided to power the end-on photomultiplier tube. An overload condition of the photomultiplier is indicated by a lit button and results in automatic power cut-off to the photomultiplier tube. Power can be restored by a "reset" function. The Y-scanning rate can be set to be 0.05, 0.1, 0.2, 0.4, and 0.8 cm/s. The position of the light beam on the particular column being scanned is indicated (000 to 999 positions) by a digital display. This feature is helpful in positioning the light beam at any particular distance in the column and also in obtaining a visual indication of beam travel. The operator may select any one of the six columns for scanning by actuating six switches on the tube selection panel. The particular column being scanned is shown by displaying digitally the corresponding column number. A digital clock counts elapsed time to 10^5 s to enable the operator to record the occurrence of a particular event. A reset button starts the clock from zero time as required. The scanning interval (cycle of scanning all selected columns in sequence) can be set in 100-s intervals from zero to 9900.

Other convenient features of the instrument include: (a) a "home" button which always positions column No. 1 in the light path, regardless of previous location, (b) a "calibrate" function which scans all columns and records in memory background data for each column, (c) a "data" function which initiates a cycle of scans and automatically subtracts the stored background data from the experimental scanning data of each column, (d) a "stop" button which stops all mechanical movements of the scanner, and (e) a "data continue" function which resumes scanning as programmed. In addition, a constant-current power supply provides adjustable current for electrophoresis. The photometer output can be directed to a strip-chart recorder or to any other data acquisition and processing system.

4. *Comments*

The TRANSANALYZER™ employs a relatively complex optical system in order to avoid the mechanical movement of the cassette itself in the Y direction. The design is elegant but it cannot entirely duplicate the scanning features of the simple mechanical stage movement. Part of the reason for this is that the light beam transcribes a shallow S-curve as it travels the length of the column. This causes considerable background noise and a

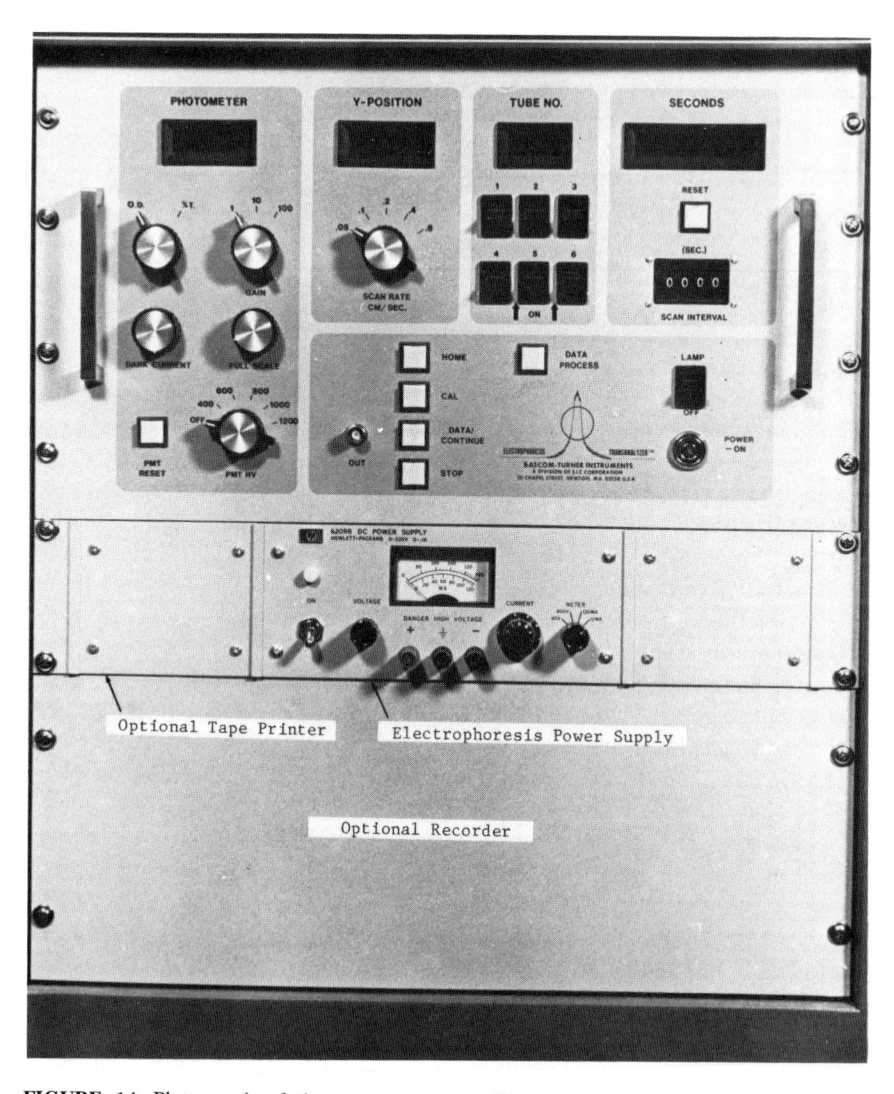

FIGURE 14. Photograph of the TRANSANALYZER™ electronic units (courtesy Bascom–Turner Instruments).

sloping irregular baseline which is fortunately constant in each scan of the same column. Thus, it is necessary to subtract the "stored" baseline of each column (obtained before sample application) from the raw data of each scan. Some small error in the absorbance measurements of the sample can occur because the path length along a cylindrical tube is not constant if the light beam does not travel exactly vertically. However, for most applications involving cells this is not a serious drawback.

III. DATA ACQUISITION AND PROCESSING

A. Data Acquisition

The analog signal from the photomultiplier during the scanning of the column is a continuous current (or voltage) whose amplitude is proportional to the absorbance being measured. In order to be processed by a computer the analog voltage must be digitized to produce a word whose number of bits after conversion is equivalent to the input voltage. To avoid large errors, the maximum input voltage has to be amplified to the maximum voltage that the analog-to-digital converter can accommodate, e.g., 10 V. A digital voltmeter can measure voltages as low as a few microvolts with as little as 0.01% error, but analog-to-digital conversion requires at least 10 ms for completion. In practice, this means that we can obtain a maximum of 100 data points from a peak 0.1 cm wide (at the base) at a scanning speed of 10 s/cm. Such slow converters act as a low pass filter and thereby smooth the data to a considerable extent. However, fast analog-to-digital converters can process an 8-bit word in less than 10 μs, which is indeed much faster than is normally required in the present system. In this case, amplification of the input signal is usually necessary.

In the present experiments with the prototype instruments the analog signal produced by the photometer is digitized by an analog-to-digital converter at preselected time intervals. Since the mechanical scanning speed v of the column is contant, the digitized values represent the photometer signal amplitude at equidistant points (i.e., center of the window width formed by the slit) (Fig. 15). This is practically possible only if the rate of analog-to-digital conversion is very fast in comparison to the mechanical transport of the column. The number of data points j obtained per peak depends on the velocity v (centimeters per second) of the scanner, the digitizing rate g (data points per second), and the total width w_t (centimeters) of the peak profile at the baseline, so that

$$j = gw_t/v \tag{1}$$

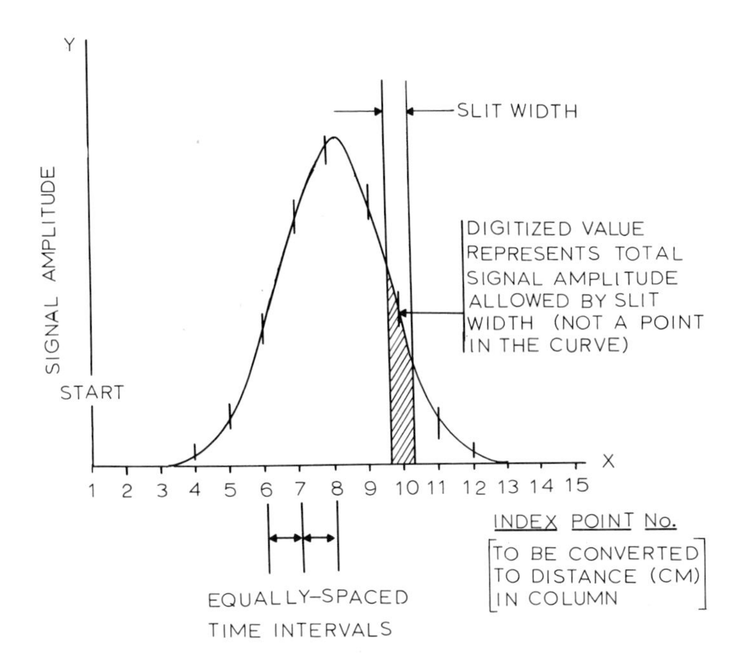

FIGURE 15. Diagram of the process of digitizing the absorbance profile of a distribution. Digitizing rate = number of index points per second.

To a first approximation, the narrower the slit width(s), the more accurately the peak profile will be recorded. However, the narrower the slit width, the larger is the random noise in the signal. A large slit width smooths the data by averaging the light absorbance over a larger window. In practice, the slit width should be approximately equal to the ratio w_t/j. Depending on baseline noise and peak shape (Catsimpoolas and Griffith, 1973) the desired value of j can be set between 10 and 100. If the peaks are of Gaussian shape, 10 data points may be sufficient to obtain their statistical moments. The more asymmetric the peak, the more data points are needed for its characterization. The total number of points k to be acquired per scan depends also on the peak capacity n which is defined as the maximum number of peaks resolvable in the column, so that

$$k = jn \tag{2}$$

The peak capacity depends primarily on the average standard deviation $\bar{\sigma}$ (centimeters) of typical peaks. Since adjacent peaks can be considered completely resolved if the peak heights are at a distance of $4\bar{\sigma}$ from each other, the value of n can be approximated by $L/4\bar{\sigma}$, where L (centimeters) is the length of the column.

After acquisition, the digitized data can be stored on punched paper tape, magnetic tape, disks, or other data-storage devices. The speed at which these devices store data must be compatible with the data-acquisition rate.

B. Smoothing of Data

The primary information from a scanning frame should be in the form of absorbance or percent transmittance of the compounds of interest versus the distance in the column. However, random errors which are characteristically described as noise are often superimposed on this information in an indistinguishable manner. Removal of the noise without degrading the underlying information can be performed by convoluted least-squares differentiation procedures (Grushka, 1975). Two important restrictions have to be taken into consideration in this type of analysis. First, the digitized data points must be at a fixed, uniform interval in the chosen abscissa (i.e., distance or time). In other words, each data point must be obtained at the same time interval from each preceding point. Second, the curves formed by graphing the points must be continuous and more or less smooth. All of the errors are assumed to be in the ordinate (absorbance, percent transmittance) and none in the abscissa.

The least-squares calculations are carried out by convolution of the data points with properly chosen sets of integers. In this procedure, we take a fixed number of points and evaluate the central point by a convoluting function (i.e., quadratic) followed by normalization (Fig. 16). Next, the point at one end of the group is dropped, the next point at the other end is added, and the process is repeated. Table 1 contains the convolution integers and their normalizing factors for smoothing (zeroth derivative) polynomials of degrees 2 and 3 from 5 to 15 fixed numbers of points. As an example, the equation for smoothing a 5-point quadratic or cubic convolute is

$$y = (-3y_{-02} + 12y_{-01} + 17y_{00} + 12y_{01} - 3y_{02})/35 \tag{3}$$

The number of fixed points that may be used for the smoothing depends on how accurately the polynomial describes the experimental curve under examination. The number of points should be chosen so that no more than one inflection in the observed data is included in any convolution interval. Data digitized at high intensities (i.e., taken very close together) offer more flexibility in the choice of the number of points to be used. Generally, the more data points included in the convoluting function, the less is the noise,

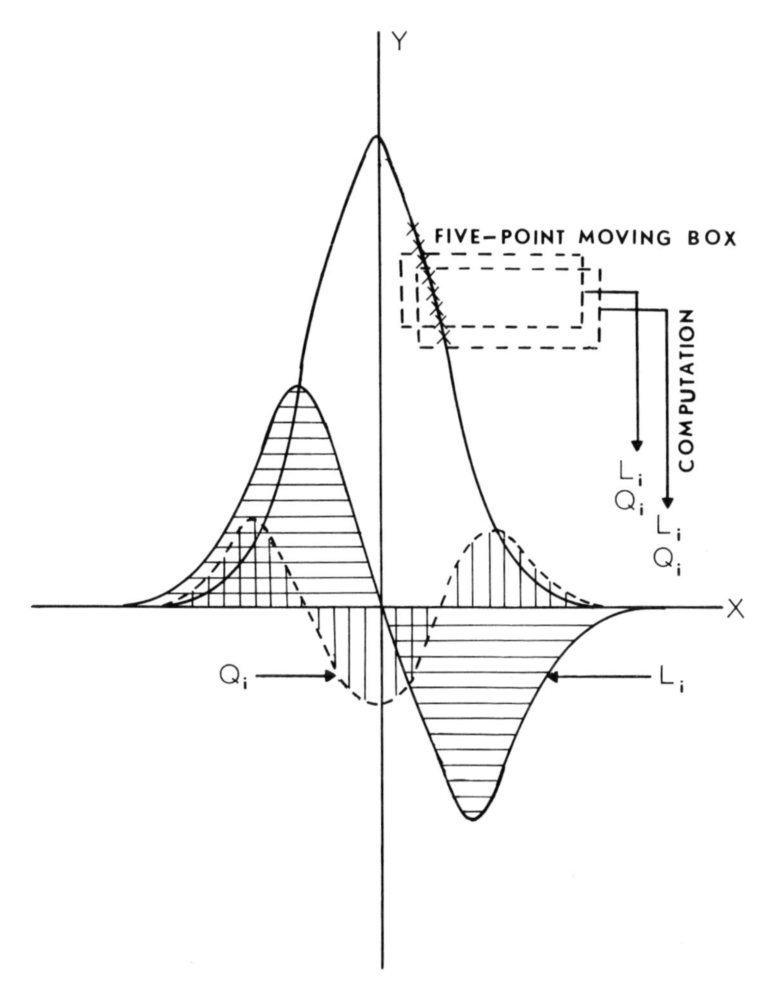

FIGURE 16. Schematic diagram of the orthogonal linear (L_i) and quadratic components (Q_i) of an approximately Gaussian distribution.

since this is reduced approximately as the square root of the number points involved. Thus, a 9-point smoothing produces approximately a threefold improvement in the signal-to-noise ratio. Although there is no way to assess the degree of distortion of recorded data introduced by the smoothing procedure, experience gained with separation of known samples may suggest compromise conditions between rate of digitizing and number of data points involved in the convolution.

TABLE 1
Smoothing (Zero-Derivative) Convolution Integers and Normalizing Factors (Quadratic or Cubic)

	Fixed number of points					
Data point	15	13	11	9	7	5
−07	−78					
−06	−13	−11				
−05	42	0	−36			
−04	87	9	9	−21		
−03	122	16	44	14	−2	
−02	147	21	69	39	3	−3
−01	162	24	84	54	6	12
00	167	25	89	59	7	17
01	162	24	84	54	6	12
02	147	21	69	39	3	−3
03	122	16	44	14	−2	
04	87	9	9	−21		
05	42	0	−36			
06	−13	−11				
07	−78					
Normalizing factor	1105	143	429	231	21	35

C. Slope Analysis

Since the distribution of a physically homogeneous population of cells can be approximated by a Gaussian curve, slope analysis can be very useful in detecting the baseline and peak shoulders and in estimating the resolution of strongly overlapping Gaussian peaks. Slope analysis can be performed by convoluted least-squares differentiation procedures (Savitzky and Golay, 1964) similar to those used for smoothing. For most work it is adequate to estimate the first- and second-derivative convolutes (Fig. 16). Tables 2 and 3 list the convolution integers and their normalizing factors for first- and second-derivative calculations for polynomials of degrees 2 and 3 from 5 to 15 fixed numbers of points. As an example, the equation for deriving the first derivative by a 5-point quadratic convolute is

$$y' = (-2y_{-02} - y_{-01} + 0y_{00} + y_{01} + 2y_{02})/10 \tag{4}$$

and for deriving the second derivative by a 7-point convolute is

$$y'' = (5y_{-3} + 0y_{-02} - 3y_{-01} - 4y_{00} - 3y_{01} + 0y_{02} + 5y_{03})/42 \tag{5}$$

The first derivative of a Gaussian curve has a maximum (+) and a

TABLE 2
First-Derivative Convolution Integers and Normalizing Factors (Quadratic)

	Fixed number of points					
Data point	15	13	11	9	7	5
−07	−7					
−06	−6	−6				
−05	−5	−5	−5			
−04	−4	−4	−4	−4		
−03	−3	−3	−3	−3	−3	
−02	−2	−2	−2	−2	−2	−2
−01	−1	−1	−1	−1	−1	−1
00	0	0	0	0	0	0
01	1	1	1	1	1	1
02	2	2	2	2	2	2
03	3	3	3	3	3	
04	4	4	4	4		
05	5	5	5			
06	6	6				
07	7					
Normalizing factor	280	182	110	60	28	10

TABLE 3
Second-Derivative Convolution Integers and Normalizing Factors (Quadratic or Cubic)

	Fixed number of points					
Data point	15	13	11	9	7	5
−07	91					
−06	52	22				
−05	19	11	15			
−04	−8	2	6	28		
−03	−29	−5	−1	7	5	
−02	−44	−10	−6	−8	0	2
−01	−53	−13	−9	−17	−3	−1
00	−56	−14	−10	−20	−4	−2
01	−53	−13	−9	−17	−3	−1
02	−44	−10	−6	−8	0	2
03	−29	−5	−1	7	5	
04	−8	2	6	28		
05	19	11	15			
06	52	22				
07	91					
Normalizing factor	6188	1001	429	462	42	7

minimum (−) at the inflection points of the curve and passes through zero (0) at peak maximum. Even in the presence of extreme baseline noise, the inflection points can be located. The distance between the maximum or minimum and the zero position corresponds to the standard deviation (σ_1, σ_2) on the front and back side of the curve, respectively. For a Gaussian distribution, $\sigma_1 = \sigma_2$. Thus, the first derivative can be utilized to detect the presence of an asymmetric peak ($\sigma_1 \neq \sigma_2$), where H is the peak height and x_m is the abscissa position of peak maximum from an arbitrary origin. In the case of a Gaussian curve, the σ estimated by slope analysis is useful in obtaining the area A of the peak from where H is the peak height.

$$A = H\sigma(2\pi)^{1/2} \tag{6}$$

The second-derivative curve of a Gaussian distribution produces a minimum (−) at the peak maximum of the original curve and two maxima (+). The magnitudes (ordinary values) of these extrema depend on the height of the peak and its variance (σ^2). However, the ratio of either maximum to the minimum (ordinates) is independent of the height and variance of the peak and in fact its value is $-2 \exp(-3/2) = -0.446$. The ratio between the two maxima is unity. Defining R_1 as the ratio of the maximum on the front side of the curve to the minimum, R_2 as the ratio of the maximum on the back side of the peak to the minimum, and R_3 as the ratio of the two maxima on the front and back sides, Grushka (1975) has suggested the following applications. In a Gaussian system, any deviation from the extrema ratios of $-2 \exp(3/2)$ and 1.0 immediately indicates the existence of double peaks. Second-derivative analysis is preferred to the first-derivative because it is sensitive to slope changes when one of the two peaks in the composite is one-tenth or less than the height of the second. In the case of two overlapping equal peaks the first-derivative ratio (maximum to minimum) is always unity. While the ratio of two maxima (R_3) of the second derivative is unity when the overlapping peaks are identical, the two ratios R_1 and R_2 increase with the resolution between the two peaks. By employing calibration curves (Grushka, 1975) with suitable standards, the R_1, R_2, R_3 ratios can indicate not only the resolution between strongly overlapping peaks in the composite but also the ratio of their heights. With single peaks, the standard deviation (σ) can be estimated from

$$\pm\sigma = (x - x_0)/\sqrt{3} \tag{7}$$

where the xs are the abscissa positions of the extrema and x_0 is the coordinate of the Gaussian's maximum (center of gravity).

D. Peak Detection and Baseline Correction

First- and second-derivative slope analysis can be utilized for distinguishing a peak maximum ($y' = 0$, $y'' < 0$) from a trough ($y' = 0$, $y'' > 0$) [baseline conditions ($y' = 0$, $y'' = 0$)], or a peak ascent ($y' > 0$, $y'' > 0$ then $y'' < 0$) from a peak descent ($y' < 0$, $y'' < 0$ then $y'' > 0$). In practice, "zero" for the y' is represented by the range of two threshold values C_1 and C_2 and that for the y'' by two additional threshold parameters C_3 and C_4. Baseline conditions are met with $C_1 > y' > C_2$ and $C_3 > y'' > C_4$. The selection of the parameters C_1, C_2, C_3, and C_4 depends on the magnitude of baseline noise in relation to the peak height. At first, a desired limit of integration *(1)* is selected such that it represents any percentage (e.g., 0.01, 0.1, 1.0%) of the peak height H. This is called an H_l increment. C_1 and C_2 have the same value but exhibit positive and negative signs, respectively. The values of C_1 and C_2 for a defined H_l are obtained from the first derivative y' of consecutive data points 5–15 (see Table 2), increasing (C_1) or decreasing (C_2) by one H_l increment. The larger the H_l increment, the higher are the values of C_1 and C_2. For example, if H_l is set at 0.1% of the peak height, baseline conditions are met within the threshold window $+C_1$ to $-C_2$ (computed for H_l of $0.1H$), even if the baseline ascends or descends by one H_l increment. Thus, the H_l values determine the sensitivity of detection of slope changes, which signify the start and end of peaks. It should be noted that detection of "peak start" by the slope increase method should be corrected by storing the data preceding the point of peak detection to set back the baseline. For a Gaussian curve, the baseline should be set back by approximately 0.3σ. Similar corrections apply to the back side of the peak where additional points are added on after the point of baseline detection. As an example, the equations for deriving the C_1 and C_2 parameters for a 7-point moving average are

$$C_{1,2} = \pm[-3(H_l) - 2(2H_l) - 3(H_l) + 0(4H_l) + (5H_l) + 2(6H_l) + 3(7H_l)]/28 \quad (8)$$

It can be seen that if the limit of integration is set at 0.1% of H the parameters C_1 and C_2 have values of $\pm 1.0 \times 10^{-2}$. The second-derivative threshold parameters C_3 and C_4 are set empirically at such levels as to avoid false triggering of peak start and end by baseline noise. Some guidelines can be obtained by entering alternate or fluctuating values of $+H_l$, $-H_l$ into the second-derivative (y'') equations of variable consecutive data points (see Table 3).

Once the baseline on both sides of the peak has been detected, the curve has to be corrected for an ascending or descending baseline by linear interpolation (Fig. 17). The method is based on the assumption that the peak is superimposed on a baseline exhibiting a linear sloping continuum. Correction of the distribution is carried out according to the equation

$$y_{corr} = y_{obs} - [(y_e - y_s)/(x_e - x_s)]\, x_{obs} - [(y_s x_e - y_e x_s)/(x_e - x_s)] \quad (9)$$

where y_{corr} is the corrected ordinate, y_{obs} is the observed ordinate, x_{obs} is the corresponding coordinate, y_s and y_e are the ordinates at peak start and end, and x_s and x_e are the corresponding coordinates.

E. Moment Analysis

After baseline correction, the nth statistical moment (m'_n) of the concentration distribution $C(x)$ of a peak is estimated by

$$m'_n = \frac{\int x^n C(x)dx}{\int C(x)dx} \quad (10)$$

Subsequently, the second, third, and fourth central moments, measured relative to m'_1, are obtained by

$$m_n = \frac{\int (x - m'_1)^n C(x)dx}{\int C(x)dx} \quad (11)$$

where x is the distance and C is the concentration.

The first moment m'_1 is the center of gravity of the concentration profile. It coincides with the peak maximum only if the peak is symmetrical (Fig. 18). The second central moment m_2 is the peak variance σ^2. The square root of m_2 corresponds to the standard deviation σ of the concentration distribution which provides a measure of peak width. The third central moment m_3 is indicative of the direction and magnitude of peak asymmetry, whereas the fourth central moment m_4 is a measure of peak flatness as compared to a Gaussian shape. Negative values of m_3 indicate a fronting shape, and positive values, tailing peaks. The zeroth moment is the normalized area of the peak.

In addition, the second, third, and fourth central moments can be used to estimate the coefficients of skewness S and excess E by

$$S = m_3/m_2^{3/2} \quad (12)$$

$$E = (m_4/m_2^2) - 3 \quad (13)$$

The skew measures the asymmetry of the peak while the excess indicates deviation from a Gaussian shape in regard to flatness. The coefficients S

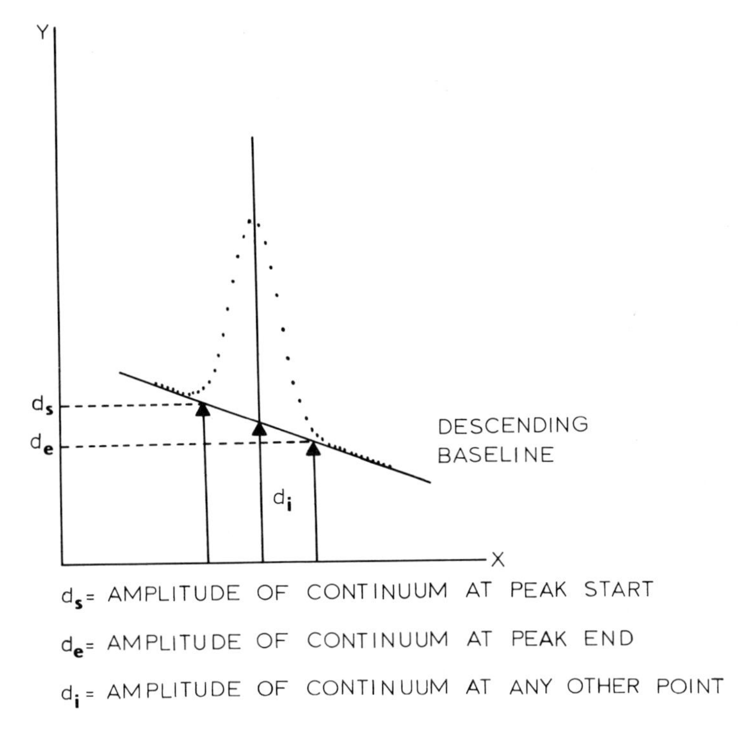

FIGURE 17. Baseline correction by assuming a linear-baseline sloping continuum under the curve of a Gaussian distribution.

and E are dimensionless quantities and therefore independent of the size of the peak (Grushka, 1975).

In practice, the moments are estimated by digitizing the absorbance A_i at the fixed time intervals which correspond to a fixed distance Δx in the column during a scan. Starting from an arbitrary origin, the coordinate at the ith interval is x_i. The moments are estimated by

$$m_0 = \Sigma A_i \Delta x \tag{14}$$
$$m_1' = \Sigma A_i x_i / \Sigma A_i \tag{15}$$
$$m_2 = \Sigma A_i (x_i - m_1')^2 / \Sigma A_i \tag{16}$$
$$m_3 = \Sigma A_i (x_i - m_1')^3 / \Sigma A_i \tag{17}$$
$$m_4 = \Sigma A_i (x_i - m_1')^4 / \Sigma A_i \tag{18}$$

It is apparent that the exact description of the peak area, position, width, and shape by moment analysis should have fundamental applica-

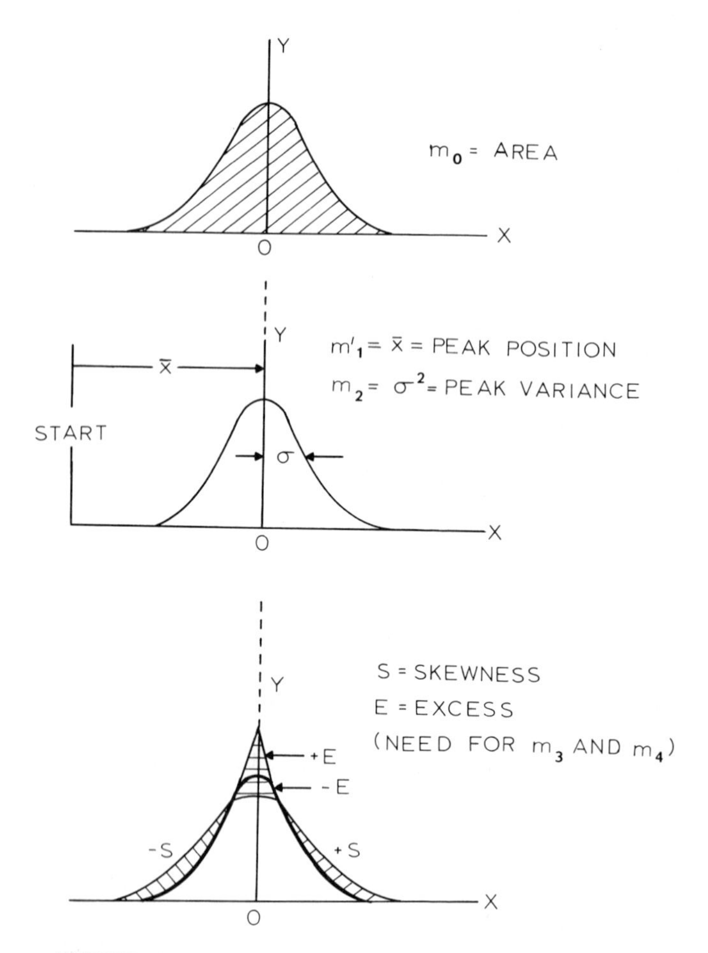

FIGURE 18. Statistical moments and their practical significance.

tions in cell analysis. The connection between the two is made by adopting mathematical models describing the cell separation process in regard to the particle transport as a function of time and also as affected by other physical factors such as viscosity, particle concentration, medium density, and osmolarity.

In this laboratory, a computer program available both in FORTRAN and BASIC languages is routinely used for processing the scanning data (Fig. 19). Scans of the distribution at different time intervals (Fig. 20) provide the values of m'_1 for the velocity plot. The velocity of cell movement under the

```
HORIZONTAL Y RANGE-          0 TO      4000.00 IN INCREMENTS OF     80.0000
VERTICAL   X RANGE-          8 TO           41 IN INCREMENTS OF      1


                    0         20        40        60        80        100
                    I....*....I....*....I....*....I....*....I....*....I
   8.0          .0 .X
   9.0           0*.X
  10.0        41.3 .+0
  11.0        75.0 . X
  12.0       130.7 .  X
  13.0       217.3 .   X
  14.0       347.0 .    X
  15.0       530.7 .       X
  16.0       778.3 .          X
  17.0      1097.0 .              X
  18.0      1483.7 .                   X
  19.0      1927.3 .                        X
  20.0      2404.0 .                              X
  21.0      2879.7 .                                    X
  22.0      3313.3 .                                         X
  23.0      3663.0 .                                              X
  24.0      3888.7 .                                                 X
  25.0      3966.3 .                                                  X
  26.0      3886.0 .                                                 X
  27.0      3657.7 .                                              X
  28.0      3305.3 .                                         X
  29.0      2869.0 .                                    X
  30.0      2390.7 .                              X
  31.0      1911.3 .                        X
  32.0      1465.0 .                  X
  33.0      1075.7 .             X
  34.0       754.3 .         X
  35.0       504.0 .      X
  36.0       317.7 .    X
  37.0        85.3 . 0+
  38.0        96.0 . X
  39.0        37.7 .0+
  40.0         1.3 .X
  41.0           0 .X
                    I....*....I....*....I....*....I....*....I....*....I
                    0         20        40        60        80        100


DATA BLOCK        1
PEAK NO.          1
VARIATION NO.     1

                                    OBSERVED        SMOOTHED

X MEAN                          =      24.91           24.91
2ND MOMENT ABOUT MEAN           =      23.45           23.48
3RD MOMENT ABOUT MEAN           =      -6.75           -6.76
4TH MOMENT ABOUT MEAN           =    1533.09         1539.50
BETA 1                          =       -.06            -.06
BETA 2                          =       2.79            2.79
STANDARD DEVIATION              =       4.84            4.85
AREA                            =   49100.33        49109.16
```

FIGURE 19. Sample computer output of a hypothetical distribution and a printed report of the estimated moments.

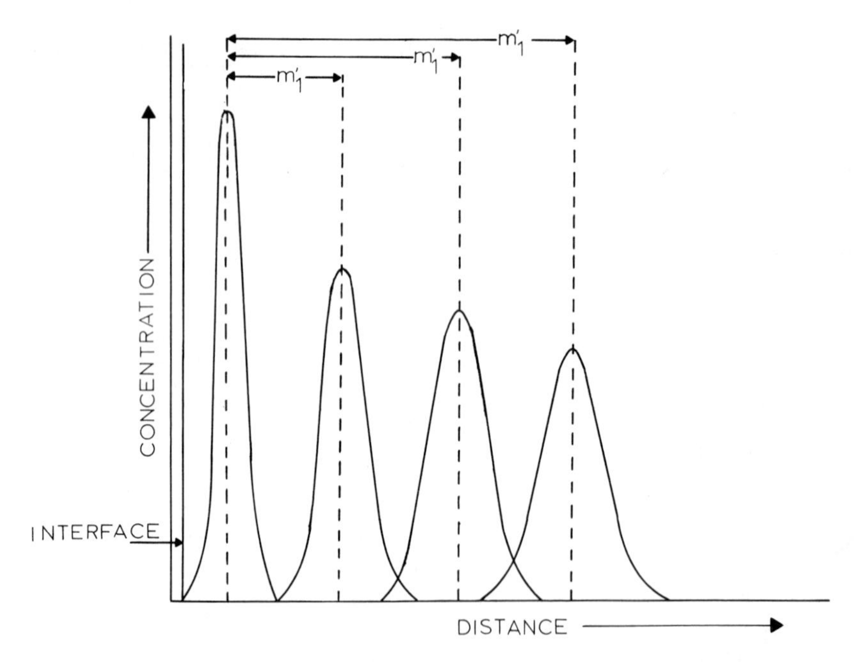

FIGURE 20. Diagram depicting the measurement of peak position as a function of time.

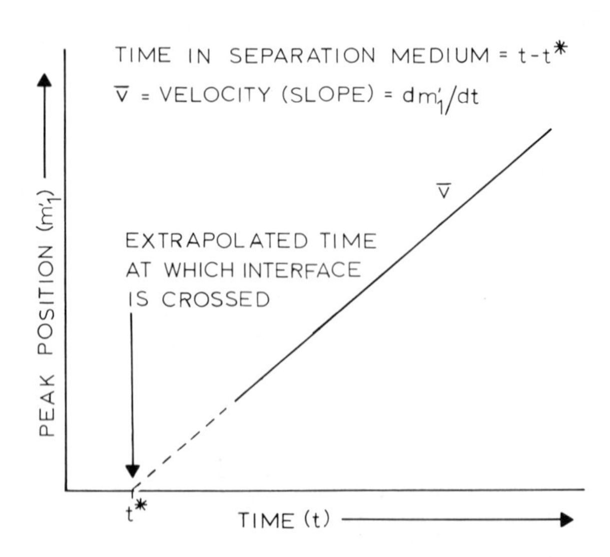

FIGURE 21. Diagram illustrating the measurement of peak velocity.

influence of the electrical and gravitational fields is measured from the slope ($\bar{v} = dm'_1/dt$) (Fig. 21) of the plot of m'_1 (cm) vs. elapsed time (s). In the case of overlapping distributions, an attempt is made to deconvolute the peaks assuming Gaussian shape.

F. Decision Boundaries

1. *Linear Categorization*

An unknown cell population is assigned by a linear categorizer to a certain category (e.g., "normal" or "abnormal") when the cell data evaluation leads to a descriptor value D_u less than a threshold T. The D_u and T values are estimated as follows: The mean sedimentation velocity ($\bar{s}$) for a particular cell population is estimated from the slope of m'_1 versus time plot. The mean skewness ($\bar{S}$) is estimated from the skewness (S) values obtained from each individual scan. Next, the mean $\bar{s}_{\mathrm{I}}$ and $\bar{S}_{\mathrm{I}}$ values of all cell populations of class I (e.g., "abnormal") and $\bar{s}_{\mathrm{II}}$, $\bar{S}_{\mathrm{II}}$ values of all cell populations of class II (e.g., "normal") are determined. The $\bar{s}_{\mathrm{I}}$, $\bar{S}_{\mathrm{I}}$ and $\bar{s}_{\mathrm{II}}$, $\bar{S}_{\mathrm{II}}$ pair values determine the centroids of the distribution of each class of cells. Subsequently, the coordinates X_{1_T} and X_{2_T} of a symmetrically placed boundary line between cell category centroids follow as:

$$X_{1_T} = (\bar{s}_{\mathrm{II}} + \bar{s}_{\mathrm{I}})/2 \quad (19)$$

$$X_{2_T} = (\bar{S}_{\mathrm{II}} + \bar{S}_{\mathrm{I}})/2 \quad (20)$$

The weight coefficients w_1 and w_2 are estimated by:

$$w_1 = \bar{s}_{\mathrm{II}} - \bar{s}_{\mathrm{I}} \quad (21)$$

$$w_2 = \bar{S}_{\mathrm{II}} - \bar{S}_{\mathrm{I}} \quad (22)$$

Consequently, the value T is given by

$$T = X_{1_T}\left[\frac{w_1}{(w_1^2 + w_2^2)^{1/2}}\right] + X_{2_T}\left[\frac{w_2}{(w_1^2 + w_2^2)^{1/2}}\right] \quad (23)$$

The discriminator value D_u of a certain cell population is computed from

$$D_u = \bar{s}\left[\frac{w_1}{(w_1^2 + w_2^2)^{1/2}}\right] + \bar{S}\left[\frac{w_2}{(w_1^2 + w_2^2)^{1/2}}\right] \quad (24)$$

2. *Ellipse of a Bivariate Distribution*

The construction of the ellipse of a given probability density (η) of a bivariate distribution of value $\bar{s}$ and $\bar{S}$ obtained from several cell populations is performed as follows: "Abnormal" cell populations are considered as class I and "normal" cell populations as class II. The variances of $\bar{s}$ and $\bar{S}$ values of class I are computed from

$$\sigma_1^2 = \frac{\sum_{i=1}^{n} (\bar{s}_i - \bar{s}_I)}{n-1} \tag{25}$$

and

$$\sigma_2^2 = \frac{\sum_{i=1}^{n} (\bar{S}_i - \bar{S}_I)}{n-1} \tag{26}$$

The covariance follows as

$$\text{cov}_{1,2} = \frac{\sum_{i=1}^{n} (\bar{s}_i - \bar{s}_I)(\bar{S}_i - \bar{S}_I)}{n-1} \tag{27}$$

The semiaxes of the wanted ellipse, a and b, are then given by

$$a = K\{\sigma_1^2 + \sigma_2^2 + [(\sigma_1^2 - \sigma_2^2)^2 + 4\,\text{cov}_{1,2}^2]^{1/2}\}^{1/} \tag{28}$$

and

$$b = K\{\sigma_1^2 + \sigma_2^2 - [(\sigma_1^2 - \sigma_2^2)^2 + 4\,\text{cov}_{1,2}^2]^{1/2}\}^{1/2} \tag{29}$$

where

$$K = \{-\ln[\eta\pi\sigma_1^2\sigma_2^2(1-\rho^2)^{1/2}]\}^{1/2} \tag{30}$$

where ρ denotes the correlation coefficient and η the desired probability density level (e.g., 0.1). Θ, the angle by which the ellipse is rotated, follows as:

$$\Theta = \tfrac{1}{2} \tan^{-1} 2[\text{cov}_{1,2}/(\sigma_2^2 - \sigma_1^2)] \tag{31}$$

The coordinates of the ellipses vertices follow as

$$\text{major axis: } \bar{s}_I + a \sin\Theta,\ \bar{S}_I + a\cos\Theta \tag{32}$$
$$\bar{s}_I - a \sin\Theta,\ \bar{S}_I - a\cos\Theta \tag{33}$$
$$\text{minor axis: } \bar{s}_I + b \cos\Theta,\ \bar{S}_I - b\sin\Theta \tag{34}$$
$$\bar{s}_I - b \cos\Theta,\ \bar{S}_I - b\sin\Theta \tag{35}$$

The above computations are repeated for the ellipse of the cell populations belonging to class II.

IV. METHODOLOGICAL ASPECTS

A. Physical Description of Cell Transport

The following equation describes downward cell velocity in a density gradient and in the presence of the electric field.

$$v(x) = \pm M \frac{i}{q\kappa(x)} + \frac{2}{9} \frac{r^2 g}{\eta(x)} [\rho_c - \rho(x)] \tag{36}$$

where $v(x)$ is instantaneous velocity of cells at any position x in the column (cm s^{-1}); M is electrophoretic mobility (cm^2 V^{-1} s^{-1}); i is current (A); q is cross-sectional area of the tube (cm^2); $\kappa(x)$ is conductivity at position x (ohm^{-1}cm^{-1}); g is acceleration of gravity (980.7 cm sec^{-2}); $\eta(x)$ is viscosity of the medium at position x (poises); ρ_c is cell density (g cm^{-3}); $\rho(x)$ is density of the medium at position x (g cm^{-3}), and r is cell radius (cm). The first term represents the velocity due to the electric field which can be positive (downward) or negative (upward) depending on the charge of the particles at the pH of electrophoresis and the position of the anode and cathode at the top or bottom of the column. Assuming that at neutral pH values most cells are negatively charged, they can be induced to migrate in the opposite direction of sedimentation by placing the anode at the top of the column. If the anode is placed at the bottom of the column—a procedure followed in the present experiments—the electrophoretic migration occurs in the same direction as the sedimentation. However, the second term of the equation indicates that if the density of the cells (ρ_c) is equal to the density of the medium (ρ) at a certain distance x in the column, the sedimentation factor becomes zero and cells should migrate downward primarily by electrophoresis. In this work, the density of the medium is just lower than that of the cells so that the sedimentation term is significantly reduced. If a strong synergistic effect of electrophoresis and sedimentation is desired, the density of the medium should be dropped to very low values. In the absence of the electric field and in the presence of a very shallow density gradient, cell migration downward will depend primarily on the radius (assuming spherical shape) and density of the cells. This is the case for the velocity sedimentation experiments at $1g$.

From the aforementioned it can be realized that the nature of the density gradient and the direction of the electric field can produce interesting variations of electrophoresis and sedimentation experiments. At present, we restricted our research activities toward the demonstration of predominantly electrophoretic and pure sedimentation-transport processes of model cell populations. In the case of isoelectric focusing, the electrophoretic velocity becomes zero when the cells hypothetically reach their "isoelectric point" (pI) and therefore at the steady state the "focused" cells should migrate downward by sedimentation alone. However, downward migration in the density gradient involves change in the pH of the environment because of the presence of the pH gradient, which should activate a restoring electrophoretic force to move the cells upward and toward their pI position.

B. Absorbance of Cell Suspensions

Optical scanning of a suspension of particles in the "absorbance" mode (i.e., the center of the detector is located at zero angle in respect to the center of the light beam) is complicated by the mutual "shading" of the particles and scattering, diffraction, and reflection effects. The observed absorbance, therefore, depends at least on the concentration of the particles in the suspension, their size and shape, and multiple-chromophore absorption at the specific wavelength used. One of the more serious sources of error is the progressive "flattening" of the absorption spectrum with increasing particle concentration (Duysens, 1956). In the course of our studies with lymphocytes from thymus and spleen, we were interested to know if there is a relationship between the number of cells per milliliter and the observed absorbance of the suspension (A_s) and if a flattening effect can be noted and be corrected for. Most lymphocytes can be considered as approximately spherical particles so that shape effects may be minimal. However, there is a significant variation in size among the various subpopulations of these cells which is more pronounced in the spleen than in the thymus. Large cells exhibit higher forward scattering than small cells. One would expect that if after separation the cells in the various fractions (or positions in the column) are not distributed at random in respect to their size, the absorption distribution profile (at a fixed wavelength) may not be representative of the cell concentration.

In order to test experimentally the various aforementioned factors involved in the optical scanning of lymphocytes, mouse (CBA/J, 14 weeks old) cells from spleen and thymus were prepared by previously described procedures (Griffith *et al.*, 1975), counted with a Coulter machine, and suspended in an isosmolar (300 mOsm) solution consisting of 6.8% sucrose in pH 7.4 phosphate buffer with KCl, sodium acetate, and glucose (Griffith *et al.*, 1975). This solution prevents the sedimentation of the cells during spectrophotometry, which was performed with a Beckman Model 25 double-beam recording instrument in 1-cm-pathlength cuvettes.

The electronic volume distribution of the spleen and thymus cells

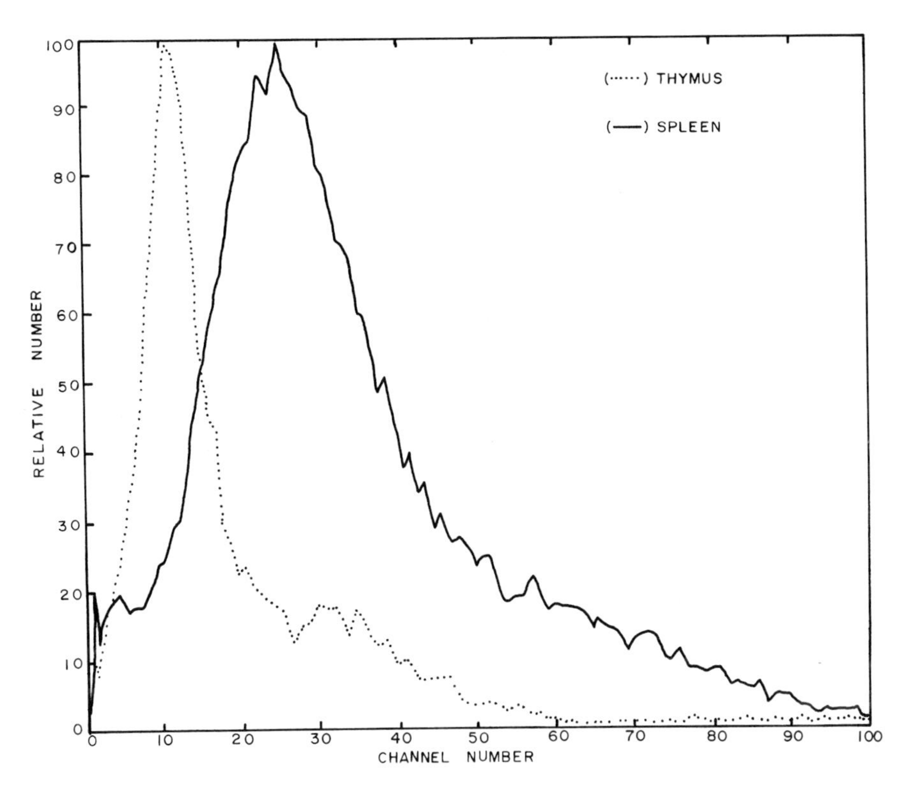

FIGURE 22. Electronic volume distribution of CBA/J mouse thymus and spleen lymphocytes obtained with the Coulter Channelyzer.

obtained with a Coulter Channelyzer instrument is shown in Fig. 22. It is apparent that the spleen cells have wider distribution of volumes and also a higher mean volume than the thymocytes. Thus, one would expect to observe size effects on the absorbance by using these two populations of cells. Figure 23 illustrates the relationship between absorbance at 400 nm and concentration of cells. The relationship is linear for up to 6×10^6 cells/ml. The magnitude of absorbance is the same for the same number of thymus and spleen cells. Thus, size distribution has no effect on the absorbance at a specific wavelength (400 nm) if the cell concentration is less than 6×10^6 cells/ml. Since the TRANS-Analyzer requires cell samples for analysis of lower concentration than the limited value, there appears to be no problem in getting a good correlation between the absorbance profile and the number of cells present in a certain position in the column. At concentrations larger than 6×10^6 cells/ml a "flattening" of the absorbance

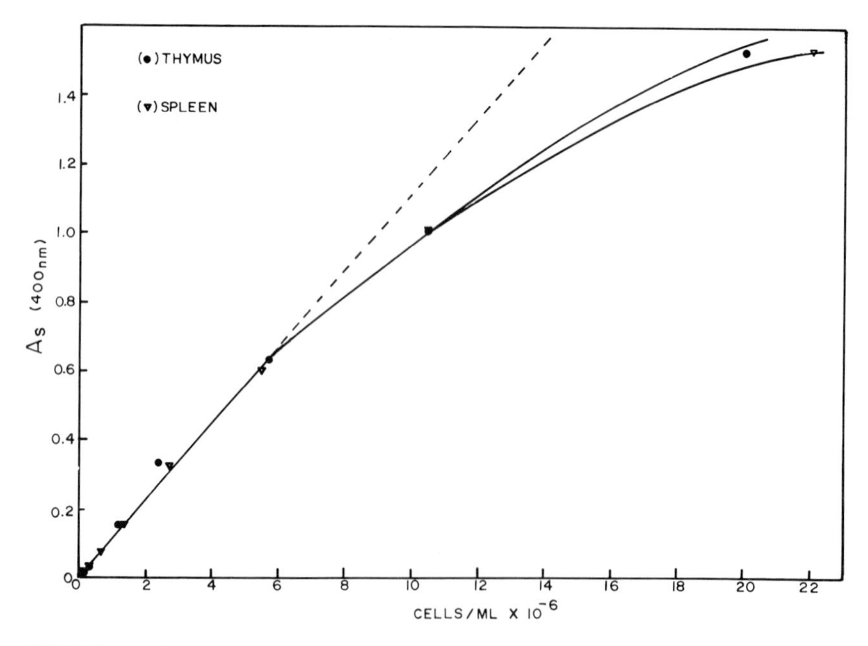

FIGURE 23. Plot of the absorbance (A_s) of cell suspensions obtained at 400 nm (1 cm pathlength). The samples were CBA/J mouse thymus and spleen lymphocytes. A straight line was obtained for up to 6×10^6 cells/ml.

was observed. When the absorbance of different concentrations of thymus and spleen cells was plotted vs. the wavelength, a linear relationship was obtained for all samples (Figs. 24 and 25). The slopes of these lines plotted vs. the concentration of the cells produced the curves shown in Fig. 26. In this particular plot the spleen cells exhibited considerably larger slope values than the thymocytes, which may be due to the increased forward scattering effect of the larger size cells. Although this phenomenon needs further investigation, it suggests the use of four detectors (each at different wavelength) for scanning so that size information can be simultaneously available. At present, the above experiments illustrate that single-wavelength absorbance measurements provide useful data in dealing with lymphocytes up to a certain limiting concentration.

C. Density Gradient Electrophoresis

Stabilization of cells during electrophoresis is achieved by a 2.5–6.25% Ficoll (400,000 mol. wt., Pharmacia Fine Chemicals) gradient, which is also an inverse 6.35–5.72% sucrose gradient (Boltz *et al.*, 1973; Griffith *et al.*,

1975). Prior to the formation of the gradient 25 g Ficoll are dissolved in 200 ml of the electrophoresis buffer and dialyzed against 5000 ml of the same buffer overnight at 4°C. Ficoll is dissolved by magnetic stirring with intermittent application of vacuum at approximately 20 mm Hg for 10 min. The dialysate is then made up to 250 ml (10% Ficoll solution) with freshly prepared buffer. Dialyzing the Ficoll dramatically reduces cell clumping. The *light solution* (2.5% Ficoll, 6.35% sucrose) is prepared as follows. Sucrose (3.175 g) is added to 12.5 ml of the stock 10% Ficoll solution and made up to 50 ml with the electrophoresis buffer. Similarly, the *dense solution* (6.25% Ficoll, 5.72% sucrose) is prepared by the addition of 2.862 g of sucrose to 31.25 ml of the stock 10% Ficoll solution and made up to 50 ml with the buffer. The *sample solution* (2.0% Ficoll, 6.44% sucrose) is made by dissolving 0.664 g sucrose in 2 ml of the 10% Ficoll solution and made up to 10 ml with the buffer. The *bottom solution* (10% Ficoll, 5.1%

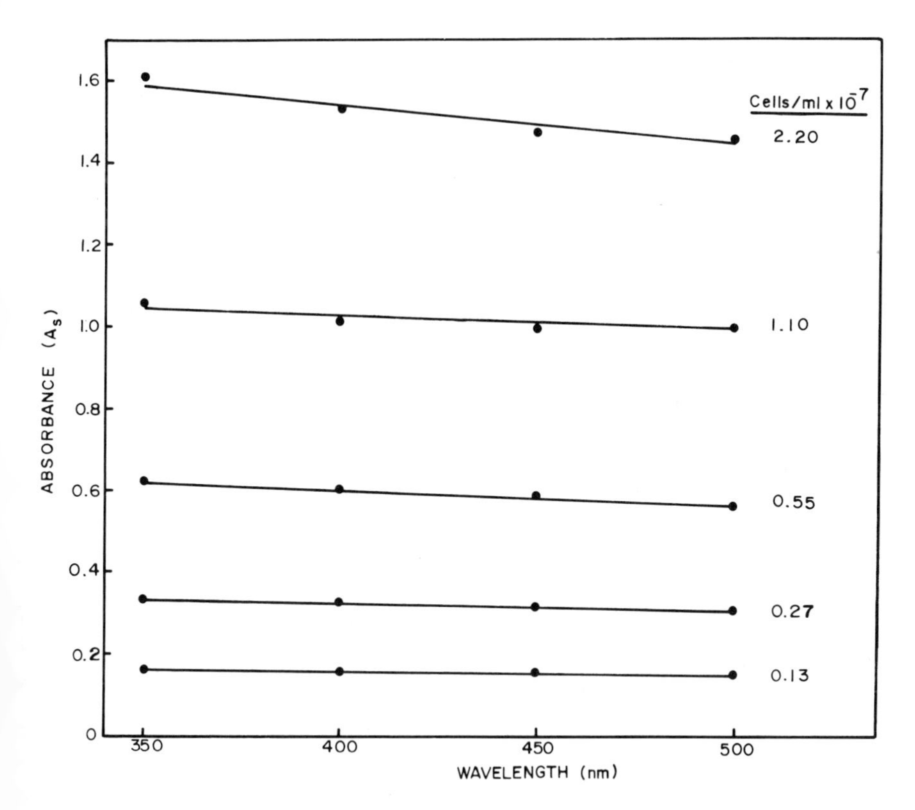

FIGURE 24. Plot of absorbance vs. wavelength for various concentrations of CBA/J mouse thymus lymphocytes.

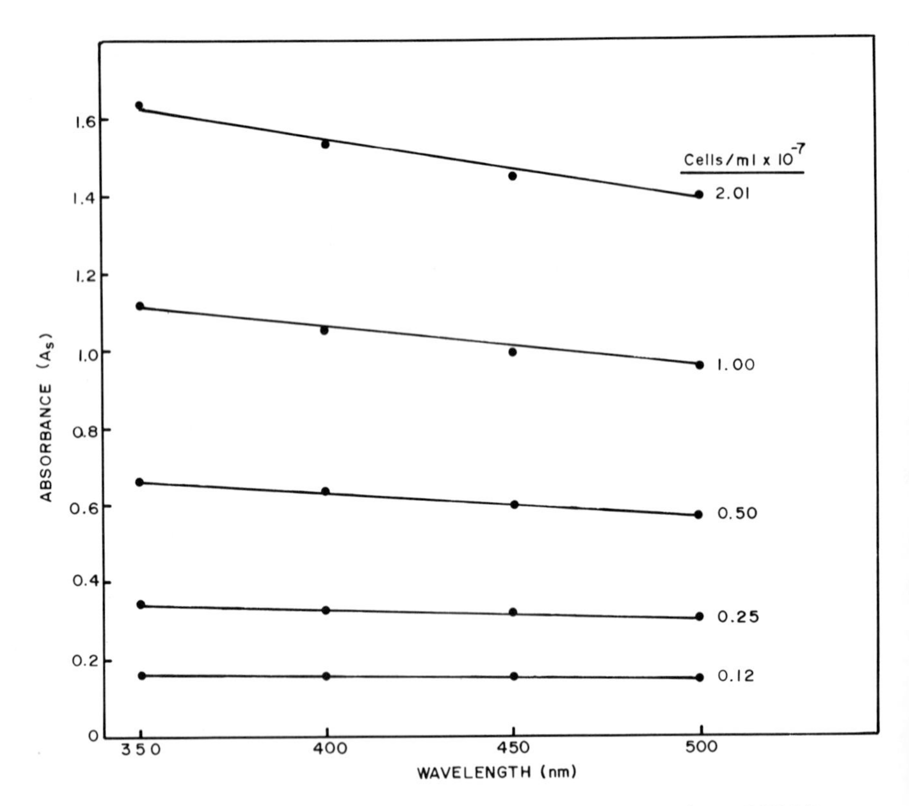

FIGURE 25. Plot of absorbance vs. wavelength for various concentrations of CBA/J mouse spleen lymphocytes.

sucrose) is prepared by dissolving 10.2 g sucrose in 150 ml of the 10% Ficoll solution and made up to 200 ml with the same stock solution. The *upper electrode solution* (6.8% sucrose) is prepared by dissolving 136 g sucrose in 1000 ml of the electrophoresis buffer and made to 2000 ml with the same buffer. The *lower electrode solution* (5.1% sucrose) consists of 76.5 g sucrose made up to 1500 ml with the electrophoresis buffer. The *electrophoresis buffer* adjusted to pH 7.4 has the following composition: 0.20 g KCl, 1.5 g Na_2HPO_4, 0.20 g KH_2PO_4, 0.12 g sodium acetate, 10.0 g glucose and is made to 1000 ml with glass-distilled water. This buffer is a modification of that described by Boltz *et al.* (1973). The specific conductivity of the buffer is 1.026 mmho/cm at 4°C and its ionic strength 0.023 M. All solutions are deaerated before use.

The experimental procedure is carried out as follows. The lower electrode reservoir is filled with *lower electrode solution* which is constantly replenished from a storage reservoir by means of a peristaltic pump (SAGE Model 375 A) at a rate of 10 ml/min. The lower part of the quartz column is filled with 5 ml of the *bottom solution* which acts as a cushion for the density gradient (Fig. 27). This is accomplished by means of a Tygon tubing attached to a syringe. The *bottom solution* is supported by a membrane attached to the lower end of the column. At this time, cooling water (4°C in the column) is circulated through the jackets of the column with a Lauda K-4/R cooler–circulator (Brinkman Instruments, Westbury, N.Y.). The *density gradient* (25 ml total volume) is then slowly layered (0.5 ml/min) on top of the *bottom solution*. The gradient is prepared from the *light* and *dense solutions* by means of an ISCO Model 570 gradient former (Instrumentation Specialties, Lincoln, Neb.). It covers the density range 1.0397–1.0480 g/cm³ at 4°C (Fig. 28) and has an osmolarity of 300 mOsM throughout. Subsequently, the cells are suspended in 0.5 ml of the *sample solution* at a concentration not exceeding 5×10^6 cells/ml and are slowly layered with a Tygon tubing–syringe combination on top of the gradient. Filling of the remainder of the column and upper reservoir is continued with

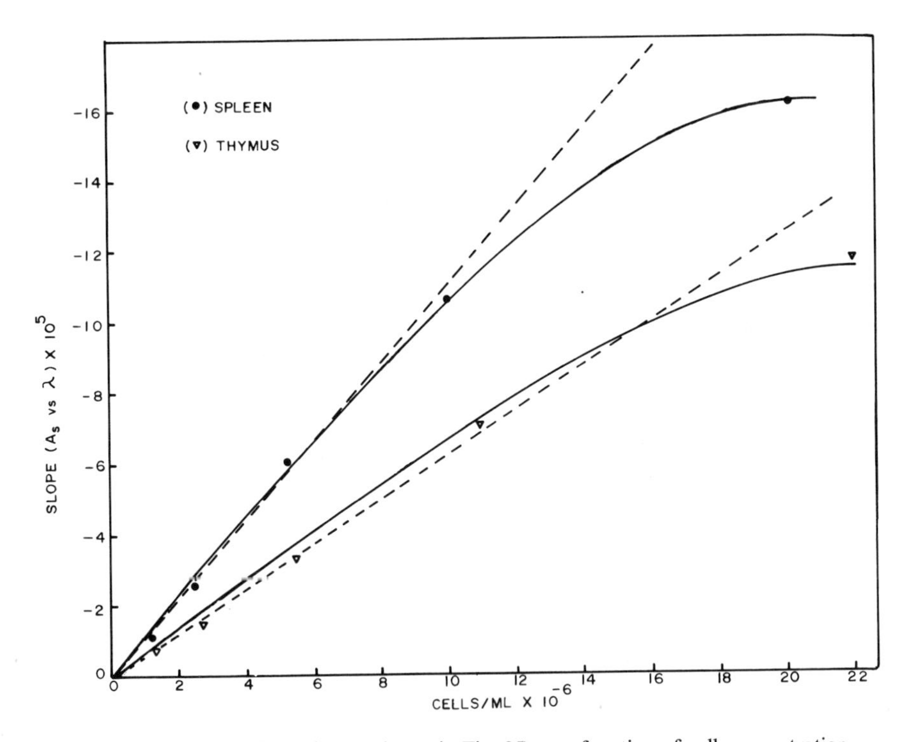

FIGURE 26. Plot of the slopes (shown in Fig. 25) as a function of cell concentration.

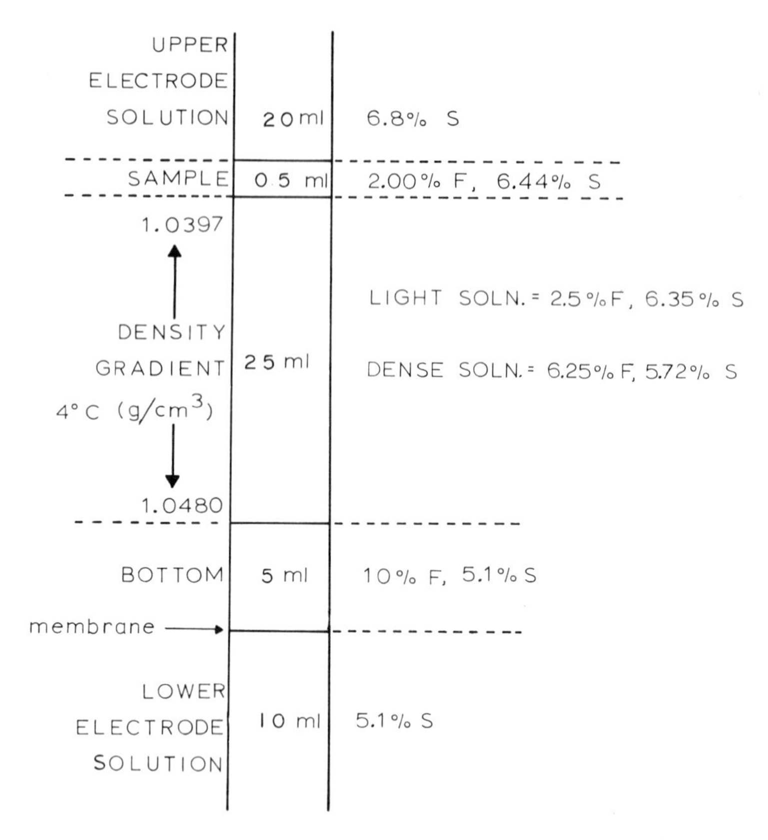

FIGURE 27. Arrangement of various solutions in the separation column for isotonic density gradient electrophoresis. F, Ficoll; S, sucrose.

upper electrode solution which circulates through the upper chamber for the duration of the experiment. Electrophoresis (toward the anode) is usually carried out at 10 mA (approximately 100 V) for a few hours.

D. Density Gradient Isoelectric Focusing

These experiments were performed in the Ficoll–sucrose gradient described above. However, in the preparation of certain solutions (i.e., *dense, light,* and *sample*) the electrophoresis buffer was replaced by a 1:1 mixture of pH 2.5–4.0 Ampholine (LKB Produkter, Bromma, Sweden) and pH 5.0–8.0 Bio-lytes (Bio-Rad, Richmond, Cal.) in 1% glucose. The total concentration of carrier ampholytes was 1% and the pH gradient at the end of the experiment covered the pH range 2.5 to 8.0 as measured at 25°C. A "protecting" solution of the carrier ampholyte–glucose mixture (see above) made 1% in Ficoll and 6.2% in sucrose was overlayered above the cell sample. The *upper electrode solution* (cathode) was 0.02 M NaOH in 6.8% sucrose and the *lower electrode solution* (anode) 5% phosphoric acid in 5.1% sucrose. The *bottom solution* was 5% phosphoric acid in 5.1% sucrose and 10% Ficoll. Some hydrolysis and alteration of the sugars in the acidic and alkaline media can be expected, but no practical interference with the isoelectric focusing process was observed. Focusing was carried out at a constant voltage (100 V) at 4°C. The initial current was 10 mA and at the steady state, 1.75 mA.

E. Velocity Sedimentation at Unit Gravity

The following solutions are prepared for these experiments. Phosphate-buffered saline (PBS) pH 7.4: 0.01 M is prepared by dissolving 1.2 g Na_2HPO_4, 0.22 g $NaH_2PO_4.H_2O$, 8.5 g NaCl in water and made up to 1000 ml volume. Seven grams of bovine serum albumin (BSA) (fraction V, lot 105C-0271, Sigma Chemical Co., St. Louis, Mo.) are dissolved in approximately 40 ml of PBS and dialyzed overnight at 4°C against 4 liters of the same buffer. The dialyzed BSA solution is made up to 70 ml volume with

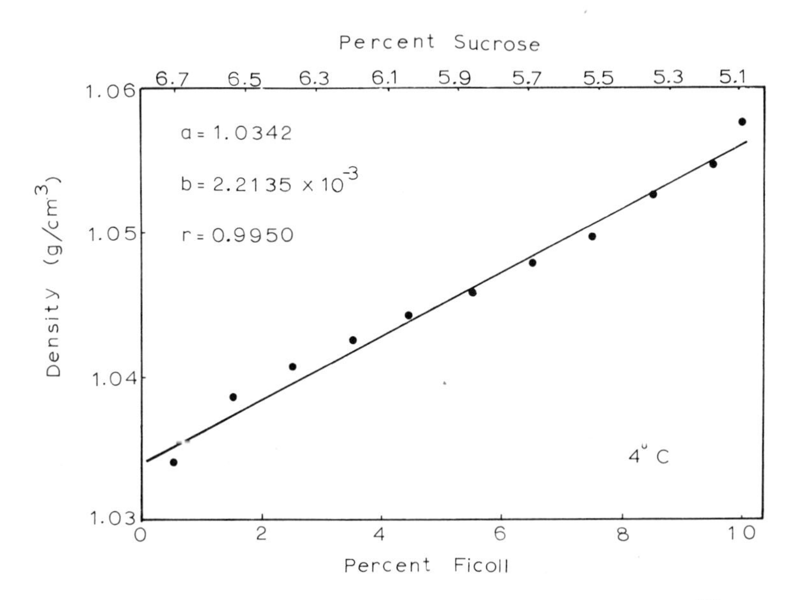

FIGURE 28. Plot of the density of the Ficoll–sucrose gradient at 4°C.

PBS and used as a stock solution to prepare 0.5%, 1%, 2%, and 3% solutions of BSA in PBS. The 3%, 2%, 1%, and 0.5% solutions of BSA in PBS are used as *bottom, dense, light,* and *sample* solutions, respectively. The cell sample is overlayered with PBS solution without BSA. The sequence of operations in filling the quartz column is: *bottom solution* (5 ml), *density gradient* (25 ml), *cell sample* (0.5 ml), and *sample overlaying solution* (0.5 ml) (Fig. 29). The concentration of the cells in the sample should not exceed 5×10^6 cells/ml. The density of the gradient covers the range of 1.009 to 1.0125 g/cm^3 at 4°C (Fig. 30). The BSA gradient has been employed previously (Miller, 1973) for preparative velocity sedimentation experiments at 1*g*.

F. Cell Samples

1. Mouse Lymphocyte Preparations

Mouse spleen and thymus lymphocytes were obtained from C57BL/6J adult mice (Charles River, Wilmington, Mass.) as described previously (Griffith *et al.*, 1975). The animals were sacrificed by cervical dislocation and the organs were dissected and placed in 10×35 mm plastic tissue

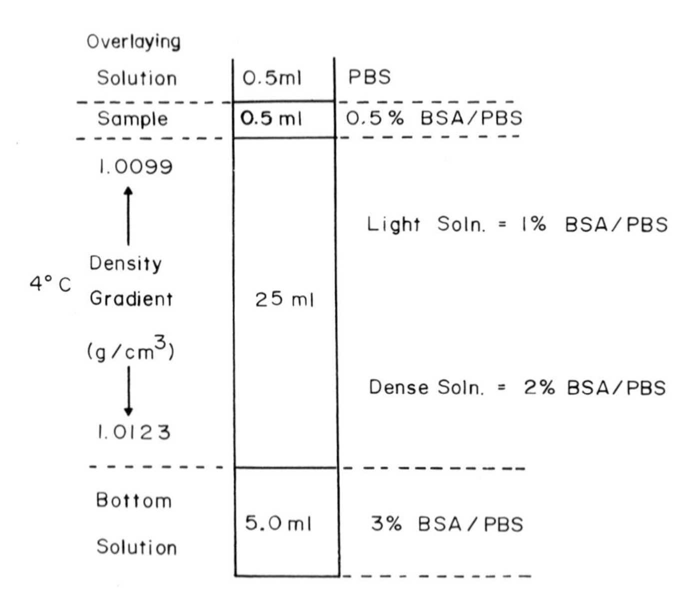

FIGURE 29. Arrangement of various solutions in the separation column for velocity sedimentation at 1*g*.

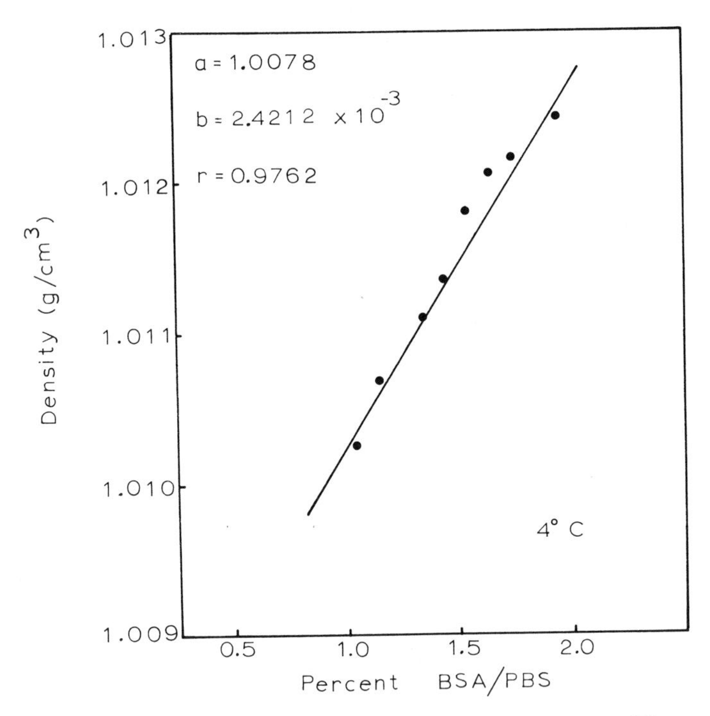

FIGURE 30. Plot of the density of the BSA/PBS gradient at 4°C.

culture dishes (Falcon Plastics, Oxnard, Cal.) containing 5.0 ml of RPMI-1640 medium with glutamine and phenol red (Grand Island Biological, Grand Island, N.Y.) and 0.5 ml anticoagulant citrate dextrose (ACD, Fenwal Laboratories, Morton Glove, Ill.) where connective tissue was removed. The tissue was transferred into additional tissue culture dishes containing the above medium. The tissue was then minced and forced through a No. 60 stainless steel mesh with a stainless steel spatula. The cell suspension was washed through the mesh with a minimum volume of RPMI-1640/ACD, layered on top of Lymphocyte Separation Medium (LSM, Bionetics, Kensington, Md.) and centrifuged for 30 to 40 min at 400 *g*. The lymphocytes were carefully removed from the LSM medium interface and washed once with Hank's balanced salt solution (HBSS, Grand Island Biological). Any remaining erythrocytes were lysed by suspending the cells in a 0.171 M tris-buffered 0.14 M NH_4Cl solution (pH 7.2) for 10 min at 4°C. The cells were washed twice with HBSS and centrifuged at 400*g*. Immediately prior to electrophoresis the cells were resuspended in the electrophoresis sample solution described below.

In cases indicated in the text, mouse spleen cells were treated with deoxyribonuclease (DNase) (Worthington Biochemical Corp., Freehold, N.J.). Cells were removed from the spleen tissue by passage through a No. 60 stainless steel screen in the tris/NH_4Cl solution mentioned above that was 0.1% in respect to bovine serum albumin (BSA) at 37°C. The cell suspension was spun at 400*g* and washed twice in HBSS containing 0.1% bovine serum albumin and 0.001% DNase. After centrifugation for 45 min on the "Lymphocyte Separation Medium" the cells remaining at the interface were washed two additional times in the HBSS/BSA/DNase solution. The cells were then incubated for 30 min at 37°C in HBSS alone. After incubation the cell suspension was washed four times with HBSS/BSA solution.

2. *Human Peripheral Lymphocytes*

These were prepared from a single donor as described previously (Ault *et al.*, 1976). Briefly, the blood sample was defibrinated by stirring with glass beads. The red cells were sedimented in 1.5% Dextran (Pharmacia Fine Chemicals, Piscataway, N.J.). The leukocyte-rich supernatant was layered onto a Ficoll–Hypaque cushion and centrifuged at 250*g* for 40 min. Prior to electrophoresis the cells were washed with the electrophoresis buffer and resuspended in the electrophoresis sample solution.

3. *Red Blood Cells*

The blood samples used for these studies were obtained from normal subjects and from patients with spherocytosis, elliptocytosis, sickle cell SC, sickle cell SS, α-thalassemia, and red blood cell aplasia (see Table 4). The blood cells were suspended in Alsever's solution and washed twice with phosphate-buffered saline (PBS) before analysis. Sheep and rabbit red blood cells were also obtained by the above procedure.

V. APPLICATIONS TO CELL ANALYSIS

A. Analysis of Lymphocytes

1. *Transient Velocity Sedimentation (TRANS-VELS) at 1g*

The capability of the TRANS-Analyzer to follow the zonal sedimentation of lymphocytes at 1*g* is illustrated in Fig. 31. A series of scans obtained

TABLE 4
Values of $\bar{s}$, $\bar{S}$, and D_u for "Normal" and "Abnormal" Human RBC

Sample number	Cell category "normal"			Cell category "abnormal"			Description[b]
	$\bar{s} \times 10^4$	$\bar{S}$	D_u[a]	$\bar{s} \times 10^4$	$\bar{S}$	D_u[a]	
1	1.70	0.48	1.58				F(20)
2	1.80	0.59	1.73				F(20)
3	1.54	0.49	1.47				F(20)
4	1.59	0.51	1.52				F(33)
5	1.64	0.51	1.56				F(20)
6	1.55	0.19	1.28				M(68)
7	1.67	0.22	1.39				M(65)
8	1.65	0.21	1.37				M(68)
9	1.65	0.42	1.51				M(20)
10	1.75	0.39	1.56				M(20)
11	1.54	0.24	1.30				M(31)
12	1.63	0.30	1.41				M(20)
13				1.65	−0.01	1.22	SPH, M(3)
14				1.40	0.00	1.04	SPH, F(7)
15				1.22	−0.05	0.87	ELL, F(1)
16				1.36	0.06	1.05	SC, F(27)
17				1.32	0.04	1.01	SC, F(5)
18				1.23	0.15	1.01	THA, M(9)
19				1.14	0.37	1.09	THA, M(29)
20				1.36	0.28	1.20	APL, F(2)

[a] T = 1.27.
[b] M, male; F, female; SPH, spherocytosis; ELL, elliptocytosis; SC, sickle cell; THA, α-thalassemia; APL, RBC aplasia; age of subject is in parentheses.

at different time intervals shows the mode of sedimentation of C57BL/6J mouse thymus lymphocytes in the BSA gradient. The right panel of the figure depicts "absorbance" (light extinction) measurements and the left, scattering at 15° angle. In the "absorbance" mode the arrows indicate the peaks resulting from the interfaces of the *sample solution* with the *density gradient* and the *overlaying solution*. These can serve as visual markers of the origin. Broadening of the interface peaks with time is due to diffusion. These marker peaks are not present in the scattering signal. The initial appearance of double peaks in the cell sample is due to the movement of the cells from the *sample solution* into the *density gradient*. There appears to be a transient concentration effect at the interface. The sedimentation distribution of the thymocytes is heterogeneous. The cells exhibit a pronounced leading edge which gives rise to a positive skewness after statistical moment analysis. Estimation of the mean (m'_1) of the distribution of the total thymocyte population as a function of sedimentation time produced

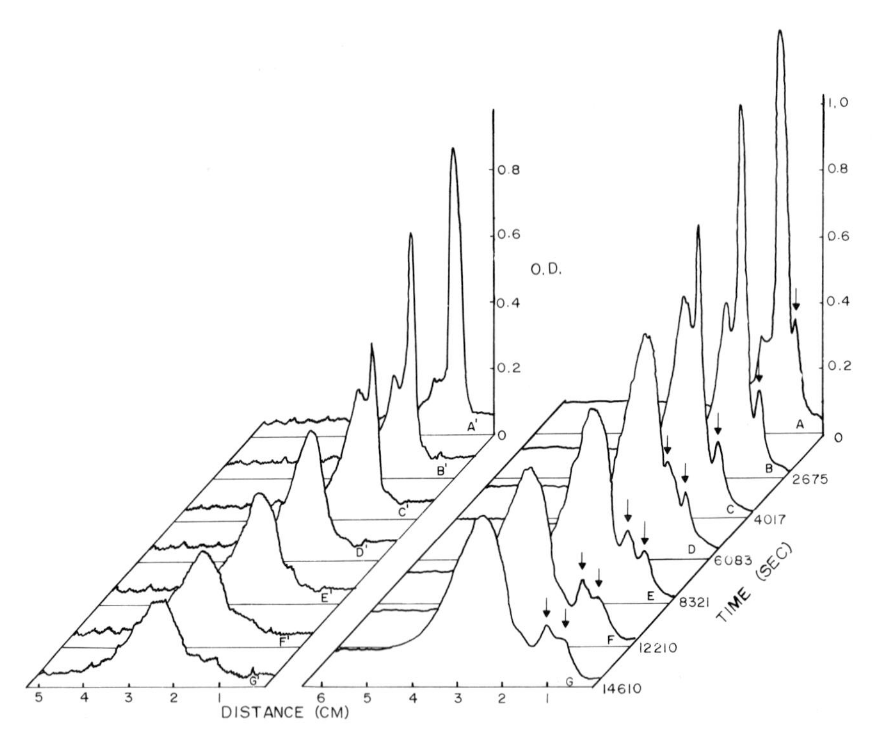

FIGURE 31. TRANS-VELS scans of CB57BL/6J mouse thymus lymphocytes. Scattering ($\theta = 15°$) and "absorbance" (light extinction) scans of the cell distributions are shown as a function of sedimentation time. The two small peaks at the sample origin indicate the interfaces of gradient/sample solution and sample solution/overlaying solution.

the plot of Fig. 32. The slope of the line corresponds to the mean sedimentation velocity ($\bar{s} = dm_1'/dt$) of the cells which was found to be 9.97×10^{-5} cm/s at 4°C. Assuming a mean density of 1.080 g/cm^3 for mouse thymus cells and taking into consideration the mean density ($\bar{\rho} = 1.0115$ g/cm^3) and mean viscosity ($\bar{\eta} = 0.0156$ poises) of the medium at 4°C, the mean volume of the thymocytes was estimated from the Stoke's equation (see above) to be 140 μm^3.

The analytical advantages of measuring sedimentation velocities at 1g by the TRANS-VELS method rather than the traditional preparative technique (Miller, 1973) are several: (a) a small number of cells (10^6) can be used for the analysis, which facilitates studies where a large sample is not available, (b) the sedimentation velocity is estimated from several experimental points of the selected position (usually mean) vs. elapsed time, (c) corrections due to apparatus geometry and fraction-collecting mode are avoided, (d) the continuous cell distribution is recorded instead of that from selected fractions, (e) several samples can be analyzed simultaneously, and (f) computer analysis provides precise statistical measurements. Therefore, the application of the method to immunological problems should provide useful information in regard to the physical features of immunocompetent cells and their alteration under certain conditions. In recent experiments we have observed that not only the shape, but also the deformability of the cell surface alters the sedimentation velocity at $1g$. The precision of the TRANS-VELS measurements allows the detection of subtle alterations in $\bar{s}$ which may not be noticed in preparative techniques.

2. *Transient Electrophoretic (TRANS-EL) Analysis*

Mouse (C57BL/6J) spleen lymphocytes were subjected to TRANS-EL analysis in the isosmolar Ficoll–sucrose gradient at 4°C. The results are

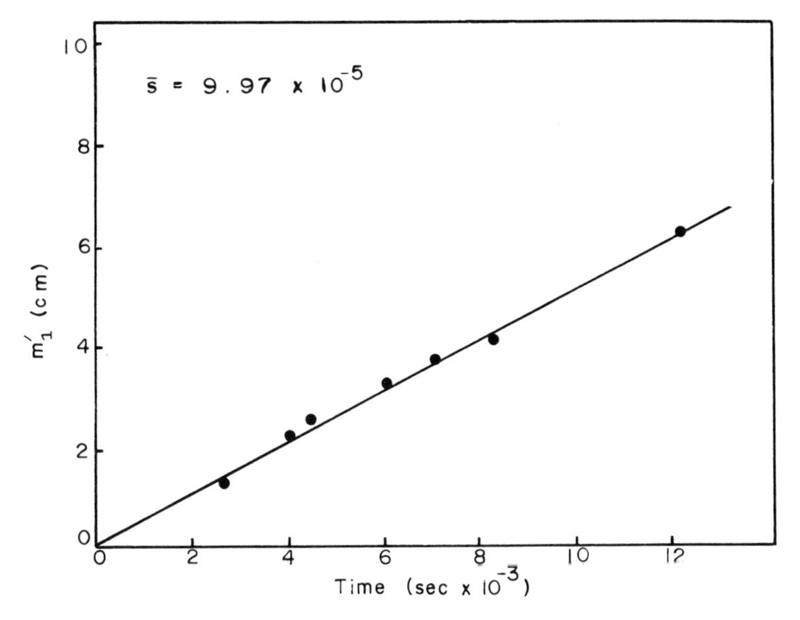

FIGURE 32. Plot of the first statistical moment m_1' (i.e., centroid of peak position) vs. sedimentation time for the cell distribution shown in Fig. 31. The slope of the lines represents the sedimentation velocity of the cells at $1g$.

illustrated in Fig. 33. Migration of the cells in the electric field resolves the population into at least three distributions, not including visibly distinguished subpeaks. The fastest and slowest peaks have been marked as HMC (high-mobility cells) and LMC (low-mobility cells), respectively. The sharp peaks near the origin represent the gradient/sample/upper-electrode-buffer interfaces. A plot of m'_1 for the HMC and LMC cells as a function of the electrophoresis time is shown in Fig. 34. The slope of each line gives a measure of the electrophoretic velocity in cm/s. Since the electric field strength can be estimated from the applied current (i), the cross-sectional area (q) of the column, and the conductivity (κ) of the buffer at 4°C, the electrophoretic mobility of the HMC cells was determined to be -10.08 TU and that of the LMC cells -6.88 TU. The Tiselius unit (TU) has been defined at 10^{-5} cms^{-1}/Vcm^{-1} (Catsimpoolas *et al.*, 1976b). Although the absolute value of these mobilities cannot be compared to those obtained in free solution, the relative values should be comparable. TRANS-EL analy-

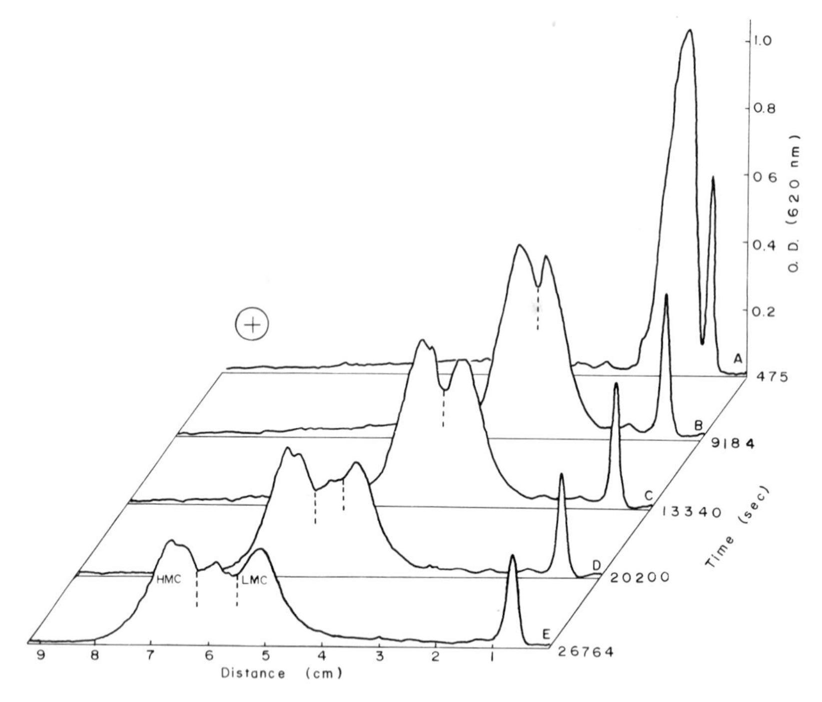

FIGURE 33. TRANS-EL scans of C57BL/6J mouse spleen lymphocytes as a function of time. HMC and LMC denote the high- and low-mobility cells, respectively. HMC represent primarily T lymphocytes and LMC the B cells. Peak(s) at the origin are due to interface(s).

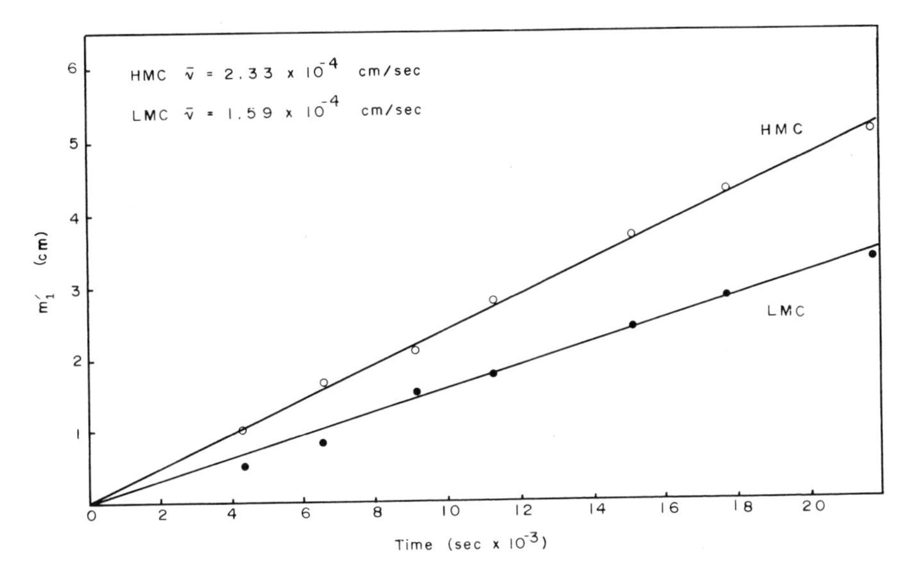

FIGURE 34. Plot of the centroid of peak position of HMC and LMC C57BL/6J mouse spleen lymphocytes as a function of electrophoresis time. $\bar{v}$ denotes mean electrophoretic velocity.

sis of C57BL/6J mouse thymus cells produced a mean mobility value of −9.88 TU, which is characteristic of HMC cells (i.e., T cells). The mean mobility of the thymus cells was somewhat lower than the HMC cells of the spleen, as expected (Griffith *et al.*, 1976). The HMC and LMC cells separated by preparative density gradient electrophoresis represent T and B lymphocytes, respectively (Platsoucas *et al.*, 1976).

Human peripheral lymphocytes from a single adult donor (normal) were analyzed by TRANS-EL. The results are shown in Fig. 35. A continuous distribution of mobilities was observed with a strong negative skewness toward the low-mobility cells. This is in agreement with previous results obtained in our laboratory by preparative electrophoretic techniques (Catsimpoolas *et al.*, 1976c; Ault *et al.*, 1976) and by others (Smith *et al.*, 1976). With certain donors the low-mobility cells can appear as a distinct peak or shoulder (Catsimpoolas *et al.*, 1967c). The majority of B cells bearing IgM and IgD are found at the tail (low mobility) of the distribution (Ault *et al.*, 1976). The mean electrophoretic mobility of the human peripheral lymphocytes was found to be −11.48 TU, almost identical to that of human red blood cells, which was −11.44 TU. Thus, it has been confirmed that human red blood cells cannot be separated from human peripheral lymphocytes by electrophoresis.

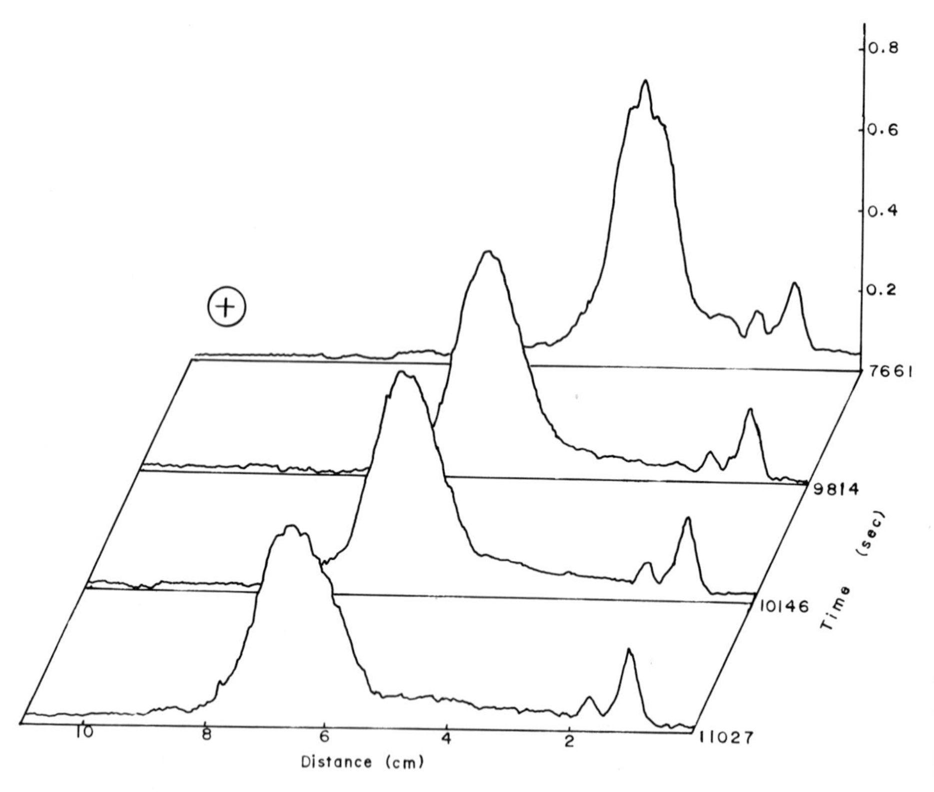

FIGURE 35. TRANS-EL scans of normal human peripheral lymphocytes. Note the asymmetric distribution of the cells exhibiting a trailing end (negative skewness).

3. *Transient State Isoelectric Focusing (TRANS-IF)*

These experiments were designed to follow the fate of lymphocytes during isoelectric focusing. More specifically, the TRANS-Analyzer was used to explore the kinetics of focusing of mouse (C57BL/6J) spleen lymphocytes. A system was chosen where the pH gradient is from pH 8.0 to 2.5 at the steady state and the cells are applied at the top of the gradient (migration toward positive electrode) under a "protective" layer of carrier ampholytes. TRANS-IF scans of the spleen cells as a function of time are shown in Fig. 36. The cells appeared to be initially "focused" and subsequently "unfocused," and finally lysed. Fig. 37 shows the kinetics of focusing and unfocusing by following the m_1' and m_2 values of the distribution with time. In the case of proteins, the m_1' reaches a steady state upon completion of focusing and m_2 (peak variance) reaches a minimum value

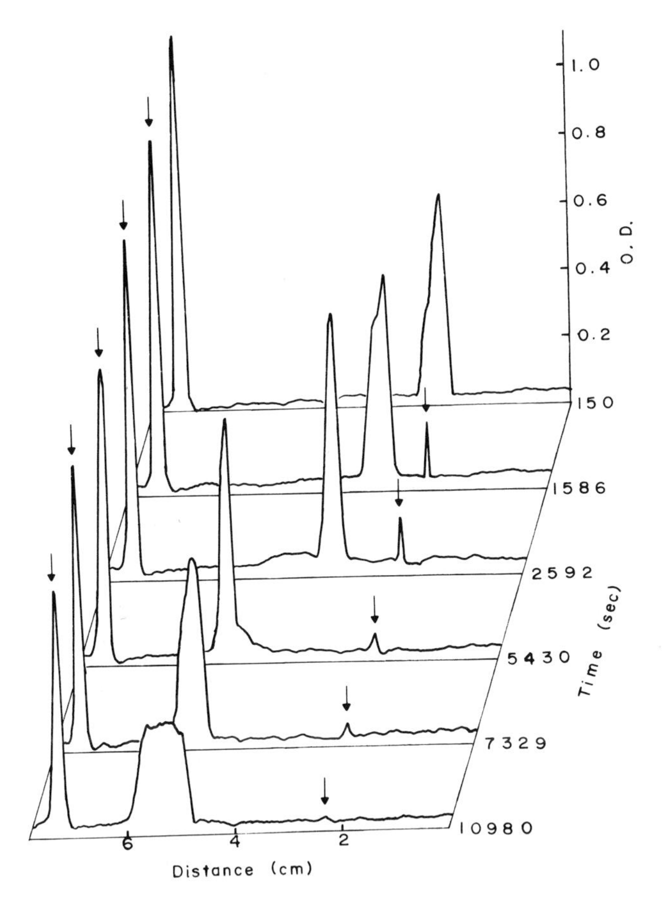

FIGURE 36. TRANS-IF scans of C57BL/6J mouse spleen lymphocytes in the pH 2.5–8.0 range (1% carrier ampholytes). The peaks marked with arrows are interfaces. Migration is toward the positive electrode. Note the unfocusing of the distribution at the 7329-s and 10980-s scans.

and remains unchanged (Catsimpoolas, 1976). With the spleen cell experiments, the m_2 value reached a minimum which indicates focusing, but then increased again indicating unfocusing. The distribution was unimodal. The m_1' value was not stabilized until the cells lysed. The above results lead to the suggestion that as the cells reach an apparent pI position in the pH gradient, they appear to be focused and exhibit minimum peak variance (m_2). At the region of the isoelectric pH, changes in the cell membrane may cause alteration of the pI toward more acidic values and therefore the m_1' is not stabilized, since the cells are now refocused in a new position. This may

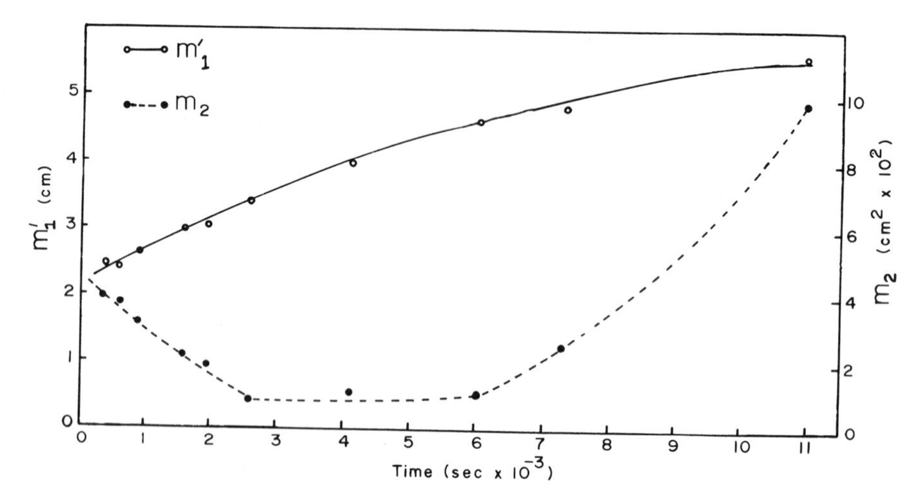

FIGURE 37. Plot of the first (m'_1) and second (m_2) statistical moments of the cell distribution shown in Fig. 36 as a function of electrofocusing time.

occur repetitively to the point where cells with a wide range of pIs exist and therefore appear "unfocused" (i.e., m_2 values are increasing with time). Finally, extensive damage to the membrane causes lysis of the cells. From the above experiments, we have concluded that electrophoresis at physiological pH values is a milder and practically more useful technique for the separation of lymphocytes and other mammalian cells than isoelectric focusing.

B. Analysis of Red Blood Cells

1. Transient Velocity Sedimentation at 1g

The superimposed velocity sedimentation profiles from two typical experiments involving normal human and sheep red blood cells as a function of time are shown in Fig. 38. As expected, the human red blood cells—being of larger volume than the sheep cells—are sedimented faster. The sedimentation velocity ($\bar{s}$ in cm/s) of the cells is estimated by linear regression analysis from the slope of the plot of the first statistical moment m'_1 vs. elapsed time (Fig. 39). By this method, the sedimentation velocity can be measured accurately with a mean correlation coefficient (r) of 0.9989 $\pm$ 0.0005 and a mean standard error of the estimate (S.E.E.) of 4.70 $\pm$ 0.75%. Characteristically, erythrocytes from two adult female subjects analyzed intermittently over a period of 2 months and at different sample loads exhibited sedimentation velocities at 25°C of $(1.66 \pm 0.08) \times 10^{-4}$ and $(1.63 \pm 0.04) \times 10^{-4}$ cm/s, respectively. Fresh sheep erythrocytes migrated with $\bar{s}$ values of $(0.98 \pm 0.07) \times 10^{-4}$ cm/s. Assuming a spherical shape for the cells, the mean volume of the human erythrocytes was estimated from the velocity sedimentation equation of 25°C to be 116 μm^3 and that of sheep red blood cells 56 μm^3. These volumes are larger than the generally accepted dimensions. This deviation is not unreasonable and may be the result of the following: (a) the erythrocytes orient themselves with the long axis of the biconcave disk aligned in parallel to the direction of sedimentation, thus exhibiting less friction than a falling sphere or spheroid at random orientation and consequently larger values of $\bar{s}$; (b) cell deformability may have influence on $\bar{s}$; indeed, glutaraldehyde-fixed human erythrocytes showed 20% higher values of $\bar{s}$ in comparison to unfixed cells; (c) cell

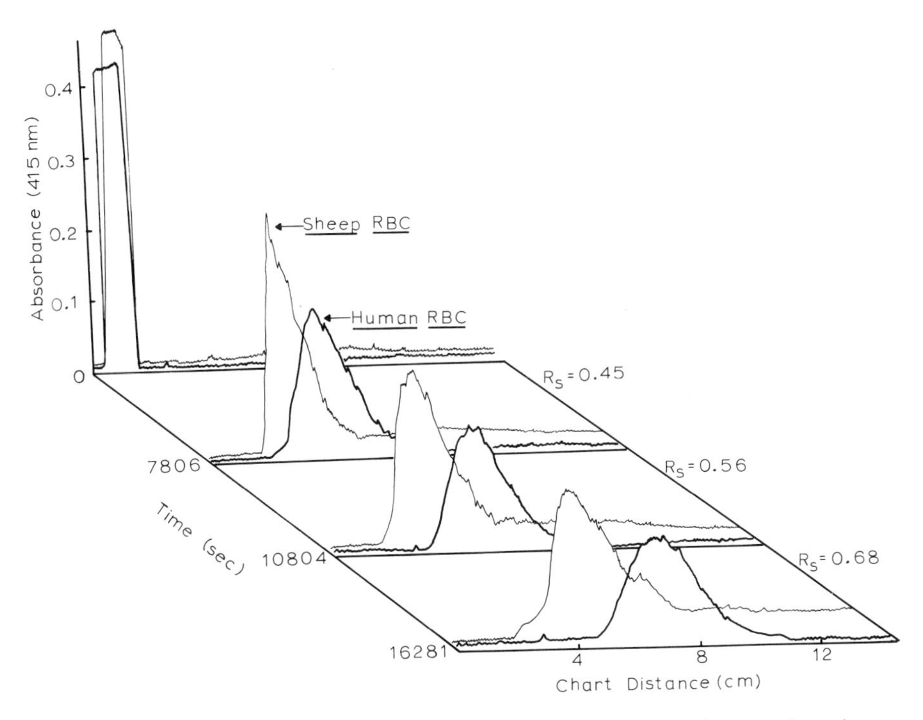

FIGURE 38. Velocity sedimentation profiles at 1g of human and sheep erythrocytes (superimposed for comparison) as a function of elapsed time. The predicted resolution (R_s) in a hypothetical separation is indicated at each scanning frame. Note that the sheep red blood cells distribution exhibits larger positive skewness than the human cells. Also note the self-correction of the distribution with time toward a more Gaussian shape; this is more obvious with the human erythrocytes.

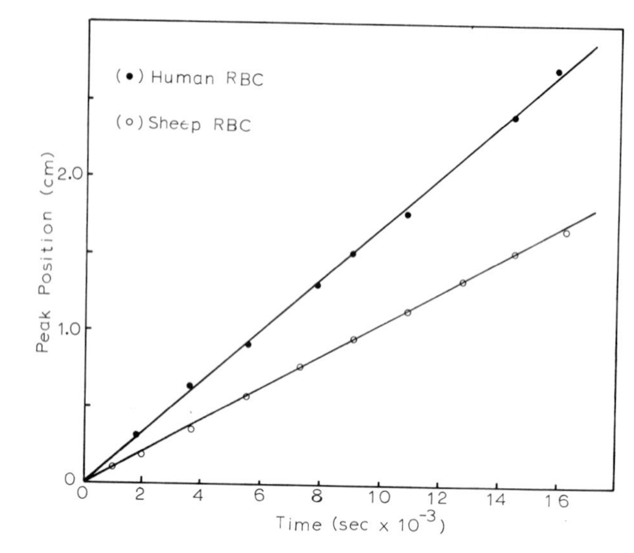

FIGURE 39. Typical plot of peak position (mean, first statistical moment) for human and sheep erythrocytes as a function of elapsed time. The slope of the straight line corresponds to the sedimentation velocity.

density may be different than the assumed literature value; and (d) presently "accepted" methods for measuring red blood cell volume operate under different physical conditions and assumptions.

Knowledge of m_1' and m_2 values has enabled us to estimate the expected resolution (R_s) directly as a function of time between the two populations of human and sheep red blood cells. Resolution of 1 is assigned to a just-resolved double peak (Catsimpoolas, 1976). It may be seen from Fig. 38 that the resolution remains lower than 1.0 even after a few hours of sedimentation; thus, complete separation is not achieved within the period shown for cells differing as much as 1.6-fold in $\bar{s}$ values. The number of theoretical plates (N) estimated from

$$N = (m_1'/\sqrt{m_2})^2$$

was found to be approximately 20–60, which signifies a low resolution system comparable to that of gel filtration of proteins.

A typical TRANS-VELS pattern of normal RBC from an elderly male and RBC from an α-thalassemia patient is shown in Fig. 40. It is evident from the diagram that normal RBC sediment at a considerably faster rate in the BSA/PBS gradient. The shape of the distribution is also different which

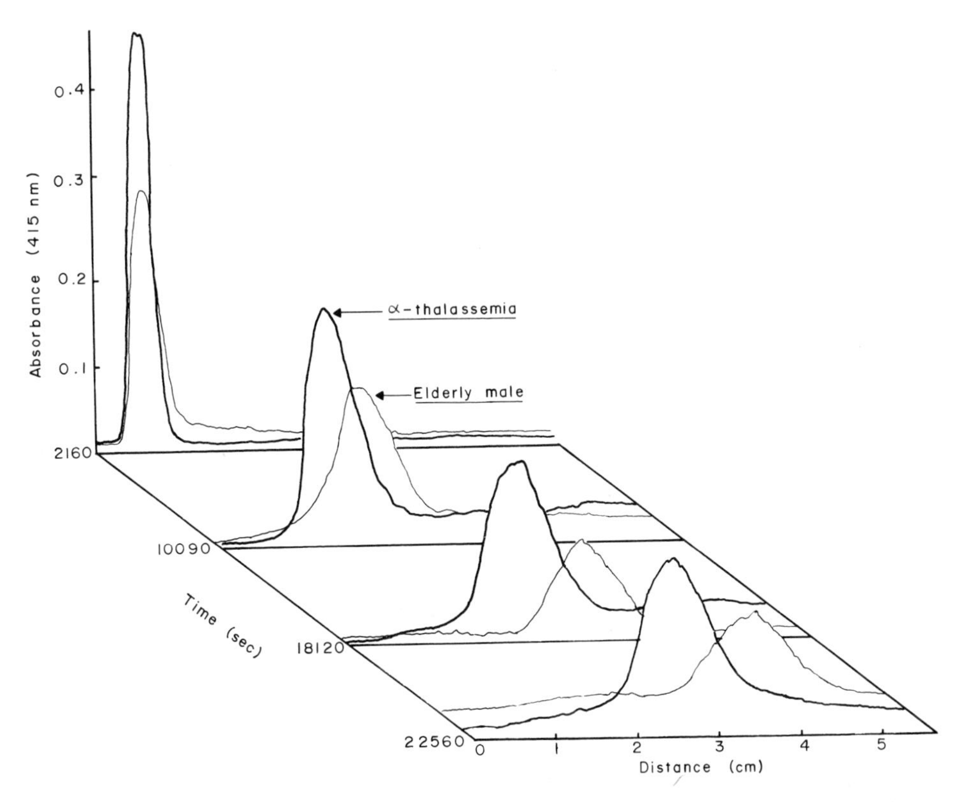

FIGURE 40. Typical TRANS-VELS profiles of erythrocytes from an elderly male subject and from a patient with α-thalassemia. Superimposed scans of the two distributions during sedimentation are shown for comparison.

is reflected in the statistical measurement of the mean skewness ($\bar{S}$). The plot of mean peak position (m'_1) as a function of sedimentation time (Fig. 41) exhibited straight lines with correlation coefficients better than 0.9990. The slope of each line produced a numerical value for the mean sedimentation velocity ($\bar{s}$) of the cells.

A series of such experiments were performed with RBC from normal subjects (11 samples) and from patients with RBC abnormalities (8 samples). A two-dimensional plot of the experimentally obtained $\bar{s}$ and S values from the individual RBC populations along with the mean values of the "normal" and "abnormal" group are shown in Fig. 42. Confidence ellipses at the 0.1 probability density level were estimated by computer for each group and are indicated by dotted lines in Fig. 42. In general, the

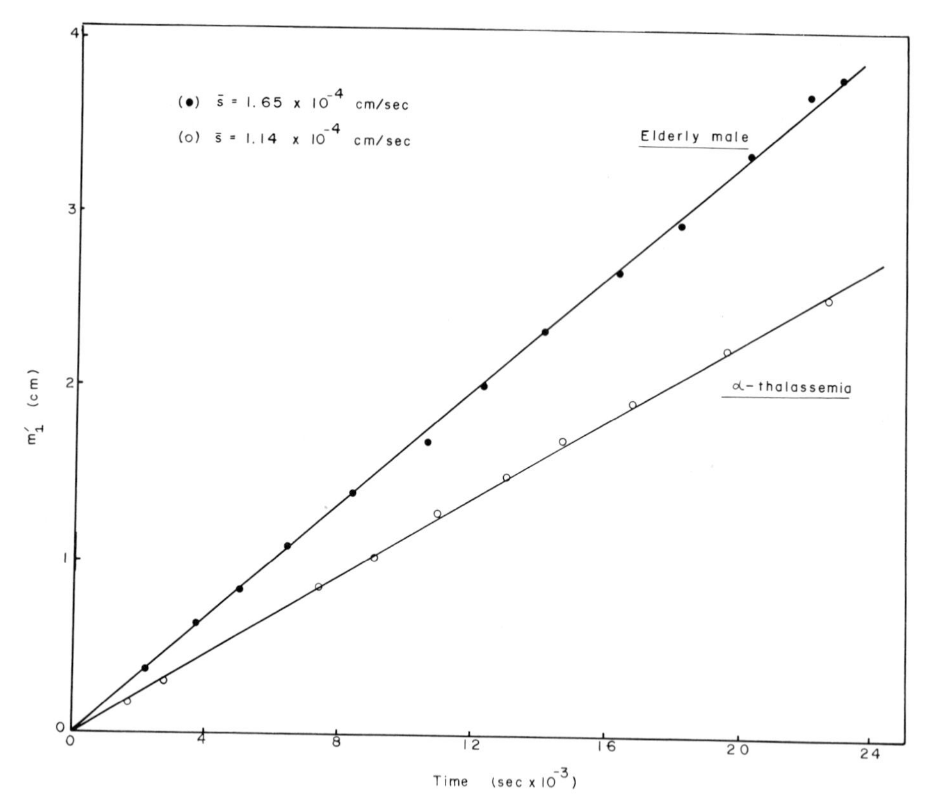

FIGURE 41. Plot of peak position (man, first statistical moment) as a function of sedimentation time for the cell populations shown in Fig. 40. The slope of the lines corresponds numerically to the mean sedimentation velocity ($\bar{s}$).

"abnormal" group of RBC exhibited lower sedimentation velocity ($\bar{s}$) values and lower $\bar{S}$ values than the "normal" group. Although the confidence ellipses were partially overlapping, the majority of the cell samples (90%) were not found in the common region. The significant difference between these groups of cells is also indicated by the fact that neither of the ellipses overlaps the center of the other. Furthermore, employment of linear categorization techniques (Wied *et al.*, 1970) allowed the determination of a threshold value T and discriminator values D_u for each cell population. A linear categorizer assigns an "unknown" cell population to a certain category when the cell data evaluation leads to a discriminator value

D_u less than a threshold T and to another category if D_u is larger or equal to T (see section III.F). Table 4 shows the D_u values obtained from $\bar{s}$ and $\bar{S}$ data for each population of cells by a computer program available in this laboratory. In all cases the cell populations were assigned to the correct group (i.e., normal and abnormal) by the linear categorizer. Therefore, we have concluded that the combined measurement of the $\bar{s}$ and $\bar{S}$ values by the TRANS-VELS technique offers two new valuable experimental parameters for the physical characterization of erythrocytes and other mammalian cells.

At present, we do not attempt to explain the possible causes for the observed differences among the cell populations examined. Changes in

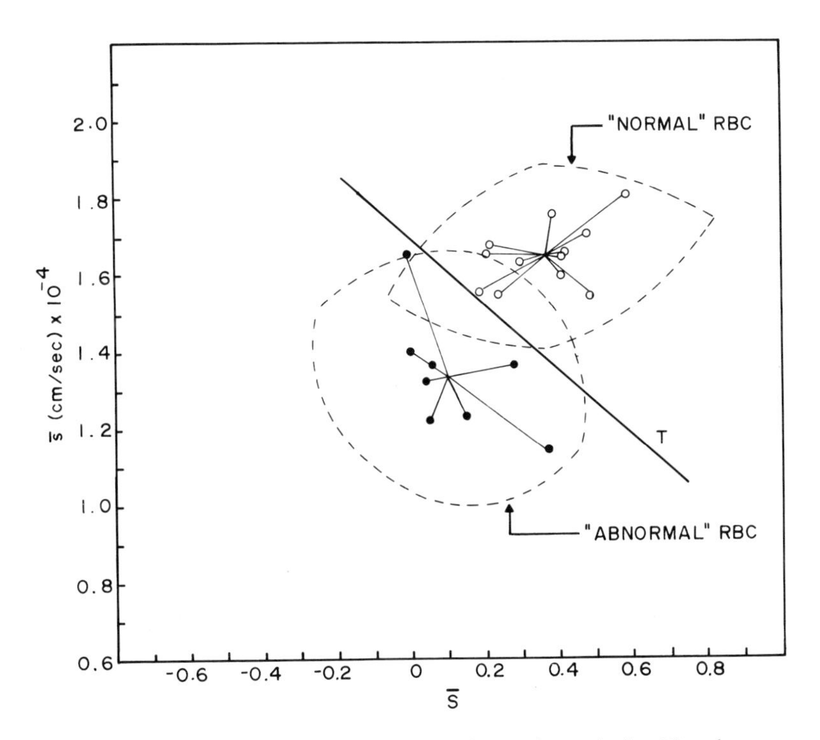

FIGURE 42. Two-dimensional plot of mean sedimentation velocity ($\bar{s}$) values vs. mean skewness ($\bar{S}$) values for a group of erythrocytes from normal subjects and a group of patients exhibiting red blood cell abnormalities (i.e., spherocytosis, α-thalassemia, sickle cell anemia, and red blood cell aplasia). The dotted line indicates computer-estimated confidence ellipses for the two groups at the 0.1 probability density level. The solid line illustrates the threshold level T for linear categorization of the two groups of cells (see section III.F).

volume, density, and shape, as well as heterogeneity of individual cells within a sample population (e.g., α-thalassemia patient) in regard to these properties, may contribute to altered sedimentation behavior. Furthermore, physical alterations are the result of even more complex biochemical events.

There is a need to examine a large number of RBC samples from healthy subjects as a function of at least sex and age to determine the normal dispersion of $\bar{s}$ and $\bar{S}$ values among various groups. In addition, a large number of patients with diagnosed red blood cell anomalies will need to be examined if biophysical criteria are to be established for the presence of certain pathological RBC conditions. Furthermore, it will be interesting

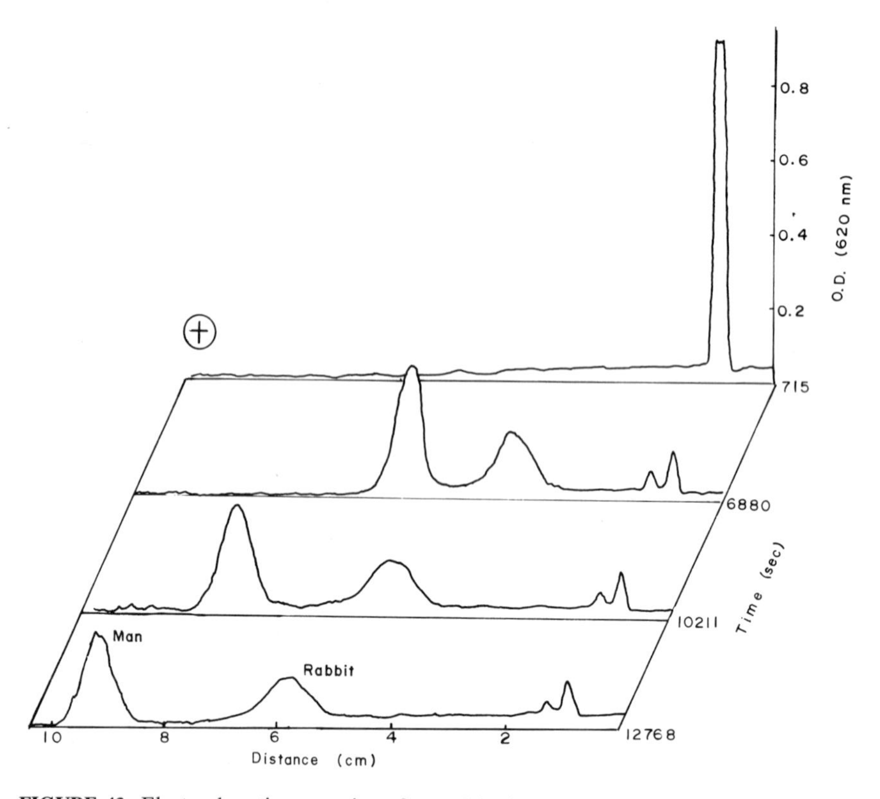

FIGURE 43. Electrophoretic separation of a model mixture of rabbit and man erythrocytes. Absorbance at 620-nm scans of the cell distributions are shown as a function of electrophoresis time. The two small peaks at the sample origin indicate the interfaces of gradient/sample solution and sample solution/buffer.

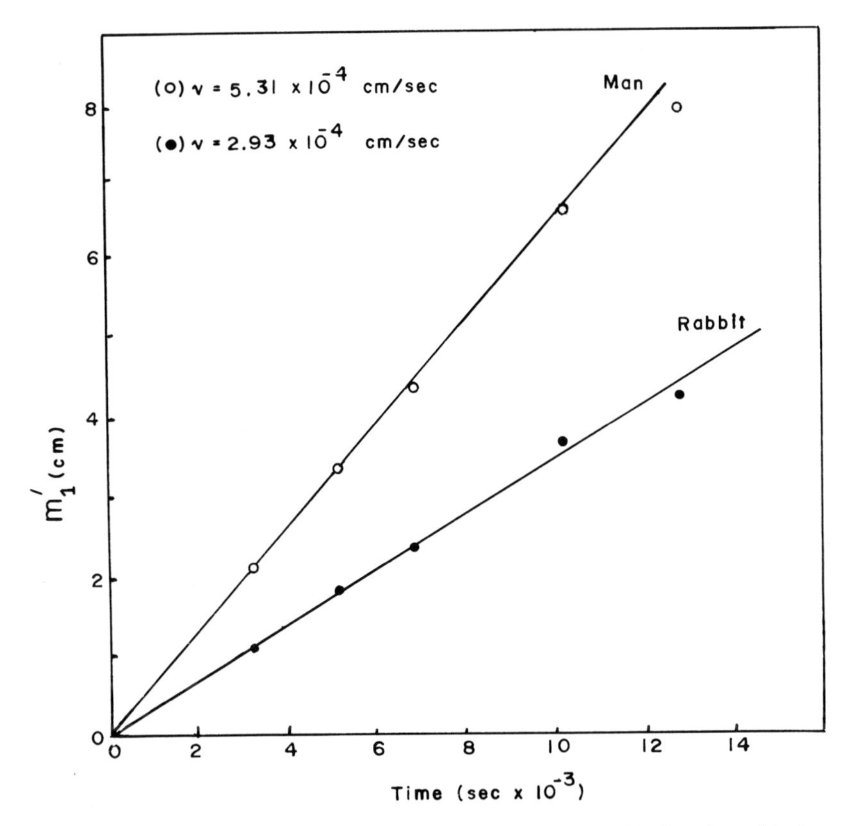

FIGURE 44. Plot of the first statistical moment, m'_1 (i.e., centroid of peak position), vs. electrophoresis time for man and rabbit erythrocytes from scans shown in Fig. 43. The slope of the lines represent electrophoretic velocity of the cells.

to know if changes in the hydrodynamic properties of RBCs under 1*g* sedimentation can be observed in cases of malnutrition and in other diseased states. At present, it appears that the TRANS-VELS technique offers a new tool for probing the physical characteristics of intact cells.

2. *Electrophoretic and Isoelectric Focusing Analysis*

A typical separation of human and rabbit erythrocytes by TRANS electrophoresis (TRANS-EL) is shown in Fig. 43. A plot of the mean position of each distribution versus elapsed electrophoretic time produces precise estimation of the velocity of the cells (Fig. 44). It can be seen that

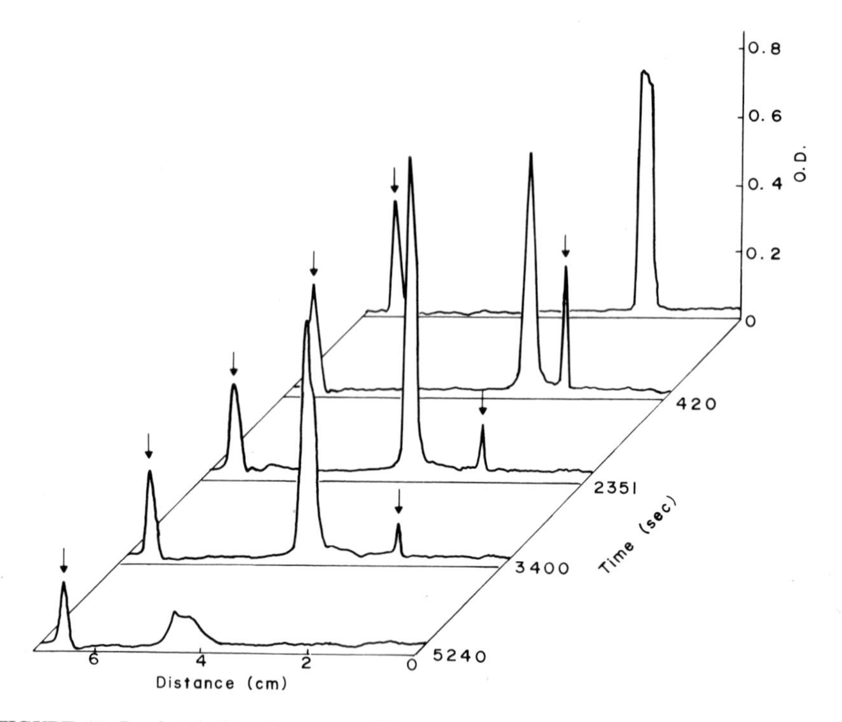

FIGURE 45. Isoelectric focusing scans of human erythrocytes in the pH 2.5–8.0 range (2% carrier ampholytes). The peaks marked with arrows are interfaces, indicating the start and end of the density gradient. Note the sharply focused peak at the 2351-s scan and subsequent unfocusing. Migration is toward the positive electrode (acidic pH).

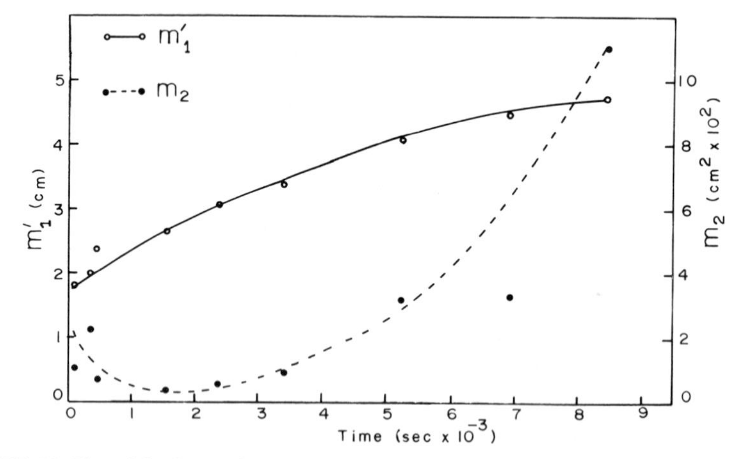

FIGURE 46. Plot of the first (m_1') and second (m_2) statistical moments of the cell distribution shown in Fig. 45 as a function of electrofocusing time.

complete separation of these two types of cells has been achieved. At 4°C the mobility of human red blood cells was 11.44 TU and that of rabbit, 6.32 TU.

TRANS-IF scans in the pH 2.5–8.0 range as a function of time for human erythrocytes are shown in Fig. 45. Similarly to the lymphocyte experiments, the cells appear to be initially focused and subsequently "unfocused" and lysed. Figure 46 shows the kinetics of focusing and unfocusing by following the m_1' and m_2 values of the cell distribution with time. The red blood cells remained "focused" for a shorter period of time in comparison to the lymphocytes, which indicates that these cells are more susceptible to isoelectric damage.

C. Conclusions

It has been demonstrated that the techniques developed for the analytical electrophoretic and sedimentation analysis of mammalian cells provide useful parameters for their characterization in terms of surface charge, volume, and density. These properties may be utilized advantageously in the future for the biophysical discrimination of different types of cells, the study of cell differentiation and transformation phenomena, and the assessment of cell–cell and cell–ligand interactions.

ACKNOWLEDGMENT

This work was supported by National Cancer Institute contract No. N01-CB-43928, National Science Foundation grant No. MPS74-19830, and Office of Naval Research contract No. NR-207-031.

REFERENCES

Agathos, S. N., Griffith, A. L., Uauy-Dagach, R., Young, V. R., and Catsimpoolas, N., 1977, Transient velocity sedimentation at unit gravity of human erythrocytes, *Anal. Biochem.* **81**:143–150.

Ambrose, E. J. (ed.), 1965, *Cell Electrophoresis,* Churchill, London.

Ault, K. A., Griffith, A. L., Platsoucas, C. D., and Catsimpoolas, N., 1976, Partial separation of human blood leucocytes by density gradient electrophoresis: Different mobilities of lymphocytes with IgG, those with IgM and IgD, T lymphocytes and monocytes, *J. Immunol.* **117**:1406.

Boltz, R. C., Todd, P., Streibel, M. J., and Louie, M. K., 1973, Preparative electrophoresis of living mammalian cells in a stationary Ficoll gradient, *Prep. Biochem.* **3**:383.

Catsimpoolas, N., 1971a, Scanning density gradient isoelectric separation of proteins on a micro scale, *Sep. Sci.* **6**:435.

Catsimpoolas, N., 1971b, Analytical scanning isoelectrofocusing: Design and operation of an *in situ* scanning apparatus, *Anal. Biochem.* **44**:411.

Catsimpoolas, N., 1974 Transient electrophoretic analysis of biomolecules and cells. Presented at the *Symposium on Recent Developments in Research Methods and Instrumentation,* National Institutes of Health, Bethesda, Maryland.

Catsimpoolas, N., 1976, Transient state isoelectric focusing, in *Isoelectric Focusing* (N. Catsimpoolas, ed.), p. 229, Academic Press, New York.

Catsimpoolas, N., and Griffith, A. L., 1973, Transient state isoelectric focusing: Computational procedures for digital data processing with a desk-top programmable calculator, *Anal. Biochem.* **56**:100.

Catsimpoolas, N., and Griffith, A. L., 1977a, New instrumentation and procedures for the analysis of mammalian cells by electrophoretic techniques, in *Electrofocusing and Isotachophoresis* (B. J. Radola and D. Graesslin, eds.), p. 469, Walter de Gruyter, Berlin.

Catsimpoolas, N., and Griffith, A. L., 1977b, Transient electrophoretic and velocity sedimentation analysis of lymphocytes. *Anal. Biochem.* **80**:555.

Catsimpoolas, N., Griffith, A. L., Williams, J. M., Chrambach, A., and Rodbard, D., 1975, Electrophoresis with continuous scanning densitometry: Separation of cells in a density gradient, *Anal. Biochem.* **69**:372.

Catsimpoolas, N., Rossi, R., and Griffith, A. L., 1976a, Transient velocity sedimentation of cells at unit gravity, *Life Sci.* **18**:481.

Catsimpoolas, N., Hjertén, S., Kolin, A., and Porath, J. K., 1976b, Unit proposal, *Nature (London)* **259**:264.

Catsimpoolas, N., Griffith, A. L., Skrabut, E. M., Platsoucas, C. D., and Valeri, C. R., 1976c, Differential ^{51}Cr uptake of human peripheral lymphocytes separated by density gradient electrophoresis, *Cell. Immunol.* **25**:317.

Duysens, L. N. M., 1956, The flattening of the absorption spectrum of suspensions as compared to that of solutions, *Biochim. Biophys. Acta* **19**:1.

Griffith, A. L., Catsimpoolas, N., and Wortis, H. H., 1975, Electrophoretic separation of cells in a density gradient, *Life Sci.* **16**:1693.

Griffith, A. L., Catsimpoolas, N., Dewanjee, M. K., and Wortis, H. H., 1976, Electrophoretic separation of radioisotopically labelled mouse lymphocytes, *J. Immunol.* **117**:1949.

Grushka, E., 1975, Chromatographic peak shape analysis, in *Methods of Protein Separation* (N. Catsimpoolas, ed.), Vol. 1, p. 161, Plenum, New York.

Miller, R. G., 1973, Separation of cells by velocity sedimentation, in *New Techniques in Biophysics and Cell Biology* (R. H. Pain and B. J. Smith, eds.), Vol. 1, p. 87, Wiley, New York.

Platsoucas, C. D., Griffith, A. L., and Catsimpoolas, N., 1976, Density gradient electrophoresis of mouse spleen lymphocytes: Separation of T and B cell fractions, *J. Immunol. Methods* **13**:145.

Savitzky, A., and Golay, M. J. E., 1964, Smoothing and differentiation of data by simplified least square procedures, *Anal. Chem.* **36**:1627.

Smith, B. A., Ware, B. R., and Weiner, R. S., 1976, Electrophoretic distributions of human peripheral blood mononuclear white cells from normal subjects and from patients with acute lymphocytic leukemia, *Proc. Natl. Acad. Sci. USA* **73**:2388.

Sturgeon, P., Kolin, A., Kwak, K. S., and Luner, S. J., 1972, Studies of human erythrocytes by endless belt electrophoresis: I. A comparison of electrophoretic mobility with serological reactivity. *Haematologia* **6**:93.

Uzgiris, E. E., and Kaplan, J. H., 1974, Study of lymphocyte and erythrocyte electrophoretic mobility by laser Doppler spectroscopy, *Anal. Biochem.* **60**:455.

Wied, G. L., Bahr, G. F., and Bartels, P. H., 1970, Automatic analysis of cell images by TICAS, in *Automated Cell Identification and Cell Sorting* (G. L. Wied and G. F. Bahr, eds.), p. 195, Academic Press, New York.

Williams, J. M., and Catsimpoolas, N., 1976, A highly regulated, recording constant power, voltage, and current supply for electrophoresis and isoelectric focusing, *Anal. Biochem.* **71**:555.

2

Electrophoretic Light Scattering and Its Application to the Study of Cells

JACK Y. JOSEFOWICZ

I. INTRODUCTION

During recent years researchers have shown that the physical properties of cells can be related to their biological function and that different cell types can be identified and separated by using appropriate physical parameters as distinguishing factors. Such properties as cell size or volume (Miller and Phillips, 1969), density (Shortman, 1968), cell surface markers (Raff, 1971; Zeiller *et al.*, 1974), and surface charge (Dumont, 1974) have been successfully used to distinguish functionally different cells. In this report, the principles of a relatively new electrophoresis technique, referred to as electrophoretic light scattering (ELS) (Ware and Flygare, 1971; Ware, 1974; Flygare *et al.*, 1976) are described. With this technique, the electrophoretic mobility distribution (refer to section II.A) can be measured for a large number of cells, in a small sample volume (0.1 ml), in a fraction of the time required by classical methods. A cell's electrophoretic mobility reflects its surface charge and thus its surface composition. For example, functional changes in a cell are often correlated with changes in the cell's electrophoretic mobility, indicating an alteration in the surface charge and possibly the composition of the membrane (Smith *et al.*, 1976). Changes made in the cell surface by the chemical removal or addition of specific membrane components have been revealed by changes in the cell electrophoretic mobility (Kaplan and Uzgiris, 1975; Josefowicz and Hallett, 1975a). Electrophoretic light scattering is a high-resolution technique which

JACK Y. JOSEFOWICZ • Xerox Research Centre of Canada, Mississauga, Ontario, Canada, L5L 1J9.

shows particular potential in distinguishing cell subpopulations which could not hitherto have been identified by other methods. These and other applications of this technique to the study of mammalian cells will be reviewed.

II. PRINCIPLES OF ELECTROPHORETIC LIGHT SCATTERING

Electrophoretic light scattering is based on a combination of two techniques: electrophoresis and laser Doppler shift spectroscopy. Because a large volume of literature is available dealing with the detailed formulation of both electrophoresis (Shaw, 1969) and light scattering theory (Watrasiewicz and Rudd, 1976), the derivation of formulas will be avoided in this chapter. Instead, an effort will be made to focus on the important physical considerations involved in electrophoretic light scattering as it applies to the study of cellular systems.

A. Electrophoresis

Surface charge is a fundamental property of the cell plasma membrane and is the most significant cellular parameter influencing the ELS technique. The charge is most likely acquired by one or more of the three possible mechanisms: ionization, ion adsorption, and ion dissolution. Because the cell membrane is composed of complex assemblies of functionally diverse, yet interacting, lipid, protein, and carbohydrate units (Rothman and Lenard, 1977), and also because cells are not smooth spheres, but rather sphere-like particles whose membranes are characterized by folds and projections (Fawcett, 1967), it is not possible to precisely determine how the individual features of a cell's surface contribute to its surface charge. However, it is the net charge of the surface components which is of significance since it can be used to distinguish different cell types and surface alterations and abnormalities. In an electrolyte solution at a pH of 7, most viable cells are electronegatively charged. This charged surface causes a redistribution of ions in the liquid medium, allowing ions of opposite charge to be attracted toward the surface. At the periphery of the resulting charged double layer, the concentration of anions will be higher than that of cations. However, at larger distances from the cell surface, the solution is electrically neutral due to the thermally induced Brownian motion of the ions. When an electric field is applied to the cell suspension, some of the weakly attracted anions outside of the double layer are stripped away by the electrostatic force, leaving the cell with a net negative charge. The resulting electrophoretic velocity which is attained by the cell is dependent primarily on three things: the concentration of electrolytes in solution, the magnitude of the applied electric field, and the cell surface charge. This velocity does not, however, reflect the charge at the cell surface. Figure 1 illustrates the actual situation. As the cell moves through its suspending fluid many of the more strongly attracted ions move with it while others are stripped away into the bulk solution. The plane in the ion atmosphere around the cell at which this occurs is referred to as the hydrodynamic slip or shear plane. Consequently, the electrophoretic velocity is a reflection of the potential difference ζ between the electrically neutral bulk solution and the slip plane, which is in turn dependent on the cell surface potential. For this reason the electrophoretic velocity should be considered as an indicator of the cell surface potential and caution should be employed when drawing conclusions about the cell surface electrochemistry based on electrophoretic data.

A useful experimental parameter often used in the electrophoresis of cells is the electrophoretic mobility U_E, which is defined

$$U_E = V_E/E \tag{1}$$

where V_E is the electrophoretic velocity and E is the applied electric field. In practice, the electrophoretic mobility for cells may be determined by the microelectrophoresis technique described by Overbeech and Wiersema (1967), Weiss (1967), and Shaw (1969). A known electric field is applied to the cell suspension by way of a pair of electrodes. As the electronegatively charged cells move toward the anode the velocity of individual cells is measured visually with a stopwatch and a microscope which has been fitted

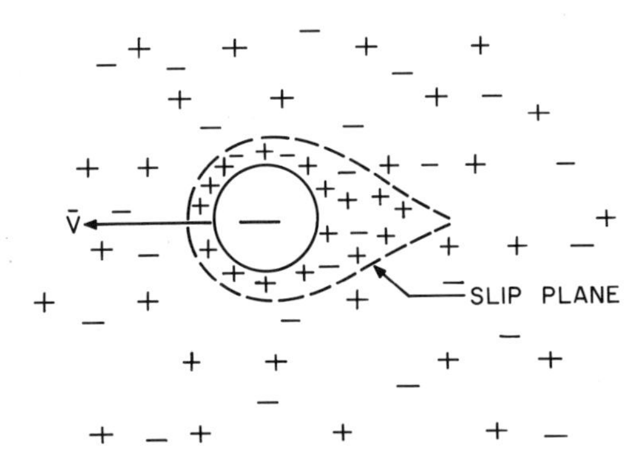

FIGURE 1. A representation of a cell moving through its suspending fluid during electrophoresis. Many of the more strongly attracted ions move with the cell while others are stripped away into the bulk solution. The plane in the ion atmosphere around the cell at which this occurs is referred to as the hydrodynamic slip plane.

with a calibrated reticule. In this way, the electrophoretic mobility may be determined for a population of cells. The disadvantages of making the measurement in this way are these: (a) Since cells within a population of the same type always exhibit a charge distribution, many of the individual cells must be measured in order to arrive at a statistically meaningful result. (b) Since the time required to measure a cell population may be as much as one hour, experiments must be limited to those where the cell suspention is stable during the time of the measurement. (c) Since cells are selected for measurement by the experimentalist, biased conclusions may result.

In contrast, the ELS technique can be used to measure the electrophoretic mobility distribution for a population of approximately 1000 cells within a matter of a minute using automated instrumentation which is independent of the experimentalist once the measurement begins.

The relationship between the electrophoretic mobility U_E and the zeta potential has been discussed in a number of works (Smoluchowski, 1914; Hückel, 1924; Henry, 1931). For particles with a diameter typical of cells ($\sim$10 μ diameter), and for suspending fluids with ionic strengths of 0.001 M or greater, the following relation applies.

$$U_E = D\zeta/4\pi\eta \tag{2}$$

D is the dielectric constant of the suspending medium, and η is the viscosity of the suspending medium. For particles in the size range of cells, this expression applies regardless of size and shape provided that the zeta potential is the same over the whole surface (Abramson and Michaelis, 1929; Abramson, 1931). However, the cell surface is likely to have a large distribution of different ionized charge groups all of which contribute to the electrophoretic mobility. Furthermore, most cells do not have smooth round surfaces, but rather have folds, indentations, and projections. Consequently, it is difficult to assign the location of the slip plane at which the zeta potential is defined. Nevertheless, the zeta potential for a cell can be roughly estimated using equation (2), and for cells of the same type, measured under similar conditions, qualitative comparisons of their surface charge densities may be made based on the calculation of ζ.

B. Laser Doppler Shift Spectroscopy

The application of laser Doppler shift spectroscopy to measure particle velocities was initially reported by Yeh and Cummins (1964). Ware and Flygare (1971) were the first to successfully demonstrate that electrophoretic velocities could be measured for charged particles in a solution, across which an electric field had been applied, using the laser light scattering method. In a typical light scattering experiment, laser light is focused into a particle–fluid suspension. The particles scatter some of this incident light at all angles. If the particles are in motion, i.e., Brownian motion or directed motion, the scattered field, which is the sum of the scattered light waves from the individual particles, exhibits characteristic fluctuations in response to this motion. An analysis of the time dependence or the fluctuation frequencies of such a scattered field provides information about the velocity distribution of the light scattering particles. To detect the fluctuations in the scattered field, two different although equivalent systems have found wide use. They are the time autocorrelation of the fluctuations in the scattered field and the determination of the frequency spectrum of the fluctuations, sometimes referred to as Doppler shift spectroscopy or laser velocimetry. A detailed analysis and review of these methods may be found in articles by Benedek (1969), Cummins and Swinney (1970), Chu (1970), as well as in the books by Cummins and Pike (1973), Chu (1974), Berne and Pecora (1976), and Watrasiewicz and Rudd (1976). The method of Doppler shift spectroscopy has been the preference of many researchers because it permits a more direct interpretation of electrophoretic light scattering data. Therefore, the principles of this light scattering technique will be described, following a brief discussion of how the fluctuations in the scattered light intensity arise as a consequence of particle motion.

Consider a typical light scattering arrangement as depicted in Fig. 2. Laser light, with incident wave vector $\mathbf{k}_0$, is scattered by particles or cells at all angles. A photomultiplier, which is positioned at an angle θ with respect

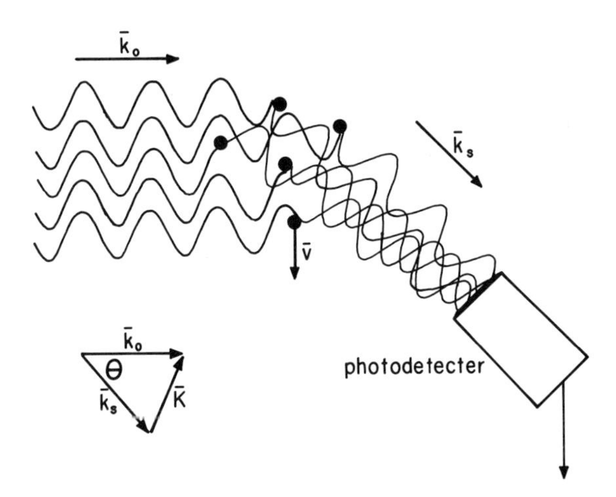

FIGURE 2. An illustration of a typical laser light scattering arrangement. The incident light is given by wave vector $\mathbf{k}_0$, the scattered light by $\mathbf{k}_s$, and the scattering wave vector by $\mathbf{K}$. The scattering angle is θ.

to the incident light, collects some of the scattered light with wave vector $\mathbf{k}_s$. The position of each particle determines the phase of the scattered light which is radiated from its surface. The resulting intensity at the detector surface corresponds to the sum of all the scattered light incident on it. Consequently, the resulting net intensity at any given time t depends on the degree of constructive and destructive interference between scattered light waves. During the ELS experiment, particles undergo a combination of two kinds of motion—Brownian motion as well as a directed motion resulting from the application of the electrostatic force. Since the particles are constantly shifting their positions as time progresses, the phases of the light scattering waves also change with time. This results in intensity fluctuations at the photodetector surface which reflect the characteristic motions of the light scattering particles.

The interpretation of the aforementioned intensity fluctuations may be easily understood by considering the Doppler model. Consider again the light scattering arrangement in Fig. 2. The incident laser light is monochromatic and can be characterized by a single frequency, w_0 ($\sim 10^{14}$ Hz). If a particle in solution is in motion, then the scattered light will be frequency-shifted relative to w_0 by an amount proportional to the velocity of the particle. This frequency shift, referred to as the Doppler shift, W_D, is given by

$$W_D = \mathbf{K} \cdot \mathbf{V}/2\pi \tag{3}$$

where $\mathbf{K}$, the scattering wave vector, is equal to $|\mathbf{k}_0 - \mathbf{k}_s|$ and $\mathbf{V}$ is the velocity vector of the particle. The magnitude of $\mathbf{K}$ is given by

$$|\mathbf{K}| = (4\pi n/\lambda) \sin(\theta/2) \tag{4}$$

where n is the refractive index of the medium surrounding the particles, λ is the vacuum wavelength of the incident laser light, and θ is the scattering angle. Consequently, using the definition for the electrophoretic mobility given by equation (1), the Doppler shift frequency which is introduced to the scattered light as a result of applying an electric field to a cell suspension is given by

$$\begin{aligned} W_D &= (2nu_E E/\lambda) \sin(\theta/2) \cos(\theta/2) \\ &= (nu_E E/\lambda) \sin\theta \end{aligned} \tag{5}$$

where E is the magnitude of the applied electric field and u_E is the electrophoretic mobility. The diffusion constant of cells is small, as they are relatively large particles, with the result that the Brownian motion contributes a negligibly small component to the cells' electrophoretic velocity. Therefore, the Doppler-shifted spectrum associated with a population of scattering cells is broadened primarily by the distribution in their electrophoretic mobilities which is a consequence of their charge heterogeneity.

The information contained in this power spectrum corresponds to the sum of the Doppler shift contributions from every particle in the scattering volume, with the magnitude of each cell's contribution proportional to its scattering cross-section.

To measure the Doppler frequencies, the scattered light, which has been frequency-shifted due to the electrophoretic velocity of the cells, is mixed with a portion of the incident reference beam at the surface of a photodetector located at a predetermined angle. The photodetector is a square-law device; i.e., the photosensitive element in the photodetector detects light intensity which is proportional to the square of the sum of the electric fields illuminating the surface. Therefore, the output signal from the photodetector contains information about the modulation frequencies (or intensity fluctuations described earlier) which correspond to the rapidly oscillating optical field.

C. The Light Scattering Apparatus

A diagrammatic representation of a typical ELS experiment is shown in Fig. 3. Since a coherent monochromatic source of light is required, a laser is employed. For light scattering experiments from cells, which are

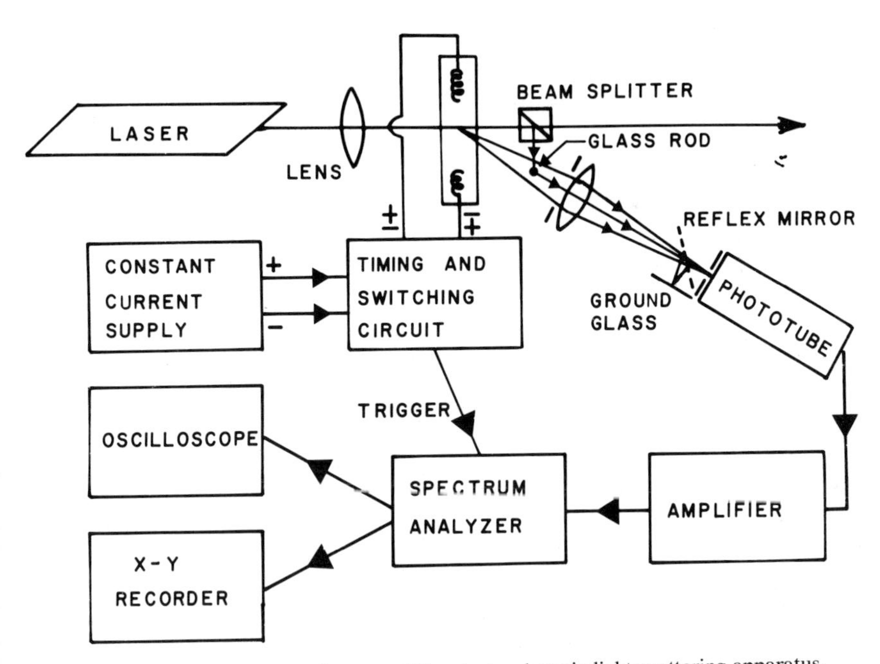

FIGURE 3. Schematic diagram of the electrophoretic light scattering apparatus.

relatively efficient scatterers, low-powered lasers in the range of 5 mV are usually sufficient. It is important however that the laser is operated in the TEM_{00} mode (i.e., the single transverse mode), since multitransverse-mode operation may result in mode hopping, which introduces unwanted intensity fluctuations that interfere with the light scattering spectrum. A lens focuses the laser light into the center of an ELS chamber. The scattering angle is defined by a pinhole and lens positioned in front of a photodetector, which focus the light from the scattering particles onto an adjustable slit located just in front of the photosensitive surface. Thus, the scattering volume size can be varied by introducing laser-focusing lenses of different focal lengths and by adjusting the opening of the slit. The ability to vary the scattering volume size is an important consideration, since one source of spectral broadening may be due to "transit-time broadening" which results from the intensity fluctuations in the scattered light associated with the time that a moving particle spends in the scattering volume. This source of broadening may be made negligibly small by defining a scattering volume large enough so that the time necessary for a moving cell to transverse it is long compared with the period of the intensity fluctuations resulting from the electrophoretic spacial repositioning of the cells.

In order to efficiently mix the scattered light from the chamber with a portion of the incident laser beam, the author as well as other researchers have found the following scheme most practical (Smith *et al.*, 1976; Josefowicz *et al.*, 1977; Luner *et al.*, 1977). A lens focuses a threefold magnified image of a portion of the light scattering chamber, through which the laser beam passes, onto the adjustable slit located just in front of the photosensitive surface of the photodetector. Using a beam splitter, the unshifted laser light is introduced by directing a portion of the beam passing through the chamber onto a 50-μm-diameter glass rod or wire (local oscillator) which is positioned along the optical axis of the photodetector. The position of this rod must be slightly out of focus at the photosensitive surface of the photodetector in order to keep to a minimum the obstruction of scattered light from the chamber. The local oscillator is aligned with the scattering volume, first by positioning one of the reference lines on the calibrated ground glass so that it corresponds with the position of the adjustable slit opening, and then by precisely superimposing their images onto the ground glass using a reflex mirror which can be swung out of the optical path during the experiment. A ratio of intensities of 1:20 is normally used between the scattered light and the local oscillator, respectively. Laser light which passes through the chamber creates an image on the ground glass which has bright spots corresponding to the positions of the front and rear windows of the chamber. Consequently, by moving the position of this image on the ground glass, using x-y-z translators upon which the chamber is mounted, and by adjusting the opening of the slit, both the location and the size of the scattering volume may be changed. This method of optical mixing is advantageous because the scattering volume can be positioned anywhere within the light scattering chamber, the ratio of intensities between the local oscillator and the scattered light can be adjusted by deflecting more or less light onto the glass rod, and the size of the scattering volume can easily be changed by varying the opening size of the adjustable slit. The other methods of mixing a reference beam with scattered light have been described by Forman *et al.* (1966a,b), Goldstein and Kried (1967), Rudd (1969a,b), Penney (1970), and Wang (1971). Either a photomultiplier tube or a sensitive photodiode can be used as the photodetector. An important consideration in this regard is that the photodetector of choice has a high quantum efficiency in the spectral range of interest so that signal-to-noise is maximized. The photocurrent which originates from the intensity fluctuations at the photosensitive surface of the detector is sent to an ammeter and then through a dropping resistor which is fixed to ground. The value of this resistance should be such that Johnson noise is small compared with the signal generated by the photocurrent. The voltage signal across the dropping resistor is sent to a preamplifier and then to the input of a real-time spectrum analyzer. The term "real time" refers to the capability of the analyzer to process an input signal in a time equal to or less than the data-acquisition time. A variety of fast-Fourier-transform real-time spectrum analyzers are now available from a number of manufacturers (Princeton Applied Research, Nicolet, Spectral Dynamics Corporation, Rockland). These spectrum analyzers allow for signal averaging, and the summed signal can be displayed on an oscilloscope and x-y recorder. The signal can also be output in digital form for computer analysis. A timing and switching circuit is used to trigger the spectrum analyzer as well as to apply voltage pulses, from a constant-current power supply, across the light scattering chamber. A duty cycle is usually chosen so that the ratio of the time during which DC voltage pulse is applied to the chamber and the time between pulses is 1/10. The polarity of the voltage is changed between sequential pulses in order to ensure that no concentration gradients are formed in solution. The duration of the voltage pulse is dictated by the time required for data acquisition, which usually corresponds to the reciprocal of the frequency window for the spectral bandwidth used. Typically, data-acquisition times are in the range of 2 and 8 s depending on the bandwidth chosen.

D. The Electrophoretic Light Scattering Chamber

One of the most important elements of the ELS apparatus is the sample chamber. A variety of chambers have recently been reported (Haas and Ware, 1976; Hartford and Flygare, 1975; Josefowicz and Hallett, 1975b). Most of these are adaptations of the chamber designs used in the classical microelectrophoresis technique (Shaw, 1969; Ambrose, 1965). The desirable features of an ELS chamber are a small sample volume, a temperature regulating system to neutralize the effects of joule heating, a method of excluding electrode contamination in and near the sample volume, the capability of applying high electric fields, and a method of eliminating or minimizing the effects of electroosmosis. One chamber design which adequately meets all of the above characteristics and which was recently used by Josefowicz *et al.* (1977) to study thymocytes is represented in Fig. 4. This chamber has three compartments: a central quartz sample chamber shown in Fig. 5, having a volume of 0.08 cm^3, and electrode chambers located at either end. The sample chamber is separated from the electrode compartments by dialysis membranes to prevent the gas bubbles produced at the electrodes from entering the sample chamber. The cylindrical ends of the sample chamber extend inside the collars of lexan blocks which contain O-rings that both seal the chamber and also hold the dialysis membranes securely in place. Semispherical platinum black electrodes are cemented (silicone) into the electrode chambers which are housed in the lexan blocks at both ends of the chamber. The lexan blocks and sample chamber are embedded in aluminum and copper blocks that are

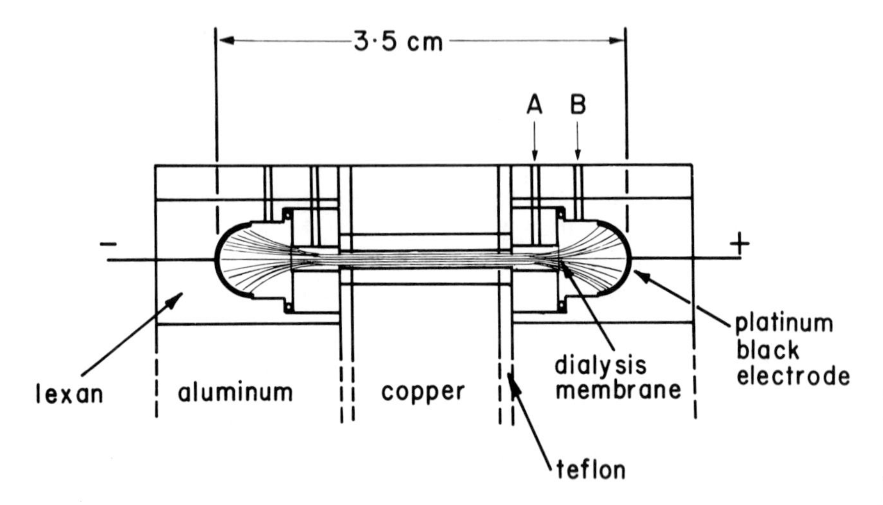

FIGURE 4. Diagrammatic representation of the electrophoretic light scattering chamber. It features platinum black electrodes which are connected to a constant-current power supply by platinum leads. Dialysis membranes are held in place over the ends of a quartz sample chamber by O-rings which also serve to seal the electrode chambers. The electric field lines between electrodes are represented by fine lines.

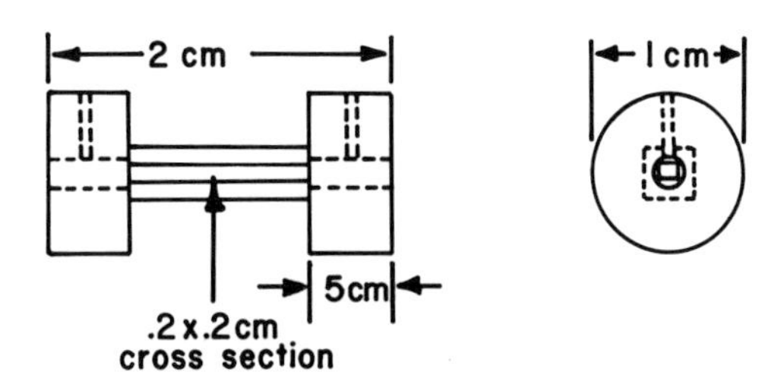

FIGURE 5. The sample chamber is composed of a quartz insert. It has a sample volume of 0.08 ml. The scattering volume is usually located inside the rectangular portion, which is indicated by the arrow, having a cross section of 0.04 cm².

temperature regulated. Using the 1-mm-diameter filling holes, labeled A, the sample chamber can be filled independently of the electrode chambers, which are filled via holes B, thereby keeping the sample volume to a minimum. Electric field lines inside the chamber are depicted between the electrodes. The electric field in the sample chamber can be calculated using

$$E = i/\sigma\alpha \tag{6}$$

where i is the current passing through the chamber, σ is the specific conductivity of the solution, and α is the cross-sectional area of the region where the field is to be determined. In cell electrophoresis experiments, one of the major sources of error in the measurement of the electrophoretic mobility is the inability to precisely calculate E. This is due mainly to the high-ionic-strength solutions required when working with cells which, at the relatively high fields used in ELS (50 V/cm), cause a substantial amount of joule heating. This heating results in a temperature increase in the solution, thereby lowering the viscosity, which increases the mobility of the charged particles (i.e., cells). Neverthelss, heating effects can be held to a minimum by using a constant-current power supply. As joule heating warms the solution the conductivity of the solution increases at approximately the same rate as the electrophoretic mobility. Maintaining a constant current causes the electric field to decrease at a rate similar to the increase in electrophoretic mobility. In this way the mobility is maintained at approximately the same value throughout the time during which the field is applied. However, if excessively high fields are used or if pulses of very long duration are applied to the chamber, the excessive heat generated can produce convection currents and turbulence which are intolerable during the measurement of Doppler shifts. Therefore, prior to an experiment, the duty cycle is adjusted so that there is sufficient time between pulses for the solution to return to the initially prescribed temperature.

Another source of error in the measurement of cell electrophoretic mobility is the electroosmotic effect. For the solutions at which cell electrophoresis experiments are normally performed (i.e., ~ pH 7), the glass walls which are in contact with the solution acquire a surface charge. Counter ions in solution concentrate at the walls so that when a field is applied across the chamber, these ions move toward the electrode of opposite charge, carrying with them some of the solution. This results in the formation of a pressure head at one of the electrode chambers which in turn causes a backflow of solution through the chamber. Depending on the nature of the charge on the walls of the chamber and the surface charge of the cells, this flow, which has a parabolic profile, contributes in an additive or subtractive manner to the electrophoretic velocity attained by the cells. This problem can be solved by coating the walls of the chamber with a neutral substance, thus neutralizing the surface charge on the chamber walls. For a solution pH of about 7, a methylcellulose coating has been found to work well. However, it is essential that the velocity profile through the sample chamber cross-section be monitored at different times during a series of experiments to ensure that the wall coating has not been removed through the action of flushing the chamber or that the walls have not been overcoated by substances in solution. Since this kind of check can only be done by moving the scattering volume through the chamber cross-section, it is important that an optical arrangement of the kind described earlier be used.

Another solution to the problem of electroosmosis has been reported by Uzgiris (1974). His ELS chamber design features a pair of parallel and closely spaced (approximately 0.5 mm) platinum black electrodes which can be immersed into any light scattering cuvette. In this arrangement the glass–water interface at the walls of the cuvette is kept far away from the electrodes, thus avoiding the effects of electroosmosis. However, this design is susceptible to a number of other undesirable effects. Since the scattering volume must be positioned between the parallel plate electrodes, the gas bubbles which are formed at their surfaces can move into the scattering volume. The parallel plate design leaves the regions above and below the electrodes open so that as joule heating occurs, the warmed lower-density solution has a tendency to rise, thereby causing convective turbulence, as has been reported by Mohan *et al.* (1976). Due to the narrow spacing of the electrodes, the applied voltage pulse must be reversed many times during a measurement in order to avoid solution inhomogeneity and electrode polarization. The switching frequency of the voltage pulses is introduced into the light scattering spectrum and consequently further data processing is required to interpret the modulated spectrum (Bennett and Uzgiris, 1973).

III. CELL ELECTROPHORETIC LIGHT SCATTERING

Since it was realized that the electrophoretic mobility distribution of a population of light scattering particles could be determined by Doppler shift spectroscopy, there has been considerable activity in applying this method to the study of viable cells (Uzgiris, 1972). Most of this work has involved the detection of cell subpopulations either to distinguish between diseased and normal cells (Smith *et al.*, 1976, 1978) or to elucidate the degree of charge heterogeneity within a cell population (Uzgiris and Kaplan, 1974; Kaplan and Uzgiris, 1975; Josefowicz and Hallett, 1975a; Kaplan and Uzgiris, 1976; Uzgiris and Kaplan, 1976; Josefowicz *et al.*, 1977). Some of this work will be reviewed in this section, following the description of an experiment that illustrates the resolution of the ELS technique in distinguishing different cell types when they are mixed in solution (Josefowicz and Ware, unpub.).

A mixture of human and rabbit red blood cells was chosen because these red blood cells, as measured by classical microelectrophoresis, have mean electrophoretic mobilities which vary by a factor of two (Abramson, 1931). The experiments were performed at solution conditions of 0.013 M NaCl, 0.290 M sorbitol, 0.010 M bis-tris, and 0.002 M HCl, with a pH of 7.1 and a conductivity of 1.34 mmho/cm at 20°C. As in most ELS cell experiments a solution with an ionic strength of approximately 1/10 physiological conditions was used to minimize joule heating and to increase the resolution of the Doppler shift measurement (cell electrophoretic mobility increases with decreasing solution ionic strength). Prior to the experiments, the quartz sample chamber was coated with methylcellulose to eliminate electroosmosis. This was confirmed by determining the mobility profile of human red blood cells. A series of experiments was performed as the scattering volume was moved vertically from the bottom to the top of the chamber while maintained in a constant central position between the front and back windows. The result of one such series is shown in Fig. 6. The mobility profile is characterized by plug flow which indicates that the coated walls were electrically neutral. The presence of electroosmosis would have resulted in a parabolic profile. The results of ELS experiments from a 1:1 mixture of human and rabbit red blood cells having a concentration of 1×10^6 cells/cm^2, as well as those from the solutions of the two individual cell types at the same concentration, are shown in Fig. 7. The x axis has been adjusted to electrophoretic mobility units of μm-cm/V-s and the y axis, which is proportional to cell number, has been normalized to facilitate comparison. The superposition of the spectra from the individual human and rabbit red blood cells with the spectrum obtained from the mixture of the two cell types indicates that ELS has excellent resolving

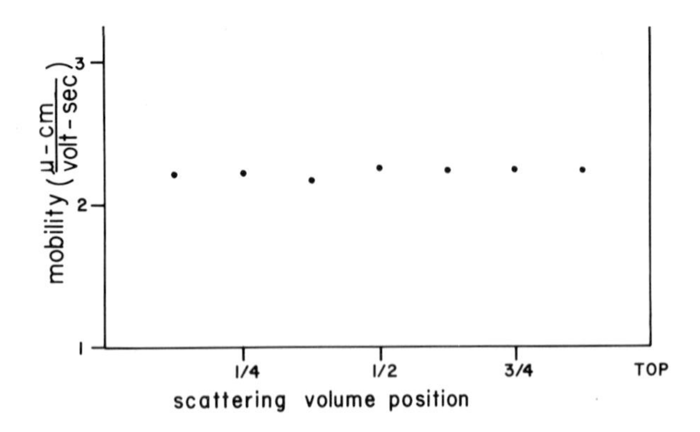

FIGURE 6. Electrophoretic mobility profile for human red blood cells through the sample chamber cross section. The flat profile indicates that coating the chamber walls with methylcellulose has essentially eliminated electroosmosis. The experiments were performed using laser light with a wavelength of 514.5 nm, a scattering angle of 11.2°, and a temperature of 20°C.

power. In addition, the characteristic form of the distributions for both cell types has been preserved. The small change in the mean mobilities of both distributions may be attributed to sample variability. The width of the distributions is primarily due to surface charge heterogeneity within the red blood cell populations. Less than 1% of the width is the result of diffusive motion.

Josefowicz *et al.* (1977) used ELS to identify and demonstrate the analytical resolution of many dynamic lymphocyte subpopulations within the mouse thymus. Previous work by other researchers, using microelectrophoresis (Dumont, 1974) and free-flow electrophoresis (Zeiller *et al.*, 1974), had identified four subpopulations of mouse thymus lymphocytes. These studies suggested that further subclasses of thymocytes exist although they could not be demonstrated by classical techniques. Josefowicz *et al.* (1977) were able to confirm and amplify these suggestions by combining a new preparative velocity sedimentation method (Catsimpoolas and Griffith, 1977) with ELS. Mouse thymus lymphocytes were obtained from CBA/J male mice, purified by Ficoll–Hypaque density gradient centrifugation, washed in PBS, and layered on top of the velocity sedimentation column which contained a 1% to 2% BSA/PBS density gradient maintained at 4°C. After the cells had sedimented for 4 h, 50 cell fractions (2.0 ml each) were removed sequentially from the bottom of the column and, using a small aliquot from each fraction, cell size and cell concentration were determined using a Coulter Channelyzer and Coulter Counter, respectively. Each fraction was then washed with the electrophoresis buffer, previously described in this section, and analyzed using ELS. The capability of the ELS technique to sample small volumes was a prerequisite in making this study feasible. In addition, the determination of the electrophoretic mobility distribution of the thymocytes in each fraction could be accomplished by the apparatus in less than 5 min, during which time approximately 10^3 cells were sampled. The profile of cells in the sedimentation column after 4 h is shown in Fig. 8. A series of ELS spectra are shown in Fig. 9. The electrophoretic-mobility distribution of the total cell sample (i.e., a portion of the cells which were not passed through the velocity sedimentation column) is shown along with the distributions of six cell fractions selected at intervals over the entire sedimentation profile. The electrophoretic mobility distribution of the total sample, which included cells in all size ranges, encompasses all the mobilities present in the distributions associated with the individual sedimented fractions. Small thymocytes had significantly lower mean mobilities than medium and large thymocytes, a characteristic also reported by Shortman *et al.* (1975) and Droege and Zucker (1975). Another most interesting finding is that these spectra provide clear evidence of at least three electrophoretically distinct

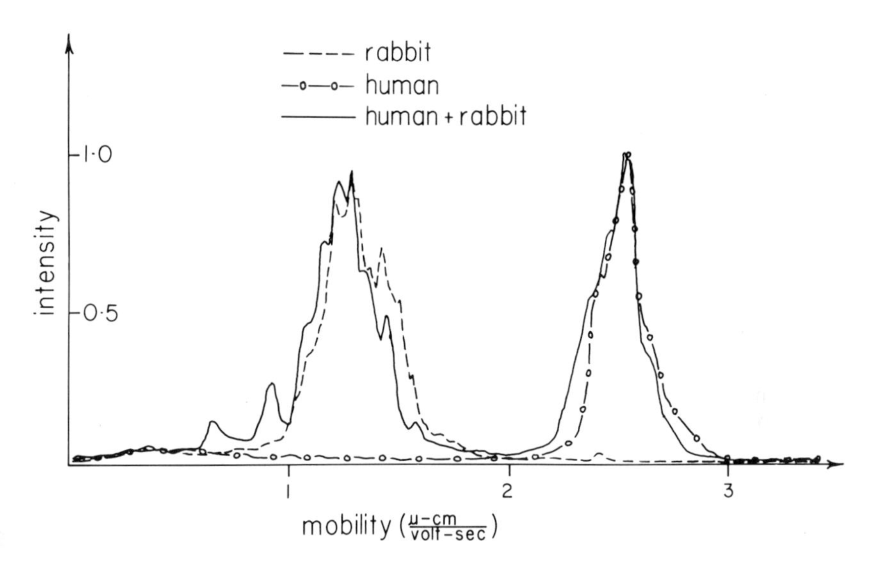

FIGURE 7. Electrophoretic mobility distributions for human red blood cells, rabbit red blood cells, and a mixture of the two at a ratio of 1:1. The cell concentration in all three cases was 1×10^6 cells/cm^3. The experiments were performed using a scattering angle of 11.2°, a laser wavelength of 514.5 nm, and a temperature of 25°C. (From Josefowicz and Ware, unpublished results.)

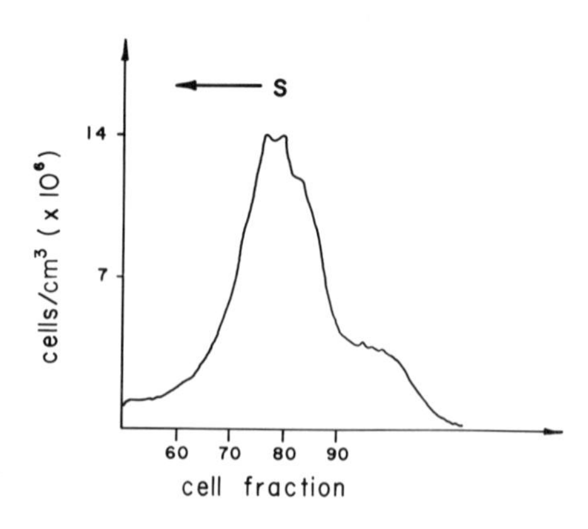

FIGURE 8. The distribution of thymocytes in the sedimentation column after 4 h as determined by the analysis of individual cell fractions using a Coulter Counter. Cell fractions were collected from the bottom of the column, the direction of sedimentation being indicated by the arrow. Measurement of the cell volume distribution in each fraction, using a Coulter Channelyzer indicated that the cells were separated primarily according to size. The analysis of low- to high-numbered fractions showed cell volume to decrease monotonically. A few fractions exhibited bimodal distributions. (From Josefowicz *et al.*, 1977.)

subpopulations in each of the cell fractions. Each of the subpopulations may represent a functionally unique subset of thymocytes. This study indicates that high-resolution electrophoretic separation would isolate a large number of physically distinct subpopulations. Once isolated, it will be possible to determine their immunological significance.

An area of cellular immunology which has recently received much attention is the cell surface effect of mitogens such as phytohemagglutinin (PHA), concanavalin A (Con A), and pokeweed. A detailed discussion of the mechanisms by which the stimulation of lymphocytes by mitogens is accomplished has been made by Edelman *et al.* (1974). Briefly, binding between the mitogen and the appropriate receptor site on the cell membrane occurs within seconds or minutes and is followed by an alteration in the chain of metabolic events within the cell which eventually lead to mitosis. Since the primary requirement for the mitogen-induced changes involves the specific binding of the mitogen to the cell surface, a measurement of the alteration in the cell surface charge using ELS provides an effective and direct observation of this initial phenomenon. Kaplan and Uzgiris (1975) have measured changes in the electrophoretic mobility and isoelectric point produced by incubating human peripheral blood lymphocytes with PHA and Con A. The lymphocytes used in their study were drawn from human blood and purified first on Ficoll–Hypaque gradients and then on nylon fiber columns. The Doppler measurements were made under conditions of low ionic strength, using an isosmotic sucrose buffer at an ionic strength of 0.005 M. The results of incubating lymphocytes with PHA-P (25 μg/ml) are shown in Fig. 10. Incubations of 1.5 and 90 h were observed to cause a decrease in electrophoretic mobility over the entire pH

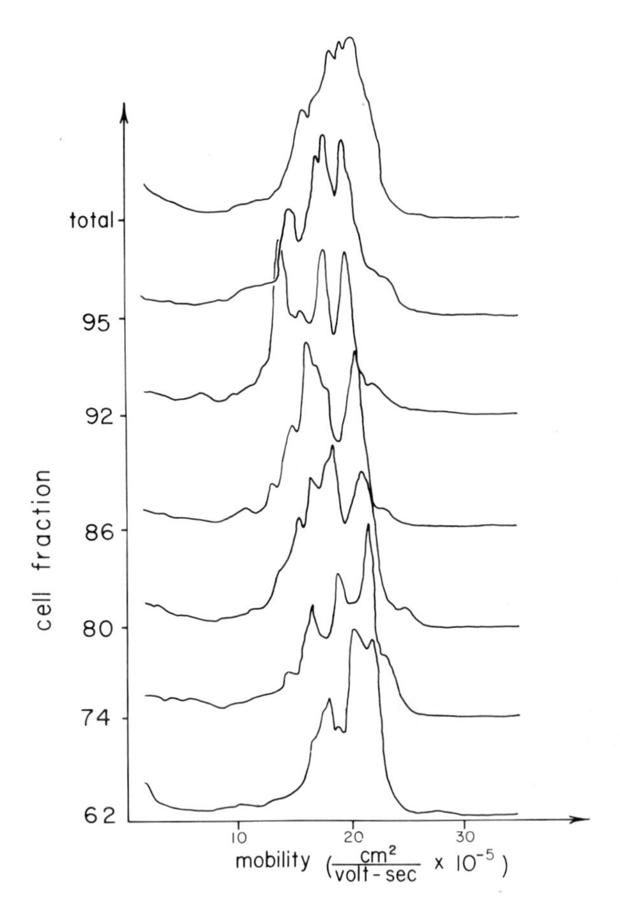

FIGURE 9. Electrophoretic mobility distributions for the total sample and six cell fractions selected at intervals over the entire sedimentation profile. The total sample was not passed through the velocity sedimentation apparatus. All electrophoretic light scattering experiments were performed at a scattering angle of 11.2° using laser light at a wavelength of 514.5 nm, an electric field of 62.5 V/cm, and a temperature of 20°C. Approximately 10^3 cells were sampled in each of the spectra shown. (From Josefowicz *et al.*, 1977.)

range studied. A similar study using Con A showed that after an initial change, no further change in mobility was detected after various periods of incubation of between 1 and 70 h. However, as the concentration of Con A was increased, a progressive decrease in mobility resulted, as shown in Fig. 11. It was also shown that cell mobilities did not change when incubation took place in the presence of the sugars methyl-α-glucoside or methyl-α-D-

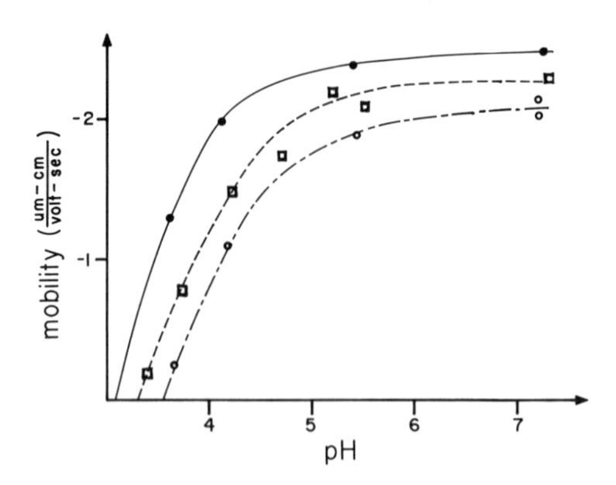

FIGURE 10. Effects of short-term (1.5 h) and long-term (90 h) incubation by PHA-P on the observed mobility of lymphocytes. PHA-P-treated lymphocytes were suspended in 0.28 M sucrose buffer of 0.005 M ionic strength. The pH was altered from 7.3 down to 3.2 by the addition of 0.005 M HCl in 0.28 M sucrose. Mobilities were measured at 25°C. ●, Control (no PHA-P); □, 1.5-h incubation with PHA-P; ○, 90-h incubation with PHA-P. (From Kaplan and Uzgiris, 1975.)

mannoside, which are specific inhibitors of Con A binding. Furthermore, the induced mobility changes could also be reversed by subsequent washing of the Con-A-incubated lymphocytes with the aforementioned sugars. This study demonstrated that specific receptor sites on the cell surface have a role in determining the overall charge density of the cell membrane, and that measured changes in electrophoretic mobility do indeed reflect the binding of mitogens to these sites. Thus, ELS has proved to be a useful technique in providing a direct assay for mitogen binding to the cell surface.

In a similar study, Josefowicz and Hallett (1975a) determined the effect of pokeweed mitogen on the electrophoretic mobility of rat thymus lymphocytes using ELS. After incubating the lymphocytes in a low-ionic-strength buffer (0.015 M) containing 50 μg/ml pokeweed for 15 min, the mean electrophoretic mobility was observed to decrease by approximately 50%.

Two separate laboratories have recently used ELS to determine the electrophoretic mobility distributions of normal human T and B lymphocytes (Kaplan and Uzgiris, 1976; Smith *et al.*, 1978). Using low-ionic-strength-solution conditions (0.005 M by the former group and 0.015 M by the latter) and rosette depletion techniques, it was shown that T cells have a greater electrophoretic mobility than B cells and that ELS can provide an assay for these two cell types in a mixture. Fig. 12 shows the electrophoretic mobility distributions of a sample of human mononuclear white blood cells and of the same sample which had been depleted of T cells by the

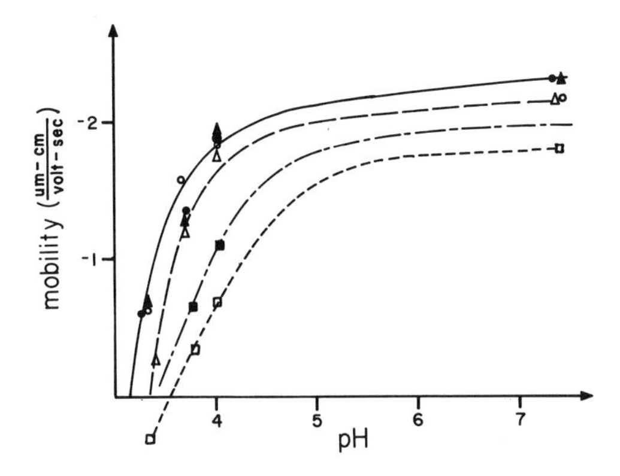

FIGURE 11. Effect on lymphocyte mobility by varying concentrations of Con A. Lymphocytes were purified on a nylon fiber column. Time of incubation with Con A was 1¾ h. ●, Control (no Con A); ▲, 60 g/ml Con A plus 0.2 M methyl-α-D-glucoside; ○, 20 g/ml Con A; Δ, 60 g/ml Con A; ■, 100 g/ml Con A; □, 200 g/ml Con A. (From Kaplan and Uzgiris, 1975.)

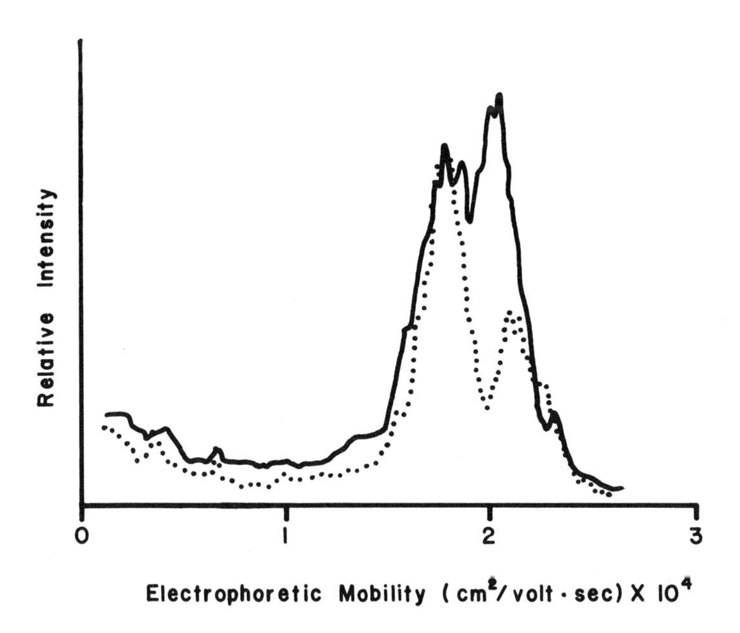

FIGURE 12. A comparison of the electrophoretic mobility distributions (at 0.015 M ionic strength) of a fresh human mononuclear white blood cell sample before (solid line) and after (dotted line) E_{AET} rosette depletion. The whole sample (solid line) contained 44% cells which form E_{AET} rosettes and 32% cells which form EAC rosettes. (From Smith *et al.*, 1978.)

E_{AET}–rosette method. Smith *et al.* (1978) also showed that by removing the B cells using the EAC–rosette method, the lower-mobility distribution was eliminated, leaving only the higher-mobility T cells, as shown in Fig. 13. After treating a mixture of B and T cells with neuraminidase (1.25 units/ml at 37°C for 70 min), the surface charge of T cells was reduced to a much greater extent than that of B cells, thus causing the relative mobilities of the two cell types to be reversed. Since neuraminidase is known to cleave *N*-acetylneuraminic acid, these results suggest that either this chemical group is more exposed at the surface of the T-cell membrane than it is at the B-cell surface or that the density of this membrane chemical component is higher on the T-cell surface. In either case, the T cells would appear to have a higher electrophoretic mobility relative to B cells before cleavage and have a relatively lower mobility after cleavage.

In comparing the results of the electrophoretic mobility distributions of normal and leukemic human mononuclear white blood cells (acute lympho-

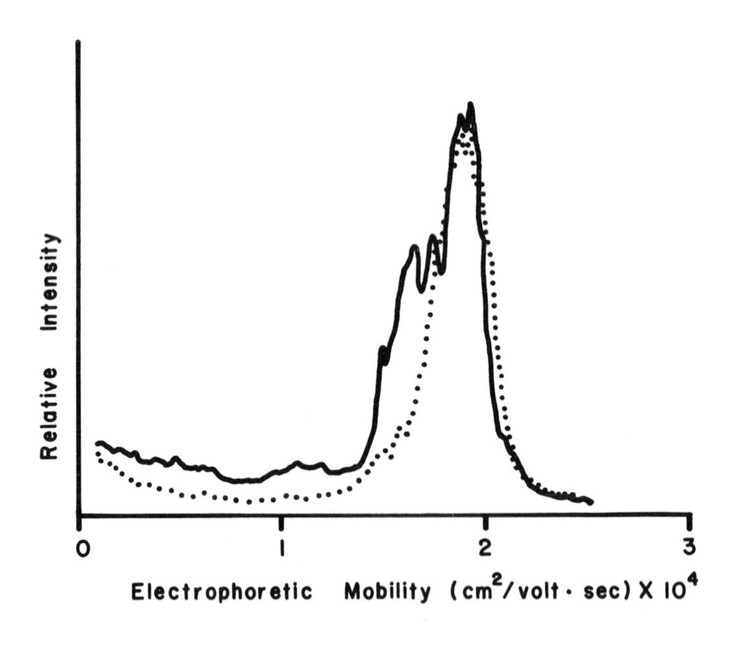

FIGURE 13. A comparison of the electrophoretic mobility distributions (at 0.015 M ionic strength) of a fresh human mononuclear white blood cell sample before (solid line) and after (dotted line) EAC rosette depletion. The whole sample (solid line) contained 63% cells which form E_{AET} rosettes and 16% cells which form EAC rosettes. (From Smith *et al.*, 1978.)

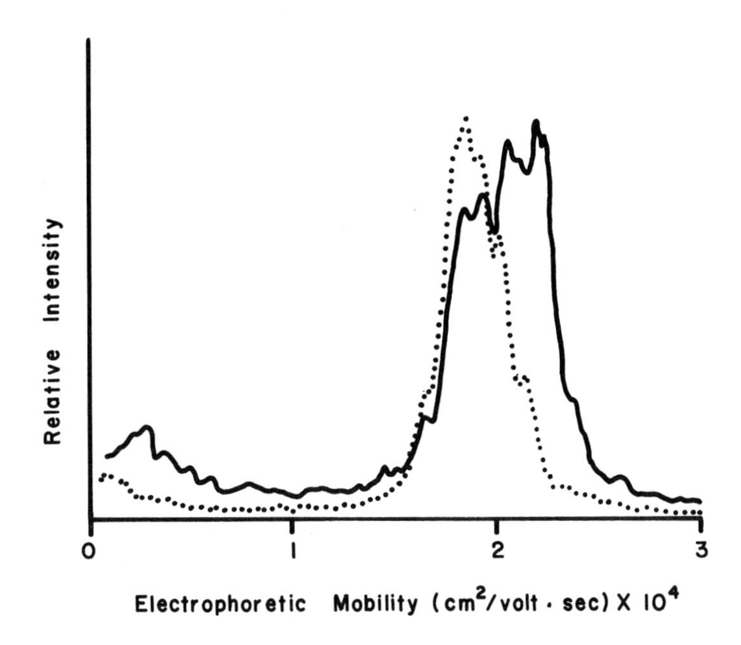

FIGURE 14. Electrophoretic mobility distributions for normal (solid line) and leukemic (acute lymphocytic leukemia, dotted line) human mononuclear white blood cells at 0.015 M ionic strength. The leukemic cells have a distinctly lower mode mobility than normal cells and their distribution nearly coincides with that portion of the normal distribution which was identified as B cells. (From Smith *et al.*, 1978.)

cytic leukemia), Smith *et al.* (1978) have shown that the leukemic cells appear to overlap with the B-cell distribution, as shown in Fig. 14. After treating leukemic cells with neuraminidase, the mode of their electrophoretic mobility distribution decreased and appeared in the same position as the neuraminidase-treated T cells. This lack of electrophoretic correspondence between leukemic and normal cells suggests that leukemic cells have a membrane composition distinct from that of either T or B cells.

IV. CONCLUSION

The electrokinetic surface of a cell provides a fingerprint of its surface chemical composition. It has been shown that, based on the measurement of electrophoretic mobility, different cell types can be distinguished, subpopulations within a cell type can be identified, and changes of the membrane surface brought about by binding of chemical agents can be revealed. Cell surface charge has been and will continue to be important in studies involving practically all aspects of cellular morphology. The new technique of electrophoretic light scattering provides a means of measuring the electrophoretic mobility distributions of cells by an automatic instrumental method which combines classical microelectrophoresis with laser Doppler shift spectroscopy. In addition to preserving all of the advantages inherent to microelectrophoresis, electrophoretic light scattering has new features which extend the capability and flexibility of electrokinetic measurements. The significant features of electrophoretic light scattering are:

1. It makes measurements quickly: the electrophoretic mobility of hundreds of cells may be measured simultaneously in a matter of seconds.
2. The resolution of an electrophoretic measurement is greater than by other methods.
3. Small sample volumes can be analyzed; i.e., 0.1 ml.
4. No concentration gradients or boundary layers are formed during the measurement which can complicate the interpretation of electrophoretic data.
5. Solution conditions of physiological to very low ionic strength can be used.
6. Both microscopic- and submicroscopic-sized particles may be analyzed.

The major disadvantage of electrophoretic light scattering is that it is strictly an analytical technique, in that, although fine differences in cell mobilities can be distinguished, the cells cannot be physically separated for further analysis. This limitation may be overcome in the near future when electrophoretic light scattering is incorporated into a preparative type of apparatus so that the subpopulations which are distinguished electrophoretically can also be simultaneously separated and analyzed for their biological significance.

ACKNOWLEDGMENTS

The author wishes to acknowledge many stimulating discussions with Ben R. Ware, Robert V. Mustacich, and Barton A. Smith. This work was supported by a Killam Foundation Scholarship of the Canada Council.

REFERENCES

Abramson, H. A., 1931, The influence of size, shape and conductivity on cataphoretic mobility, and its biological significance. A review, *J. Phys. Chem.* **35**:289.

Abramson, H. A., and Michaelis, L., 1929, The influence of size, shape and conductivity of microscopically visible particles on cataphoretic mobility, *J. Gen. Physiol.* **12**:587.

Ambrose, E. J., 1965, *Cell Electrophoresis,* Churchill, London.

Benedek, G. B., 1969, *Polarization, Matiere and Rayonnment,* Presses Universitaire de France, Paris.

Bennett, A. J., and Uzgiris, E. E., 1973, Laser doppler spectroscopy in an oscillating electric field, *Phys. Rev. A* **8**:2662.

Berne, B. J., and Pecora, R., 1976, *Dynamic Light Scattering,* John Wiley and Sons, New York.

Catsimpoolas, N., and Griffith, A. L., 1977, Preparative density gradient electrophoresis and velocity sedimentation at unit gravity of mammalian cells, in *Methods of Cell Separation,* Vol. 1 (N. Catsimpoolas, ed.), pp. 1–23, Plenum, New York.

Chu, B., 1970, Laser light scattering, *Annu. Rev. Phys. Chem.* **21**:145.

Chu, B., 1974, *Laser Light Scattering,* Academic Press, New York.

Cummins, H. Z., and Pike, E. R. (eds.), 1973, *Photon Correlation and Light Beating Spectroscopy,* Plenum Press, New York.

Cummins, H. Z., and Swinney, H. L., 1970, Laser light scattering, in *Progress in Optics* (E. Wolf, ed.), American Elsevier, New York.

Droege, W., and Zucker, R., 1975, Lymphocyte subpopulations in the thymus, *Transplant Rev.* **25**:3.

Dumont, F., 1974, Electrophoretic analysis of cell subpopulations in the mouse thymus as a function of age, *Immunology* **26**:1051.

Edelman, G. M., Spear, P. G., Rutishauser, U., and Yahara, I., 1974, Receptor specificity and mitogenesis in lymphocyte population, in *The Cell Surface in Development* (A. A. Moscona, ed.), John Wiley and Sons, New York.

Fawcett, D. W., 1967, *The Cell,* W. B. Saunders, Philadelphia.

Flygare, W. H., Hartford, S. L., and Ware, B. R., 1976, Electrophoretic light scattering, in *Molecular Electro-Optics,* Part I (C. T. O'Konski, ed.), pp. 321, Marcel Dekker, New York.

Forman, J. W., Jr., George, E. W., and Lewis, R. D., 1966a, Fluid flow measurement with a laser doppler velocimeter, *IEEE J. Quantum Electron.* GE-2, 260.

Forman, J. W. Jr., Lewis, R. D., and Thornton, J. R., 1966b, Laser Doppler velocimeter for measurement of localised fluid velocities in liquids, *Proc. IEEE* **54**: 424.

Goldstein, R. J., and Kried, D. K., 1967, Measurement of laminar flow development in a square duct using a laser Doppler flowmeter, *J. Appl. Mech.* **89**: 813.

Haas, D. D., and Ware, B. R., 1976, Design and construction of a new electrophoretic light scattering chamber and applications to solutions of hemoglobin, *Anal. Biochem.* **74**:175.

Hartford, S. L., and Flygare, W. H., 1975, Electrophoretic light scattering of calf thymus deoxyribonucleic acid and tobacco mosaic virus, *Macromolecules* **8**:80.

Henry, D. C., 1931, The cataphoresis of suspended particles. Part I, The equation of cataphoresis, *Proc. Roy. Soc.* **A133**:106.

Hückel, E., 1924, Die Kataphorese der kugel, *Physik. Z.* **25**:204.

Josefowicz, J., and Hallett, F. R., 1975a, Cell surface effects of pokeweed observed by electrophoretic light scattering, *FEBS Lett.* **60**:62.

Josefowicz, J., and Hallett, R. R., 1975b, Homodyne electrophoretic light scattering of polystyrene spheres by laser cross-beam intensity correlation, *Appl. Optics* **14**:740.

Josefowicz, J. Y., Ware, B. R., Griffith, A. L., and Catsimpoolas, N., 1977, Physical heterogeneity of mouse thymus lymphocytes, *Life Sci.* **21**:1483.

Kaplan, J. H., and Uzgiris, E. E., 1975, The detection of phytomitogen-induced changes in human lymphocyte surfaces by laser Doppler spectroscopy, *J. Immunol. Methods* **7**:337.

Kaplan, J. H., and Uzgiris, E. E., 1976, Identifications of T and B cell subpopulations in human peripheral blood: Electrophoretic mobility distributions associated with surface marker characteristics, *J. Immunol.* **117**:115.

Luner, S. J., Szklarek, D., Knox, R. J., Seaman, G. V. F., Josefowicz, J. Y., and Ware, B. R., 1977, Red cell charge is not a function of cell age, *Nature* **269**:719.

Miller, R. G., and Phillips, R. A., 1969, Separation of cells by velocity sedimentation, *J. Cell Physiol.* **73**:191.

Mohan, R., Stiener, R., and Kaufmann, R., 1976, Laser Doppler spectroscopy as applied to electrophoresis in protein solutions, *Anal. Biochem.* **70**:506.

Overbeech, J. Th. G., and Wiersema, P. H., 1967, The interpretation of electrophoretic mobilities, in *Electrophoresis: Theory, Methods and Application,* Vol. 2 (M. Bier, ed.), Academic Press, New York.

Penney, C. M., 1970, Differential Doppler velocity measurements, *Appl. Phys. Lett.* **16**:167.

Raff, M. C., 1971, Surface antigenic markers for distinguishing T and B lymphocytes in mice, *Transplant. Rev.* **6**:52.

Rothman, J. E., and Lenard, J., 1977, Membrane asymmetry, *Science* **195**:743.

Rudd, M. J., 1969a, Measurements made on a drag reducing solution with a laser velocimeter, *Nature* **224**:587.

Rudd, M. J., 1969b, A self aligning laser Doppler velocimeter, ICO-8, *Proc. Optical Instruments and Techniques, Opel,* 58.

Shaw, D. J., 1969, *Electrophoresis,* Academic Press, New York.

Shortman, K., 1968, The separation of different cell classes from lymphoid organs. II. The purification and analysis of lymphocyte populations by equilibrium density gradient centrifugation, *Aust. J. Exp. Biol. Med. Sci.* **46**:375.

Shortman, K., von Baehmer, H., Lipp, J., and Hopper, K., 1975, Sub-populations of T-lymphocytes, physical separation, functional specialisation and differentiation pathways of sub-sets of thymocytes and thymus-dependent peripheral lymphocytes, *Transplant. Rev.* **25**:163.

Smith, B. A., Ware, B. R., and Weiner, R. W., 1976, Electrophoretic distributions of human peripheral blood mononuclear white cells from normal subjects and from patients with acute lymphocytic leukemia, *Proc. Natl. Acad. Sci. U.S.A.* **73**:2388.

Smith, B. A., Ware, B. R., and Yankee, R. A., 1978, Electrophoretic mobility distributions of normal lymphoblasts in acute lymphocytic leukemia: Effects of neuraminidase and of solvent ionic strength, *J. Immunol.* **120**:921.

Smoluchowski, M., 1914, in *Handbuch der Elektrinzitat und des Magnetismus,* Vol. 2 (B. Graetz, ed.), pp. 366, Leipzig, Germany.

Uzgiris, E. E., 1972, Electrophoresis of particles and biological cells measured by the Doppler shift of scattered laser light, *Optics Commun.* **6**:55.

Uzgiris, E. E., 1974, Laser Doppler spectrometer for study of electro-kinetic phenomena, *Rev. Sci. Instrum.* **45**:74.

Uzgiris, E. E., and Kaplan, J. H., 1974, Study of lymphocyte and erythrocyte electrophoretic mobility by laser Doppler spectroscopy, *Anal. Biochem.* **60**:455.

Uzgiris, E. E., and Kaplan, J. H., 1976, Laser Doppler spectroscopic studies of the electrokinetic properties of human blood cells in dilute salt solutions, *J. Colloid. Interface Sci.* **55**:148.

Wang, C. P., 1971, New model for laser Doppler velocity measurements of turbulent flow, *Appl. Phys. Lett.* **18**:522.

Ware, B. R., 1974, Electrophoretic light scattering, *Adv. Colloid Interface Sci.* **4**:1.

Ware, B. R., and Flygare, W. H., 1971, The simultaneous measurement of the electrophoretic mobility and diffusion coefficient in bovine serum albumin solutions by light scattering, *Chem. Phys. Lett.* **12**:81.

Watrasiewicz, B. M., and Rudd, M. J., 1976, *Laser Doppler Measurements,* Butterworths, Toronto.

Weiss, L., 1967, *The Cell Periphery, Metastasis and Other Contact Phenomenon,* North-Holland, Amsterdam, and Wiley, New York.

Yeh, H., and Cummins, H. Z., 1964, Localized fluid flow measurements with a He–Ne laser spectrometer, *Appl. Phys. Lett.* **4**:178.

Zeiller, K., Pascher, G., Wagner, G., Leibich, H. G., Holzberg, E., and Hannig, K., 1974, Distinct subpopulations of thymus-dependent lymphocytes, tracing of the differentiation pathway of T cells by use of preparatively electrophoretically separated mouse lymphocytes, *Immunology* **26**:955.

3

Cell Separation by Endless Fluid Belt Electrophoresis

ALEXANDER KOLIN

I. THE OBJECTIVE

The objective of endless fluid belt electrophoresis (Kolin, 1960, 1964, 1966, 1967a, b), is roughly analogous to the objective of mass spectroscopy. In the latter, a continuous stream of particles is to be split into discrete nonparallel streams carrying corpuscles differing from each other in the value of a physical parameter (e/m). In the case of the electrophoretic method considered here, the separation parameter is the electrophoretic particle mobility μ.

In both cases the particles have to move through an electric field and are subject to the force of gravity. Because of the very short transit time of the particles in a mass spectrograph, gravitational deviation is imperceptible. On the other hand, the force of gravity introduces a major experimental obstacle in the case of cell electrophoresis in free solution. The problem is not sedimentation of the cells, which is rather slow and could be effectively suppressed by adjusting the density of the solution so that it is close to that of the cells. The difficulty lies in generation of thermal convection which develops only in the presence of a gravitational or centrifugal inertial field (Kolin, 1964).

While the presence of an electric field in the vacuum of a mass spectrograph presents no problem, the maintenance of an electric field in the conductive solution of an electrophoretic column is necessarily accompanied by an electric current which heats the solution. In the central region

ALEXANDER KOLIN • Molecular Biology Institute, University of California, Los Angeles, California 90024.

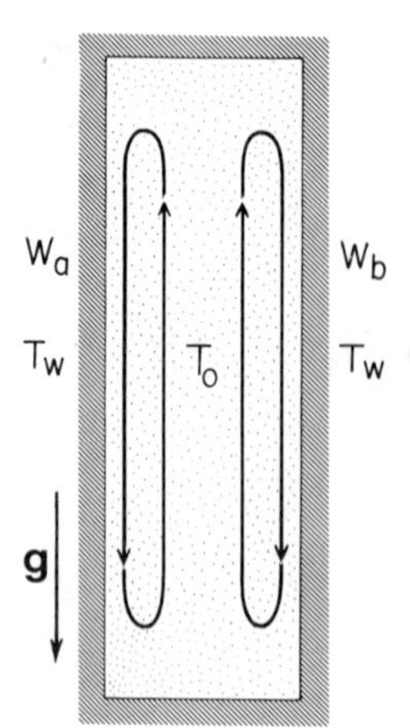

FIGURE 1. Thermal convection pattern in a rectangular channel. The fluid in the channel is heated uniformly by a current perpendicular to the page and cooled at the vertical walls Wa, Wb. The maximum temperature is at the center (T_0) and the lowest temperature at the walls T_W. **g** represents the gravitational field intensity.

of a tall vertical column, for instance, the heat will be escaping mainly through the lateral walls of the column. This will give rise to horizontal temperature gradients in the fluid column which, as a rule, will be linked with horizontal density gradients. Due to the specific gravity differences between the cool and warm masses of fluid in these gradients, thermal convection will develop in the electrophoretic separation column due to action of gravity. This convection will tend to remix the particles which might have been separated in the apparatus. Figure 1 illustrates such a convection pattern engendered between vertical walls which act as a heat sink for the fluid between them. The suppression of such fluid convection is considered to be indispensable for successful electrophoretic separations in a free solution.*

II. ROTATIONAL SUPPRESSION OF THERMAL CONVECTION

To visualize how thermal convection in a confined fluid volume could be suppressed, let us consider Fig. 2A. An annular volume of liquid is trapped between two concentric horizontal cylinders. (The direction of the gravitational field is indicated by the vector **g**.) Imagine now the inner cylinder to be at a higher temperature than the outer cylinder. There will thus be a horizontal temperature gradient in the fluid in the horizontal midplane of symmetry. To the right of the inner cylinder, the fluid elements adjacent to it will be warmer and less dense than the ambient fluid remote from the inner cylinder. The buoyant force experienced by each fluid

*It was recently shown, however, that thermal convection can be used in conjunction with a suitable laminar flow to increase throughput and resolving power (Kolin, 1979).

element near the inner cylinder wall will exceed the fluid element's weight and the fluid will rise near the inner cylinder. The situation will be converse near the low-temperature outer cylinder and the cooler fluid near the outer wall will descend. As a result, a clockwise fluid circulation will be formed which is indicated by the closed solid line on the right of the inner cylinder. We should keep in mind that a certain amount of time is required to build up the rotational kinetic energy of a fluid vortex in the steady state (Kolin, 1964).

Let us now perform an imaginary experiment. We assume that somehow the annular fluid column between the cylinders has been rotated counterclockwise (as indicated by the upper curved arrow) by 180°. Our solid vortex shown on the right will thus be transposed to the left of the inner cylinder as indicated by the closed *dotted* line. The inner fluid masses which were previously moving upward (on the right) will now be moving downward. However, this downward motion is now *opposed* by the resultant of the gravitational and buoyant forces. Since the upward force of buoyancy still predominates over the weight of each fluid element near the inner cylinder, the fluid elements are subjected to a net upward force which tends to retard the fluid motion near the inner cylinder. Under the converse conditions near the outer cylinder the upward motion of the fluid on the extreme left is retarded because the weight of the cooler outer-fluid ele-

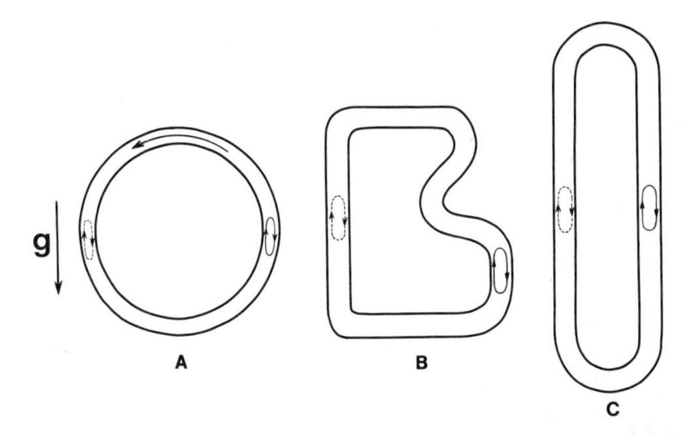

FIGURE 2. Thermal convection patterns in channels of different cross-section. The channels are perpendicular to the page. The inner wall is warmer than the outer wall. The fluid density diminishes with increasing temperature. **g** represents the gravitational field intensity. The solid closed line represents the circulation in a thermal convection vortex engendered on the right-hand side of the channel. The dotted vortex on the left-hand side of the channel represents in all diagrams the vortex shown on the right-hand side after its relocation (as indicated by the top arrow in part A) to the left side of the channel. (A) Circular annular channel; (B) noncircular quasi-annular channel; (C) endless fluid belt "annulus."

ments surpasses the force of buoyancy acting on them. The fluid vortex generated on the right-hand side of the cylinder (solid line) will thus come to a standstill when inverted to assume the position shown by a dashed line on the left-hand side. If we wait long enough after this inversion, the fluid circulation will be restored by the same mechanism, but now the fluid motion next to the inner cylinder on the left will be directed upward, as would be expected from the higher temperature of the fluid elements in this location. The same reasoning shows that the outermost fluid elements on the left will now be moving downward. In other words, we have reversed the sense of circulation in our original vortex by inverting it in its final position and leaving it there long enough to establish a new steady-state motion after a brief temporary standstill.

Since the accumulation of an appreciable angular momentum by the fluid vortices requires time, we can expect that generation of disturbingly high thermal convection could be avoided by rotating the annular fluid column of Fig. 2A as indicated by the upper curved arrow at a suitable rate.

Since our objective is a periodic inversion of nascent vortices, there is no reason why the fluid column should be a *circular* annular cylinder, as shown in Fig. 2A. We would achieve the same result in an arbitrary closed fluid path indicated in Fig. 2B or in a fluid volume resembling an elongated vertical endless belt shown in Fig. 2C (Kolin, 1964, 1966).

III. THE CIRCULAR ENDLESS BELT APPARATUS

Our next objective will be to find the simplest and most reliable way to achieve a constant circulation of fluid in an endless circulation path. Let us

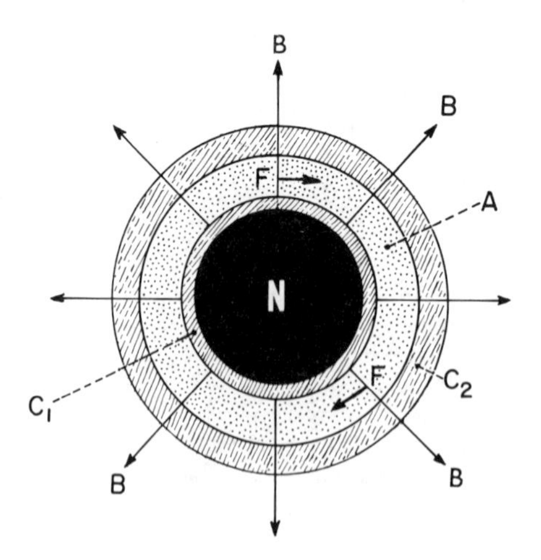

FIGURE 3. Radial magnetic field (B) surrounding a cylindrical magnetic north pole inside a buffer-filled annulus: C_1, C_2, dielectric cylinders confining the buffer (dotted shading); F, electromagnetic force produced by an electric current flowing through the annulus away from the reader. The engendered fluid rotation in the annulus has the direction of F.

assume that the fluid confined between the two horizontal cylinders of Fig. 2A is an electrolyte solution, say a horizontal annular electrophoretic buffer column shown in cross-section in Fig. 3 between the plastic cylinders C_1 and C_2. To maintain electrophoretic migration in this buffer column, we must pass an electric current through it. Let us say that this current is flowing at right angles to the page away from the reader. If we now introduce a cylindrical magnetic north pole N into the cylinder C_1, its radial magnetic field B (only two of the radial magentic field vectors are labeled in Fig. 3) will interact with the axial electric current in the electrophoretic column so as to generate the tangential electromagnetic force F which will set the fluid annulus in rotational motion. Combination of a permanent magnet with a constant-current power supply will produce a very constant rate of fluid circulation (Kolin, 1960).

Figure 4 shows how an extended cylindrical source of a radial magnetic field can be satisfactorily approximated in practice. A short soft-iron

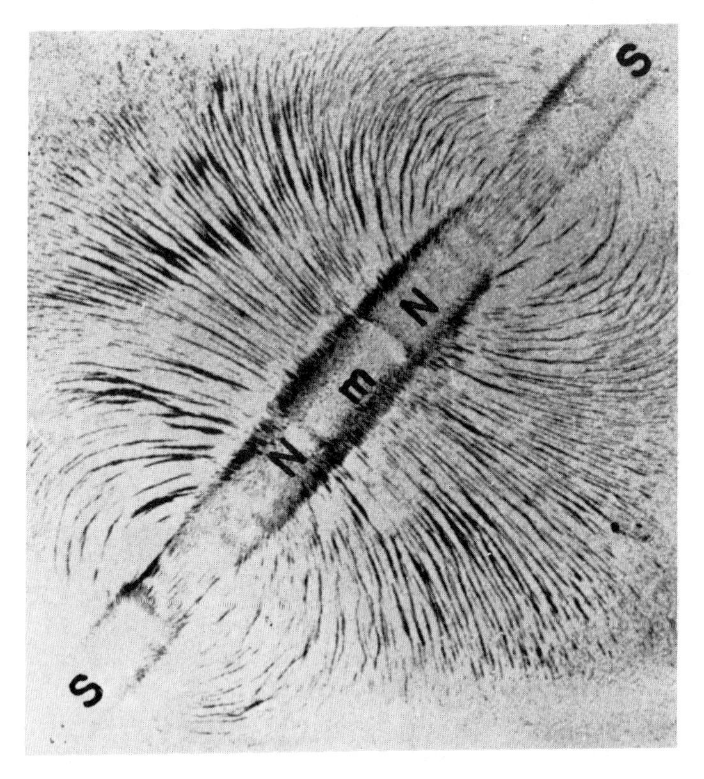

FIGURE 4. Magnetic field distribution about two cylindrical magnets: N, S are their north and south poles, respectively; m is an intermediate soft-iron cylinder. (From Kolin, 1967a,b.)

cylinder m (1020 cold-roll steel) is sandwiched between two cylindrical Alinco magnets facing each other with like poles (N-poles in this example). As the iron filing pattern of Fig. 4 shows, the region close to the surface of m between the two N-poles is a close approximation to a radial magnetic field.

Figure 5 shows in perspective a simple arrangement (Kolin, 1960) for continuous-flow electrophoresis in a horizontal annular buffer column maintained in steady-state electromagnetic rotation by the electrophoretic current. The outer cylinder C_2 joins the inner walls of the electrode chambers EC_1 and EC_2. The longer inner cylinder C_1 passes concentrically through cylinder C_2 so as to emerge through the outer walls of the electrode chambers. The lumen of the electrode chambers is thus linked by the annular cylindrical space between the cylinders C_1 and C_2. The bar magnets and the iron piece glide into the inner cylinder C_1 as illustrated in Fig. 5. The length of m is a little shorter than the distance between the electrode chambers which harbor the electrodes E_1 and E_2.

If we now pour buffer solution into chamber EC_1, it flows eventually through the annulus between C_1 and C_2 into compartment EC_2 until the cell is filled. Connecting the electrodes to a current source results in an axial current flowing through the annulus between C_1 and C_2 and the horizontal annular buffer column begins to rotate in the radial magnetic field. In the case shown in Fig. 5, the rotation is counterclockwise when viewed from the right.

Let us now imagine that we inject through a glass capillary IN, terminating at the midpoint between C_1 and C_2, a fine streak of a suspension of electrically neutral particles from the reservoir R. The particles will go into a circular orbit (assuming absence of electroosmosis and axial streaming) in which they will accumulate. Negatively charged particles will migrate toward the anode as they perform their circular orbital motion. The result will be a helical path—a left-handed helix. On the other hand, positive particles will migrate toward the cathode following a right-handed helical path. Figure 5 shows two helical paths for negatively charged particles differing in electrophoretic mobility. The faster particle path is depicted by a solid helix while the dashed helix pictures the path of the low-mobility particle species. W is a window milled out in the soft-iron core m, which permits visualization of the particle streaks by dark-field illumination.

We can see at once that this simple apparatus has potential for preparative as well as analytical work involving characterization of the particles by their electrophoretic mobilities. The electrophoretic mobility can be determined from the pitch of the helix (pitch is the distance between two consecutive helical turns). If we know the rate of revolution of the

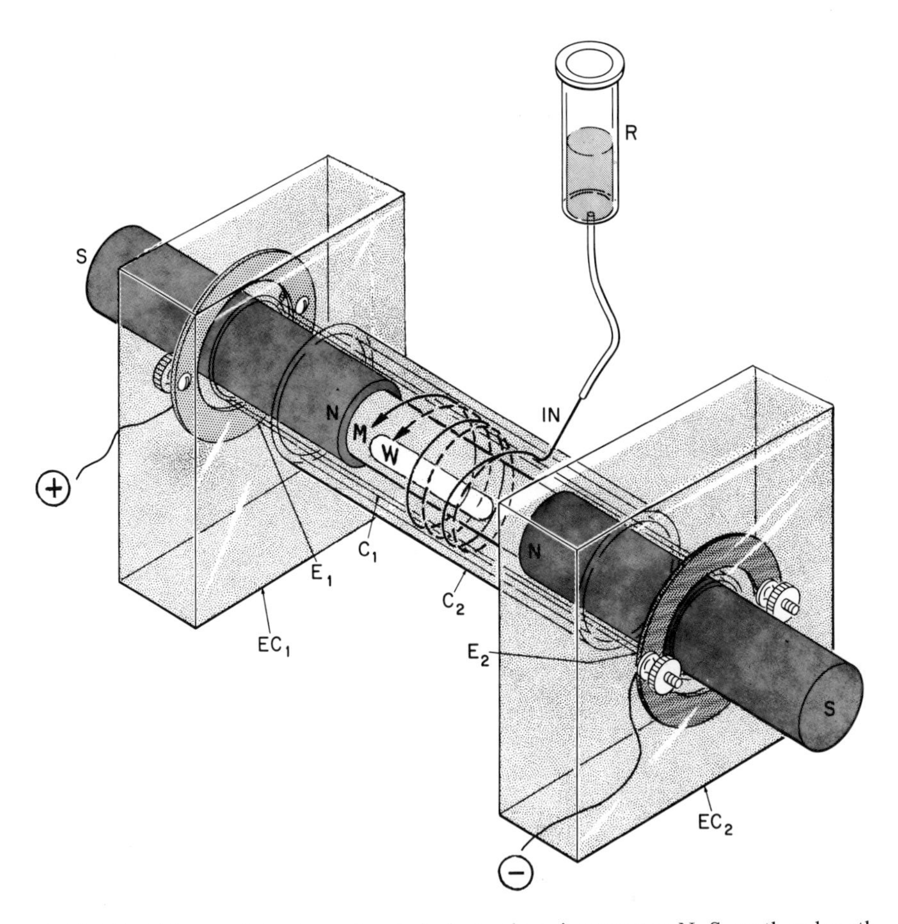

FIGURE 5. Scheme of circular endless belt electrophoresis separator: N, S, north and south poles, respectively, of cylindrical magnets; m, intermediate soft-iron cylinder; W, window in m; C_1, C_2, plastic cylinders which enclose buffer-filled annulus; EC_1, EC_2, electrode compartments which communicate through the annulus, E_1, E_2, electrodes; IN, injector; R, sample reservoir.

particles in the rotating buffer column, the pitch divided by this time interval will give the electrophoretic particle velocity. From the current density in the annulus and the buffer conductivity we know the electrical potential gradient, which permits us to find the electrophoretic mobility from the velocity of electromigration. Because of electroosmosis this procedure can lead us to errors. We shall later discuss a reliable method for mobility determination.

For preparative purposes, a collector can be installed in the annulus at the end of the helical particle path to collect the isolated particle species as separate fractions. We shall discuss the instrumental details of such fraction collection in connection with a more advanced version of the apparatus considered below.

IV. THE NONCIRCULAR ENDLESS VERTICAL BELT APPARATUS

The circular endless belt scheme has a drawback which is illustrated in Fig. 6A. It would be too cumbersome to have to adjust the density of the buffer solution to equal that of the particles emerging from the injector IN. Besides, if mixtures of particles of different densities are to be fractionated, the density adjustments will apply to only one of the components of the mixture. No effort is made therefore to match the buffer density to the particles. In Fig. 6A the emerging particles are assumed to be denser than the buffer. Although they emerge at the center of the annulus (position a), they are seen to sediment as they circle around the inner cylinder C_1. Thus, instead of remaining midway between the cylinders C_1 and C_2, they come close to the cylinder C_1 at b due to sedimentation. For the same reason they recede from this position of closest approach as they move toward c and, at d, come close to the outer cylinder C_2. From there their path gradually approaches the midpoint as they move toward position a. The close approach to the cylinder walls is undesirable because of the steep velocity gradients near C_1 and C_2 (see section XV for discussion) which reduce the resolving power of the separation. The situation is much worse if the particle density is greater than illustrated in Fig. 6A. In this case the particles can actually sediment on the walls of the cylinders C_1 and C_2 and thus be removed from the streak and never reach the collector at the end of the helical path. What has been said about the path of dense *particles* can also be said about a dense *streak* of molecular solutes emerging from the injector IN.

This drawback is easily remedied by resorting to a noncircular path (Kolin, 1966) shown in Fig. 6B (cf. also Fig. 2C). In this endless belt, the particle path is vertical during most of its period of revolution. The sedimentation rate is slow as compared to the fluid velocity in the endless belt. On the way down it is added to the endless belt velocity and on the way up, subtracted from it, so that the particles' revolution time is the same as it would have been without sedimentation.

The effect of sedimentation at the bottom of the endless belt in Fig. 6B tends to deviate the particles below the dashed midline shown between the endless belt confines C_1 and C_2. As they come around the lower semicircu-

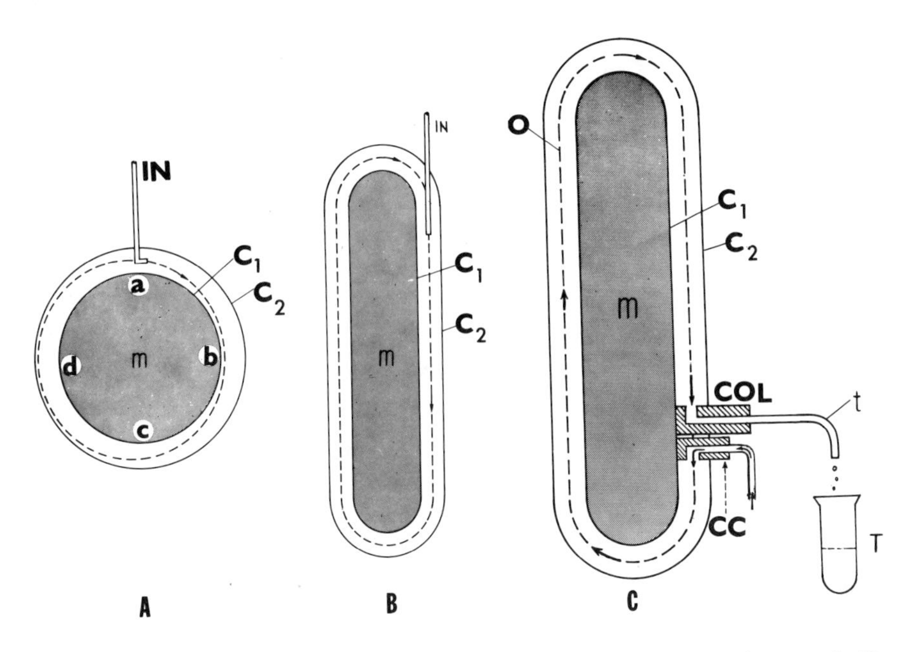

FIGURE 6. Circulation of injected particles in annuli of different shapes: m, iron core inside annulus; IN, injector; C_1, C_2, walls confining the annulus; COL, collector; t, collector tubing; CC, collector compensator; T, test tube. (A) Circular annulus; (B) noncircular endless belt annulus with injector; (C) noncircular endless belt annulus with collector and collector compensator. (Redrawn from Kolin, 1966.)

lar path section they will rise somewhat to the left of the dashed vertical midline and will move above the midline as they enter the upper semicircular path section of the vertical endless belt. Sedimentation in the semicircular top portion of their path will move them back toward the midline. Thus, particles injected from the capillary IN into the central portion of the revolving endless fluid belt near the top will oscillate slightly about the (dashed) central path due to sedimentation in the substantially horizontal portions of their path. This oscillation will have the effect of making even an infinitely thin particle streak behave as if it had a thickness delineated by the amplitude of the oscillation. The significance of this effect will become clear during the subsequent discussion (section XV) of the effect of the velocity distribution in the annulus on the resolution of the separation.

Figure 6C shows how a particle streak can be trapped at the end of its helical path in a collector COL which guides the separated fractions to individual test tubes. Under the collector COL is seen the opening of the collector compensator CC. Like the collector, it comprises several openings. Buffer is injected into the endless belt downward through the apertures of CC at the same rate at which it is removed from the endless belt by entering the openings of the collector COL.

The scheme of the vertical endless belt apparatus (Kolin, 1966, 1971) is illustrated more clearly in the perspective drawing of Fig. 7. (The collector compensator is omitted.) The particles emerging from the capillary Cap of the injector IN are seen to follow noncircular helical paths terminating in the collector COL. The intercepted particle fractions are guided by fine polyvinylchloride (PVC) tubes t to the fraction collector (not shown). The window W permits observation of the particles not only as they pass in front of the insulated soft-iron core C but also as they pass behind it. The

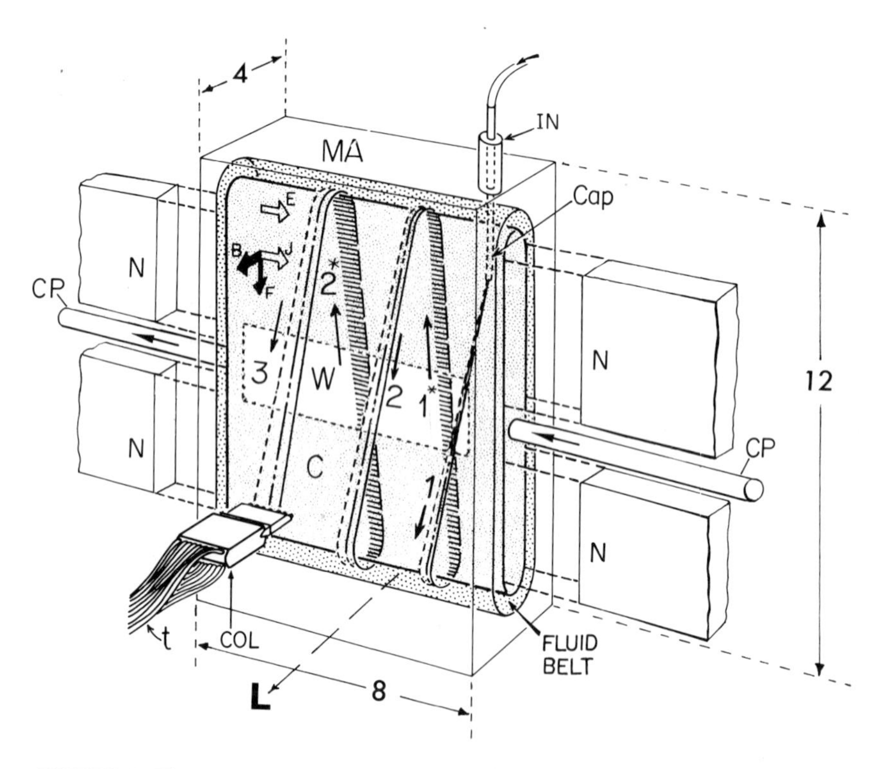

FIGURE 7. Electrophoretic separation space of noncircular endless belt apparatus: N, north poles of magnets; C, hollow iron core; CP, cooling pipes carrying cooling fluid circulating through C; W, window in C; MA, mantle surrounding annulus (fluid belt); IN, injector; Cap, capillary; COL, collector; t, collector tubing; **E**, electric field vector; **B**, magnetic field vector; **J**, current density vector; **F**, electromagnetic force vector, 1*, 2* are first and second ascending streaks (behind the core C); 1, 2, 3 are first, second, and third descending streaks (in front of the core D); L, light beam passing through the bottom of the annulus.

first descending triplet of streaks is labeled 1 in the figure. The first ascending streak 1* is seen in the back through the core window. After completion of the first turn, the particles form the second descending set of streaks (labeled 2) in front of the window W and rise again behind it (2*). The third descending set of streaks (3) is shown intercepted by the collector COL.

The vector **E** indicates the direction of the electric field in the annulus which contains the buffer confined on the inside by the insulated soft-iron core C and on the outside by the mantle MA. The **B** vector shows the direction of the magentic field at the front surface of the core C. **J** is the current density vector and **F** the electromagnetic force driving the fluid belt in front of the core C. The magnetic field is perpendicular to the surface of the core and is directed on the side of the core facing the reader as shown by vector **B** in the figure. Its direction is reversed on the back surface of the core C. Hence, the electromagnetic force **F** is also reversed and points upward in back of core C so that the endless fluid belt revolves counter-clockwise as seen from the right side.

The soft-iron core C is hollow and is perfused by cooling water via the tubes CP and CP (cf. Fig. 21). The mantle is also cooled by circulating water. This outer cooling system is omitted for clarity in this figure. The magnetic field is provided by four flat Alinco magnet bars which actually contact the core C but are shown, for clarity, out of contact with C in Fig. 7. Further details of the apparatus will be considered in section IX.

V. ENDLESS BELT ELECTROPHORESIS AS A FORM OF DEVIATION ELECTROPHORESIS

Before proceeding with further description of the endless belt electrophoresis (EBE) apparatus, it will be useful to consider the relationship between endless belt electrophoresis and fluid curtain electrophoresis (FCE). Both are special cases of the general method of deviation electrophoresis. Since the configuration of the fluid curtain electrophoresis is the simplest form of deviation electrophoresis, it lends itself best for exploration of theoretical relationships. It is thus convenient to consider a straight portion in the annulus of the EBE apparatus as a section of the FCE apparatus (cf. section XV).

An early form of deviation electrophoresis was filter paper curtain electrophoresis (Grassmann and Hannig, 1950). Buffer flow descended down a vertical rectangular filter paper curtain terminating laterally in vertical electrodes on the right and left side of the curtain. A downward flow of buffer solution confined to the paper curtain by capillary retention descended toward the curtain bottom cut in sawtooth fashion so as to cause the buffer to escape in a rain of drops released from the sawteeth. A streak of dye released in central location from the top of the curtain will be entrained in the downward buffer flow and will eventually leave the curtain in drops released from the saw teeth located under the point of application.

If we now establish a horizontal electric field across the curtain by connecting the electrodes to an electrical power source, the dye ions will migrate toward the electrode of opposite polarity as they descend in the curtain toward a new exit point at the bottom. The angle of deviation of the streak will depend on the ratio of the ion velocity in the electric field to the downward flow velocity of the buffer. A dye mixture will give rise to a multiplet of streaks which will escape at different points. This is, of course, a greatly simplified description which does not take into account electroosmosis, heating and evaporation of the buffer, electrolysis, and other complications. As far as our objective of cell separation is concerned, this attractively simple method is unsuitable because of impediment of cell movement through the filter paper pores and cell adsorption. The same criticism will apply to any method making use of a "supporting medium" which could interact with the cells in a similar fashion. Thus, the fluid curtain employed for cell separation must ideally contain no macroscopic or microscopic ingredients besides the cell.

The first fluid curtain of this type was described by Barrolier, *et al.* (1958). Their paper was followed closely by two independent publications which described electrophoresis in freely flowing buffer curtains, each relying on a different principle of curtain propulsion and stabilization (Kolin, 1960; Hannig, 1961, 1964). While Kolin's paper described the principle of endless belt electrophoresis with magnetohydrodynamic propulsion, Hannig employed the classical configuration of deviation electrophoresis in a rectangular fluid curtain shown schematically in Fig. 8.

In his first apparatus Hannig used a fluid curtain which was horizontal or, like that of Barrolier *et al.*, was somewhat inclined against the horizontal plane. For cell separations, this is disadvantageous because of cell sedimentation. This drawback was eliminated in a later apparatus using a fluid curtain sandwiched between vertical plates (Hannig, 1964), according to the scheme of Fig. 8. The buffer solution ("separation buffer" B_1) enters the narrow space (0.5 mm) between the plates which confine the fluid curtain from the top through a manifold (MF). The buffer escapes at the bottom through the collector tubes CT. M_1, M_2 are ion exchange membranes which separate the electrophoretic separation space from the electrode compartments EC_1 and EC_2. A buffer solution ("electrode buffer" B_2, which need not be of the same concentration as the "separation buffer" B_1) is circulated through the electrode compartments EC_1, EC_2 containing

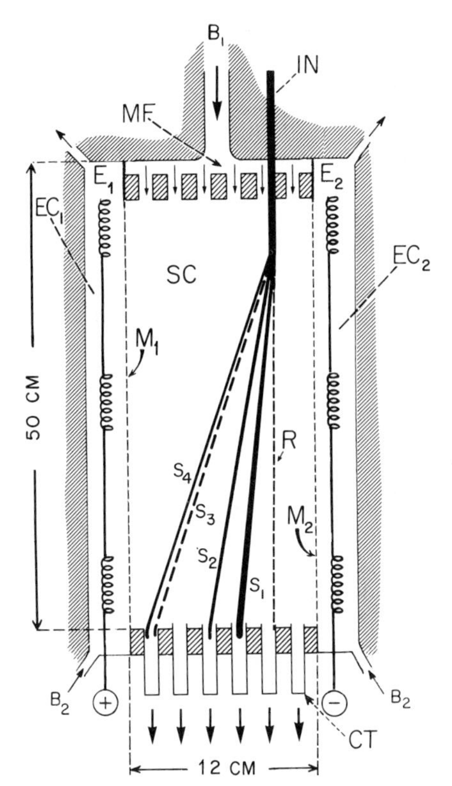

FIGURE 8. Scheme of fluid curtain "free-flow" electrophoresis: EC_1, EC_2, electrode chambers, M_1, M_2, membranes; B_2, buffer inflow tubes of electrode chambers; SC, separation chamber; E_1, E_2, electrodes; MF, manifold; B_1, buffer inflow tube of manifold; CT, collector exit tubes; IN, injector; R, zero-deviation reference line; S_1–S_4, streaks of components of different electrophoretic mobilities.

the electrodes E_1, E_2. The cell mixture is injected into the buffer stream through the injector IN. The cell components of different electrophoretic mobilities are deviated at different angles against the reference line R (injection axis). Since the cell populations are not necessarily of equal electrophoretic homogeneity, the streaks carrying them may diverge to different extents and may be of different widths when they reach the collector tubes CT. This rudimentary schematic description will suffice for purposes of reference and comparison in subsequent discussions. For instrumental details refer to Hannig's publication (1972).

If we compare Fig. 7 with Fig. 8, we see that the front and back segments of the endless belt can be considered as vertical fluid curtains similar to Hannig's (Fig. 8), the fluid flow being downward in the front curtain and upward in the rear curtain. As in Fig. 8, the electric field is transverse to the fluid motion in the endless belt seen in Fig. 7. The fluid trapped between the cylinders C_1 and C_2 of the circular endless belt (Figs. 3 and 5) can be also *roughly* regarded as a flat fluid curtain if we consider a small angular segment and if the difference between the radii of cylinders C_1 and C_2 is negligible as compared to the mean radius. This approximation has been made in theoretical treatments (Kolin, 1960, 1967b).

In the previous descriptions as well as in the following ones preceding the theoretical considerations of section XV, certain simplifying assumptions are made about the operation of fluid belt or curtain electrophoresis. There are, however, certain complications which are common to both, the Hannig-type fluid curtain as well as the endless fluid belt. The most important one is due to the disparity between the uniform distribution of the electrophoretic velocity relative to the buffer and the distribution of the electroosmotic streaming velocity in the direction of the electric field on one hand and the superimposed transverse curtain velocity profile on the other hand.

Neglecting the temperature gradients in the fluid curtain (or belt) we can assume, as a first approximation, the electrophoretic mobilities and velocities to be constant within the belt or curtain. On the other hand, the horizontal electroosmotic velocity profile will be parabolic with a *nonzero velocity at the walls*. On the other hand, the profile of the vertical curtain velocity (or tangential velocity in the fluid belt) will be parabolic with a *zero velocity at the walls*. As will be shown in section XV, these circumstances lead to a deformation of the cross-section of the injected particle streak (Kolin, 1960, 1967b) which has a decisive limiting effect on the resolving power of the electrophoretic separator. A streak of circular cross-section containing large nondiffusing particles will remain neither constant nor circular in cross-section but will have diverging boundaries and its cross-section will be distorted into a crescent as shown in Fig. 9 (Luner, 1969; Kolin and Luner, 1971). This photograph has been taken at the top of the endless belt in a manner suggested by the line of sight L at the bottom in Fig. 7. One can see a short portion of the ascending and of the descending streaks on either side of the crescent. As we recede from the origin of the streak (the tip of the capillary cap of Fig. 7), the separation between the peak of the crescent (at the center of the fluid curtain or belt) and its "horns" (the streak portion closest to the walls) increases; i.e., the streaks grow broader. Two neighboring particle streaks will thus tend to overlap eventually when they reach the collector slots (Kolin, 1967b).

As we shall see below, the same means that can alleviate this drawback in endless belt electrophoresis can also be effective in fluid curtain electrophoresis (Kolin, 1960, 1967b). In fact, the performance of the fluid belt system during the first half-turn of the streak on its way around the belt (cf. streak 1 in Fig. 7) is equivalent to that of the streak in the fluid curtain. The main points of distinction between the two systems are (1) the possibility of allowing the streak to wind itself repeatedly around the iron core in the endless belt, (2) the absence of membranes separating the electropho-

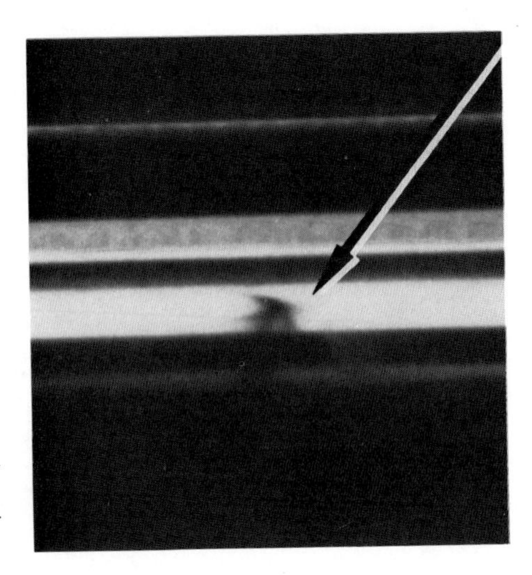

FIGURE 9. "Crescent" distortion of an originally circular streak cross-section. End-on view of streak at the top of endless belt annulus. (From Luner, 1969.)

retic separation space of the endless belt system from the adjacent buffer compartments, (3) the maintenance of laminar buffer flow parallel to the electric field, and (4) the mode of propulsion of the buffer at right angles to the electric field. The consequences of these differences will become apparent in subsequent discussions.

VI. PROPERTIES OF THE ENDLESS BELT SYSTEM

The streak of particles undergoing electrophoresis and simultaneous electromagnetic revolution in the endless belt is wound up into a coil as shown in Fig. 10 (Kolin, 1967a). This photograph shows 15 turns of human erythrocytes injected at the extreme right from the injector IN and migrating toward the left in physiological saline solution. The uniformity of the helical path (i.e., the distance between consecutive turns) demonstrates the uniformity of the radial magnetic field in the annulus. The pitch of the helix is a measure of the electrophoretic mobility of the particles, provided the lateral movement is due exclusively to electrophoretic migration! The measurement of electrophoretic mobility in the presence of lateral streaming will be discussed in section XIII.

It is of special interest to note an important property of endless belt electrophoresis which makes it very insensitive to fluctuations of the voltage applied to the electrophoretic column (Kolin, 1960). Figure 11A shows five helical turns of the dye Evans blue spiraling toward the left at a voltage of 75 V between the cell electrodes at a cell current of 25 mA. Figure 11B shows the same number of turns obtained after doubling the cell

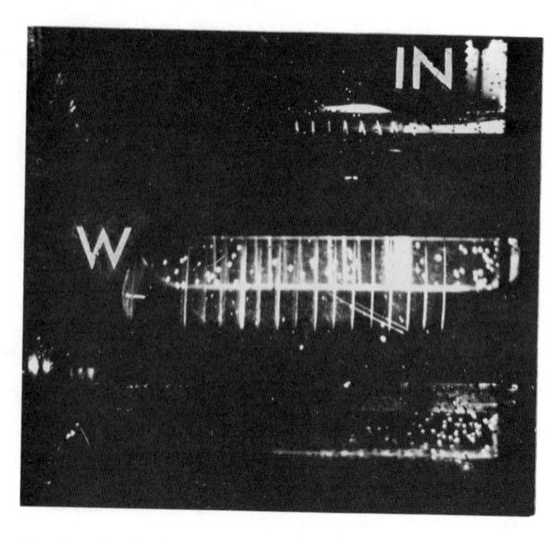

FIGURE 10. Visualization by light scattering of 15-turn streak of erythrocytes in a circular endless belt: IN, injector; W, window in core of central iron cylinder. The illumination is directed toward the reader (forward scattering). (From Kolin, 1967a,b.)

voltage and current. There is no perceptible change in the pitch of the helix. Although doubling the electric field intensity increases the electrophoretic velocity by a factor of two, the helical pitch is not doubled because the rate of revolution of the circular endless belt is also doubled due to increase of the current to 50 mA. This cuts the period of revolution by 50% and the particles migrate a correspondingly shorter time to the left.

On the other hand, the helical pitch is quite sensitive to changes in the electrical conductivity of the buffer solution at constant current. Figure 11C shows the helical pitch somewhat more than doubled at the same current of 25 mA as used in Fig. 11A after dilution of the buffer 1 : 2.

Figure 11D illustrates the speed with which electrophoretically distinct components can be separated. The photograph shows the splitting of a streak containing a mixture of the dyes Evans blue and rose Bengal at a voltage of 700 V between the electrodes. The dye reached the bottom of the photograph within 4 s, but a clear-cut separation is seen about 1.5 ss, suggesting the possibility of obtaining rapid analytical information.

Figure 12 shows another important property of endless belt electrophoresis exhibited in a separation of two fungi: *Saccharomyces cerevisiae* and *Rhodotorula*, a mixture of which emanates from injector IN (Kolin, 1967a). The consecutive descending turns in the front part of the annulus are labeled a, b, c, d. (The ascending turns visible in the rear through the window W are unlabeled.) The separated particle species gain equal increments in separation with each consecutive revolution around the iron core (i.e., with each helical turn).

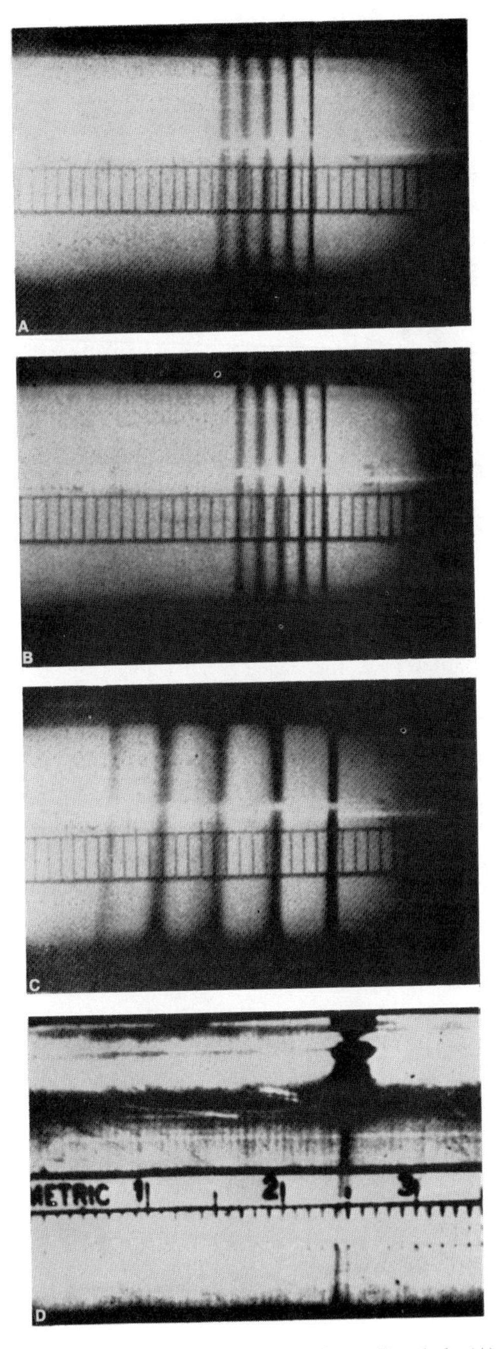

FIGURE 11. Effect of voltage on helical pitch in circular endless belt: (A) Helix of Evans blue obtained at a voltage of 75 V across the cell and a cell current of 25 mA. (B) Helix of Evans blue after raising the voltage to 150 V using the same buffer as in (A). (C) Change in helical pitch under conditions used in (A) after diluting the buffer 1 : 2. (D) Illustration of separation speed. Separation of rose Bengal (slower component) from Evans blue achieved within about 4 s at a cell voltage of 700 V. (From Kolin, 1960.)

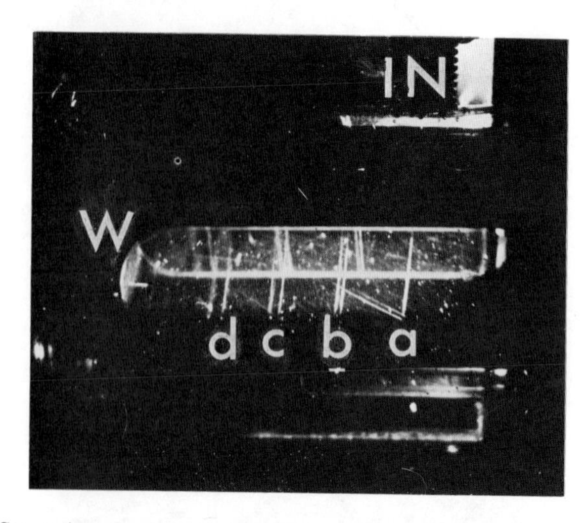

FIGURE 12. Separation of two microorganisms visualized by light scattering. Separation of the yeasts *Saccharomyces cerevisiae* and *Rhodotorula* in circular endless belt. The labels a, b, c, d represent consecutive helical turns; IN, injector (the arrow marks the point of entry of the sample); W, window in iron core. The source of parallel light was behind the core directed toward the camera so as to miss the lens. (From Kolin, 1967a,b.)

It is important to emphasize that the separation between the two streaks in any turn is independent of whether there is horizontal fluid streaming parallel to the electrical field superimposed upon the electrophoretic migration. In both endless belt as well as fluid curtain electrophoresis, there will be, as a rule, horizontal streaming superimposed upon electrophoresis due to electroosmosis (cf. sections XIII and XV). However, in endless belt electrophoresis, an additional horizontal laminar fluid flow is superimposed for the following reason.* Let us consider the two helices (the solid and the dashed one) represented for a slow and a fast electrophoretic component in the circular endless belt of Fig. 5. The pitch p_1 of the solid helix (faster component) is larger than the pitch p_2 of the dashed helix. The separation S between the solid and the dashed helix increases with each turn so that after n turns it will be $S = n\Delta p$, where Δp is the separation after one turn. When the separation becomes $S = p_1$, the nth turn of the dashed helix will coincide with the $(n - 1)$th turn of the solid helix and the two components which were previously separated will unite again.

This limitation of separability between the two components of the mixture can be easily removed by superimposing a lateral streaming toward

*Superposition of such a flow is neither necessary nor possible (due to the sealing of the fluid curtain by the membranes) in fluid curtain electrophoresis (cf. Fig. 8).

the left upon the electrophoretic migration. If the streaming displaces the particles by the distance d during one period of revolution, the pitch of the solid helix will now be $(p_1 + d) > n\Delta p$ and the solid and the dashed helix will now be separated at the point of previous coincidence. Since we can make d as large as we please, we can always easily avoid remixing of separated components.

In practice, lateral streaming toward the anode is always used in endless belt electrophoresis (Kolin, 1967a,b). This has the additional advantage of bringing constantly cool fresh buffer into the endless belt. In the cell separation shown in Fig. 12, lateral streaming toward the left has been used. In the simple apparatus shown in Fig. 5 such lateral streaming can be generated by permitting the buffer to leak out of the left compartment EC_1 at the rate of n drops per second and by simultaneously adding buffer at the same rate to the right compartment. Normally the volume rate of transverse flow is about 1 drop/s. Figure 13 illustrates the effect of axial streaming on helical pitch (Kolin, 1967a). Figure 13A shows a tight helix of dye without axial streaming; streaming is introduced in Fig. 13B and increased in Fig. 13C. The point of dye injection is indicated by an arrow.

In the presence of transverse streaming, the pitch of the helix is no longer independent of the magnitude of the electrophoretic current. The pitch decreases as the current is increased. On the other hand, the distance between two separated components after n turns is not changed by the current because the period of revolution is shortened so as to compensate for the increase in the electrophoretic velocity difference.

The collector placed at the end of the helical path represents an obstacle to the electromagnetic circulation of buffer in the annulus as long as it is not activated (i.e., as long as it is not draining the buffer solution at an appropriate rate). This is clearly illustrated in Fig. 14A (Kolin, 1967a). A mixture of three dyes (Evans blue, rose Bengal, and "Brush" green recording ink, from right to left) is injected into the annulus at the arrow. We see the dye separation in successive helical turns. As the separated streaks approach the collector C, they begin to follow a curved path, indicating a deviation of the buffer circulation around the collector.

This streamline picture changes drastically as soon as the collector is activated. The buffer solution enters the collector C shown in Fig. 15 and leaves from the ends of the plastic (PVC) tubes T (Kolin, 1967a). If the rate at which the buffer flow enters the collector C in Fig. 14B is such that the tangential buffer velocity just above the collector is about the same as it would have been in the collector's absence, the separated streaks enter the collector roughly parallel to each other. If the rate at which the collector drains the buffer is too high, the streaks converge as they approach the collector; i.e., the separation achieved by electrophoresis is diminished by the flow pattern. (This does not necessarily impair the resolution, because the streaks become proportionately thinner as they converge.) If the rate of

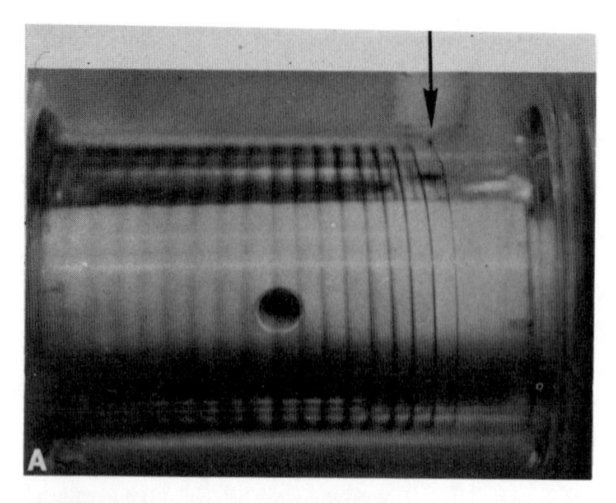
A

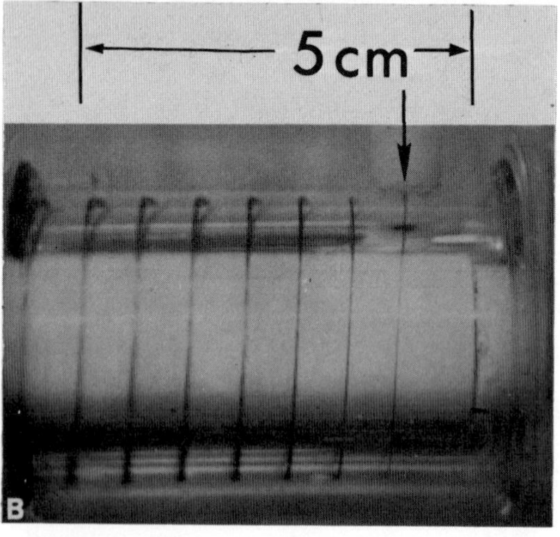
5 cm
B

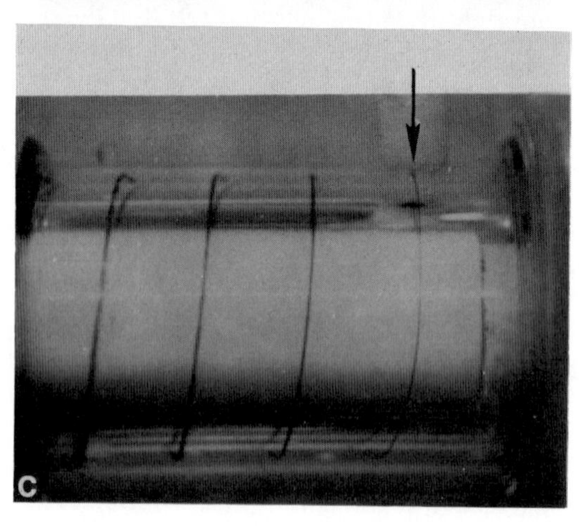
C

buffer drainage from the collector is less than the illustrated optimum, the streaks diverge as they enter C and become proportionately wider.

As mentioned before it is advantageous to introduce a collector compensator to establish a compensatory buffer flow as follows. Imagine a set of rectangularly bent tubes like those for the collector shown in Fig. 15, except that the vertical tubes point down instead of up as in Fig. 15. Place this bundle of tubes exactly under the tube configuration shown in Fig. 15. The vertical tubes of the original bundle C point upward and those of the added bundle C* underneath point downward. Imagine now that you expel buffer solution downward through C* at the same rate as you aspirate it through the upward vertical tubes of C. This will make the combination C and C* "hydraulically transparent," so to speak. The fluid would move in the annulus above and below this structure as if C and C* were not in the path of the fluid flow. This arrangement is equivalent to the collector compensator and collector scheme shown in Fig. 6C.

Visualization of the particle streaks is accomplished most simply by dark-field illumination, i.e., by light scattering (Kolin, 1967a). It is most advantageous to use forward scattering. The streaks of erythrocytes and yeasts shown in Figs. 10 and 12 have been photographed in this fashion. We have to picture a source of parallel light behind the page aiming its beam at right angles to the page toward the reader or the camera (cf. Fig. 7). If we now incline the camera angle somewhat upward to avoid direct entry of the illuminating beam into the lens, we will be able to form an image of the separation pattern on the film by focusing the camera on the light scattering streaks. All of the subsequently shown photographs of cell separations have been obtained in this fashion. For this purpose, a window is milled out in the iron core m and filled out with a glass or quartz plate for a flat core (cf. Fig. 7) or by a cylindrically curved glass or lucite inset for a circular endless belt (cf. Figs. 5 and 12).

VII. MODES OF OPERATION

The flexibility of the endless belt system permits operation in several different modes as follows (Kolin, 1967a).

A. Single-Order Collection

We shall designate the separation pattern obtained after n helical turns of the injected particle mixture as "nth-order separation." Since the collec-

←

FIGURE 13. Effect of lateral flow on helical pitch. The lateral flow is from right to left. The arrow marks the entry point of sample. The rate of lateral flow is increasing as we progress from A to C. (From Kolin, 1967a, b.)

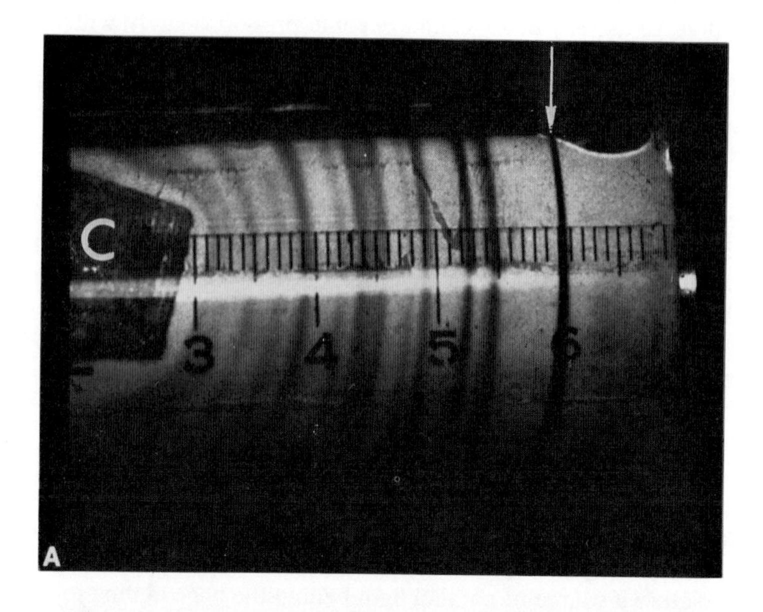

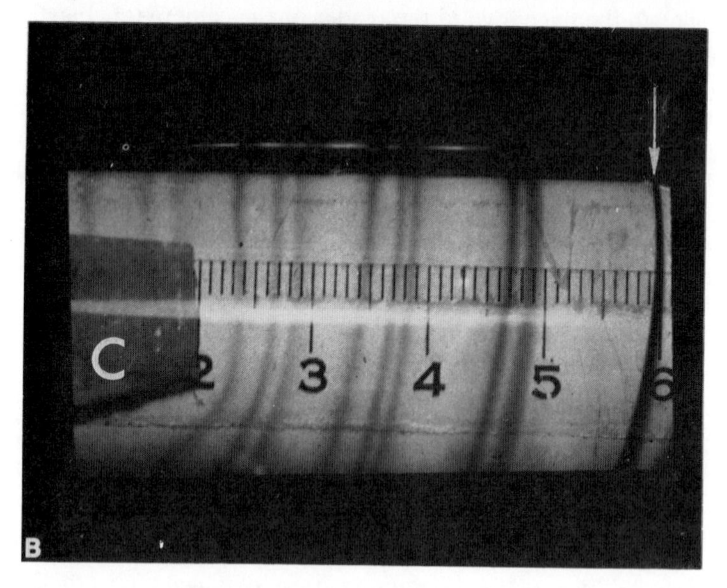

FIGURE 14. Effect of collector activation on streak pattern. The sample enters the circular endless belt at arrow. We see five helical turns of three separating dye components (from right to left: Evans blue, "Brush" recording ink, rose Bengal). (A) The collector is not activated and acts as an obstacle to flow so that the streaks are moving around it. (B) The collector is activated and receives the three separated streaks in their fifth turn. (From Kolin, 1967a,b.)

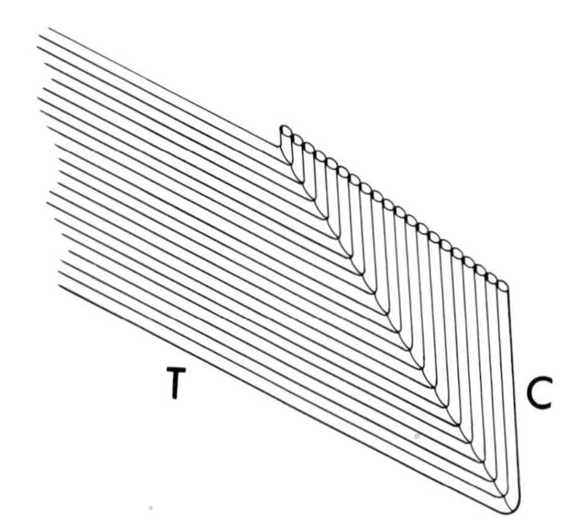

FIGURE 15. Removable collector: T and C are mutually perpendicular PVC tubes cemented with tygon cement. A collector of this type is shown inserted into the annulus in Fig. 14. The buffer flow is intercepted at the top of tubes C and escapes outside the cell at the end of the long exit tubes T. (From Kolin, 1967a,b.)

tor tubes are about 1 mm apart, we would want the separated streaks to be at least this far apart in order to be collected as separate fractions. This may require several helical turns. There is however an optimum number of turns beyond which the separation between two given streaks begins to diminish in the absence of lateral streaming. This optimum number of turns is at hand when the streak of component A is located midway between two adjacent turns of component B at the collector entrance. In the preceding and subsequent helical turns the deviation of the component A from this central location places it closer to either of the two adjacent turns of the component B.

If lateral streaming is used, the above limitation does not apply. One can use as many turns as desired to maximize streak separation, provided the lateral streaming velocity is properly adjusted.

B. Split-Order Collection

It is not necessary to collect *all* of the separated components after the same number of helical turns. In fact, it is sometimes advantageous not to do so, as can be seen from the following concrete example. Figure 14B shows the collection of three components after completion of four turns (fourth-order collection). Let us suppose that the two slowest components are so close to each other that they tend to enter an intermediate collector tube and emerge mixed in a tube of the fraction collector. In this case, we can slow down the axial streaming until the slowest component just misses the collector C. It will perform an additional revolution and enter the collector after five turns (fifth-order collection) far to the left of the two components which remain intercepted by the collector. Thus, two streaks which were too close to each other have been maximally separated by "split-order" collection.

C. Isoelectric Accumulation

An electrically neutral species of particles could be accumulated, in principle, in a circular orbit in the absence of electroosmotic streaming and at zero imposed lateral flow. This is, however, not a practically significant situation since electroosmosis is difficult to suppress, and it is even less likely that this suppression will occur at a pH corresponding to the isoelectric point of the component to be accumulated in a stationary orbit.

D. Nonisoelectric Accumulation

The accumulation of injected particles in a stationary orbit in an endless belt outlined above for an ampholyte at its isoelectric pH can actually be achieved with nonampholytes as well as for ampholytes at any pH. This can be accomplished by injecting a thin streak at the center of the annulus and superimposing upon the electroosmotic streaming a lateral streaming velocity of such magnitude that the sum of these two latter streaming velocities is equal and opposite to the particles' electrophoretic velocity. Such an axial counterflow makes it possible to detect particles present in a very dilute suspension by accumulation in a stationary orbit at an enriched concentration. Fig. 16A shows a helix of india ink injected into the annulus at the arrow in the presence of lateral streaming to the left. Fig. 16B shows the accumulation of this material in a stationary orbit after establishing a suitable lateral counter flow.

E. Zonal Separation

Microanalytical separations can be accomplished through what could be designated as "orbiting zone electrophoresis." The required volume of the suspension need not exceed a few tenths of a microliter. A fine streak, about 0.1 mm in diameter and 1 cm long, is injected at the center of the annulus and allowed to revolve around the iron core m as an "orbiting" zone. The original streak breaks up, due to electrophoresis of its components, into individual zones which land in different collector tubes. One can maximize the width of the separation pattern by imposing an axial flow immobilizing the axial migration of the slowest component. Then, the separation pattern can be spread over the entire width of the window W. (The collector may be removed if no fraction collection is intended.)

F. Multiple Separations

As we shall see in section XV, an increase in the width of the injected streak for the purpose of increasing the scale of separation impairs the

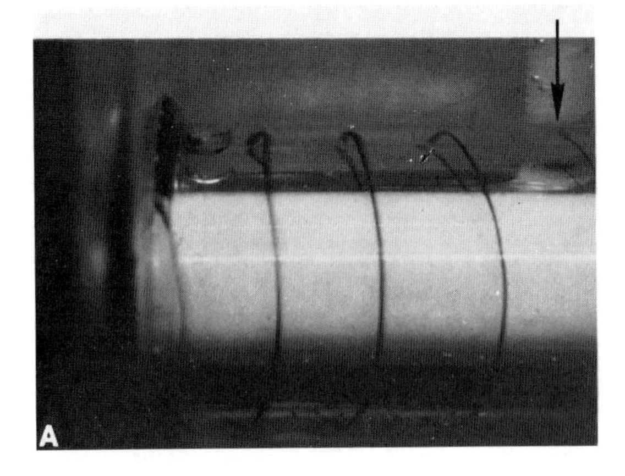

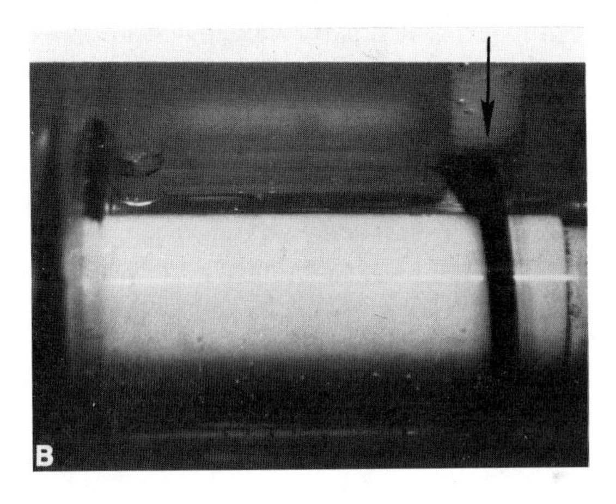

FIGURE 16. Nonisoelectric accumulation in stationary orbit: (A) Helix of india ink injected at arrow. (B) Lateral flow is adjusted to accumulate india ink in a zero-pitch helix, i.e., circular orbit. (From Kolin, 1967a,b.)

resolving power. One could, without impairment of resolution, double or treble the separation scale by placing two or three thin injectors side by side, provided the separation pattern of the mixture is not too wide. In this case the separation pattern repeats itself in the fraction collector for each of the injector outputs.

VIII. THERMAL CONVECTION ARTIFACTS

Thermal convection is caused by horizontal temperature gradients in the electrophoretic column (Kolin, 1960, 1964, 1967a). Section II dealt with temperature gradients perpendicular to the walls of the endless belt (and to the electrophoretic current) and with the suppression of thermal convection produced by them. In addition, there are horizontal temperature gradients which are parallel to the electrophoretic current in the vertical endless buffer belt of Fig. 7 or annular buffer column of the apparatus of Fig. 5. Due to the fact that the temperature in the annulus, which is heated by the electrophoretic current, is higher than in the buffer compartments (cf. Fig. 5) where the heating is minimal due to low current density, there is a sharp change in temperature at the ends of the annular buffer column at the boundaries of the buffer compartments. This gives rise to thermal convection with fluid circulation about a horizontal axis perpendicular to the current.

Figure 17 illustrates the consequences of such thermal convection (Kolin, 1967a). The direction of the current and magnetic field in the annulus are such that the fluid is moving downward in the rotating buffer column on the side facing the reader. In Fig. 17A the cooling of the buffer solution is normal while the current density is very low. As a result, the temperature in the electrophoretic column falls below the temperature of the electrolyte in the buffer compartments. The thermal convection thus developed involves downward movement of the cooled buffer in the annulus and an upward movement near the boundaries of the adjacent warmer buffer compartments. The sense of circulation is thus clockwise on the left-hand side and counterclockwise on the right-hand side. The downward movement of the rotating buffer column is thus accelerated by the thermal convection on the side facing the reader. This leads to the distorted (converging) streak pattern shown in Fig. 17A. (The pattern on the opposite side is a converse one showing streak divergence.)

Figure 17B illustrates a case where the electrophoretic current has been increased so as to raise the temperature in the annulus above the temperature in the buffer compartments. This tends to develop convection at the ends of the horizontal buffer column in a pattern opposite that encountered in the case of Fig. 17A. The streaks of the dye helix are seen to diverge as they descend on the right-hand side. The asymmetry of the streak pattern is due to appreciable lateral streaming: cold buffer enters the annulus from the right, creating an extended region of horizontal temperature gradient to the right of the center, while a relatively uniform temperature distribution is established left of the center.

A comparison of the distortion patterns of Figs. 17A and B obtained at a low and a high current density, respectively, suggests that there may be an intermediate current density at which the helical turns will show no distortion. Fig. 17C shows a helical streak obtained at a suitably adjusted intermediate current density, confirming that there is an optimum value of current at which the distortion of the helical path is minimized.

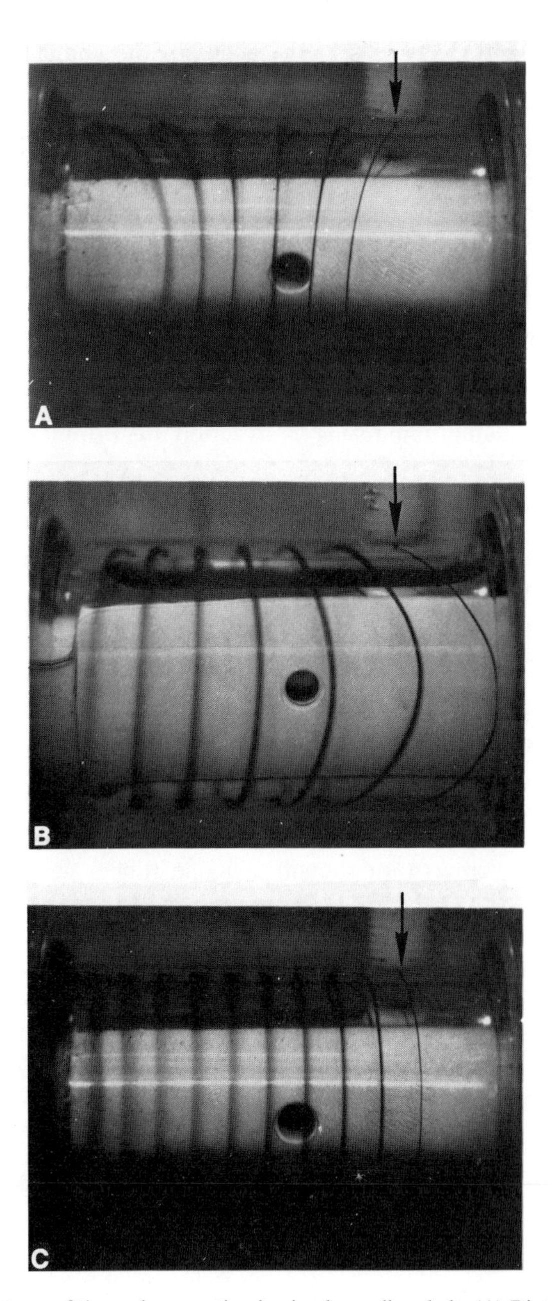

FIGURE 17. Patterns of thermal convection in circular endless belt: (A) Distortion of helical pattern under normal conditions of cooling at a low current density. (B) Change in distortion pattern obtained by replacing cooling fluid by warm water. (C) Rectification of distorted helical pattern by adjustment of current. (From Kolin, 1967a,b.)

Convective disturbances at the edges of the endless belt where the buffer belt contacts the lateral buffer compartments can be rather effectively suppressed by anticonvection baffles. These can take different forms, but typically they are thin (about 3 mm wide) corrugated ribbons inserted into the endless belt at the ends of the annulus. The corrugations have the effect of subdividing the circumference of the endless belt at its ends into short segments, thus inhibiting formation of large-scale convection (cf. Fig. 20).

An additional precaution against convection disturbances is the placement of the injector not too close to the right edge of the endless belt. Placing it about 1 cm away from the right end of the annulus is a satisfactory compromise between the objectives of maximizing the electrophoretic migration path and minimizing convection distortion of the emerging streak.

IX. PREPARATIVE INSTRUMENT WITH REMOVABLE EXTERNAL MAGNETS

A. Major Components of the Cell

Figure 18 shows a perspective drawing of a partly disassembled endless belt electrophoresis cell omitting some details to avoid overloading the diagram.* The left side of the cell is fully assembled. The electrode chambers EC on the right-hand side are shown detached revealing the end plate of the right buffer compartment BC against which the electrode chambers are pressed by screws (not shown); silicone rubber gaskets (not shown) insure a leak-proof seal.

Because of the cell's symmetry, it is sufficient to consider only the center section and the left-hand section. The magnets are omitted. Their mode of incorporation is illustrated in Fig. 20. We begin with the soft-iron core C (cf. Figs. 7 and 19) that is surrounded by the revolving buffer belt which is sandwiched between the core C and the surrounding plastic mantle MA. A gap is milled into the iron core C to accommodate a window W_c (made of glass or quartz) which is cemented in place with "silastic" cement (General Electric Co. RTV 112 or similar material). The core is insulated with a layer of Epoxylite 6001-M cement (Epoxylite Corp., South El Monte, Cal.), about 0.2 mm thick, which is applied and treated as described elsewhere (Kolin and Luner, 1969). The core is centered within the mantle

*This cell has been constructed under funding of Medical Testing Systems, Inc. of Fountain Valley, Cal. I am indebted to MTS for a long-term loan of this instrument and accessories. This instrument evolved from earlier models (Kolin, 1966; Kolin and Luner, 1969, 1970).

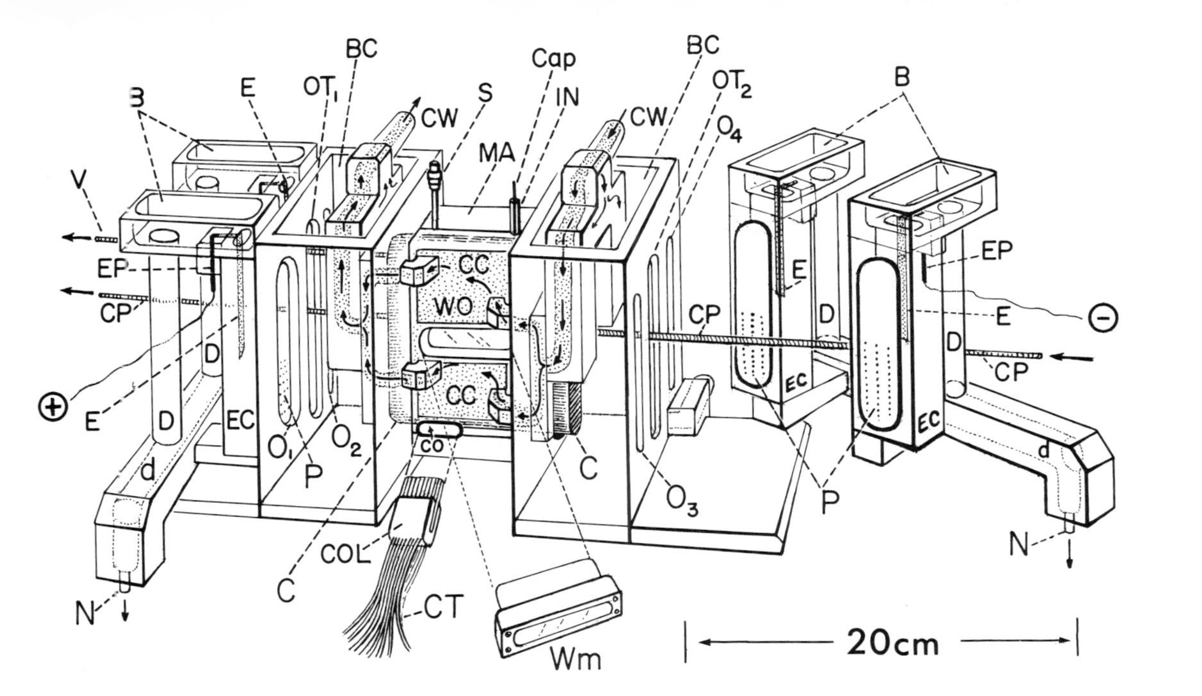

FIGURE 18. Endless fluid belt apparatus with removable magnets. (The magnets are removed and are seen in position in Figs. 20, 24A, and 24B.) C, iron core; WO, window opening; MA, mantle surrounding iron core; S, syringe needle for removal of bubbles from top of annulus; IN, injector mount; Cap, injector capillary; CC, cooling chambers in mantle; CO, gasketed opening for insertion of collector; COL, collector; CT, collector tubing; Wm, gasketed plug-in quartz window which fits into opening WO; CW, cooling water tubes (The arrows indicate the path of cooling water through these tubes and cooling chambers CC. The construction is the same on the back side of the mantle which is not seen.); BC, buffer chambers; OT_1, OT_2, openings for passage of magnet tunnel TU seen in Fig. 20 (The opening OT_2 is sealed by the plate TP of the tunnel of Fig. 20.); O_1–O_4, openings in the outer walls of the buffer chambers against which the four perforated gasketed plates P are pressed; CP, cooling pipe conveying coolant to core C; V, vent for removal of air bubbles from core C; E, electrodes; EC, electrode compartments; EP, electrode connection posts; B, the four "balconies"; D, drainage tubes; d, continuation of drainage tube; N, terminal nipple of drainage tube for attachment of tubes dt of Fig. 22. The balconies are shown in place on the left side of the cell and removed on the right.

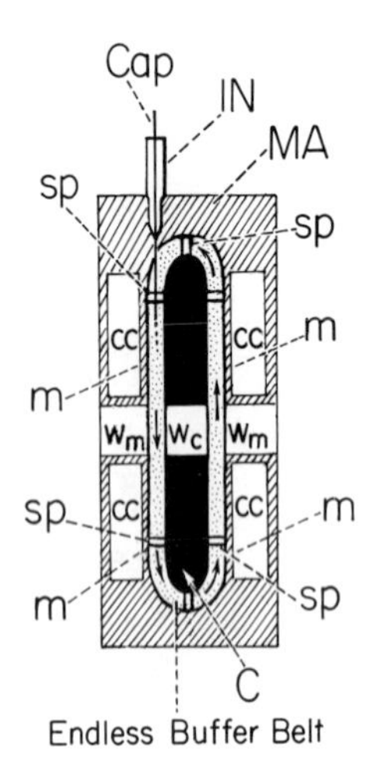

FIGURE 19. Cross-section of core and mantle: MA, mantle; IN, injector mount; Cap, injector capillary; cc, cooling chambers; m, membranes (thin plastic walls) separating cooling water from buffer in annulus; Wm, windows in mantle; Wc, window in core; C, core; sp, centering pins which align and center the core within the mantle tunnel. The arrows indicate fluid circulation in the annulus.

by means of small plastic cylindrical spacers SP shown in Fig. 19, which offer a negligible resistance to the circulation of the buffer indicated by arrows.

The end points of the iron core C are located in air, while the remainder of the core is in contact with buffer. This is accomplished as shown for the right side of the core C in Fig. 20. A plastic "tunnel" TU equipped with a silicone rubber gasket G is fitted over the end portion of the core C so that the gasket forms a water-tight seal. Thus the buffer which is on the left-hand side of the gasket is prevented from leaking into the air space on the right-hand side of the gasket, i.e., into the tunnel TU through which the magnets MG are inserted with their north poles abutting against the core C. Silicone rubber sheeting cemented to the magnets' surfaces, which face the core, protect the core insulation against damage by impact of the magnets. The tunnel TU has an end plate TP which is screwed onto the end plate of the buffer compartment BC in water-tight fashion. The magnets can thus be easily removed and reinserted on both sides of the cell.

The electrode compartments EC are then screwed onto the end plates of the buffer compartment BC as indicated in Fig. 18. The tunnel TU is located between them. It has been omitted in Fig. 18 partly to avoid overcrowding the diagram and partly because it would have been largely concealed in the assembled left-hand portion of the drawing.

CB in Fig. 20 is an anticonvection baffle. It is a plastic noncircular ring conforming to the shape of the core C with milled-out corrugations (indicated by arrows). These corrugated rings are sandwiched in gasket fashion between the left end of the tunnel TU and the left wall of the buffer chamber BC. The openings in CB permit the flow of buffer and of electric

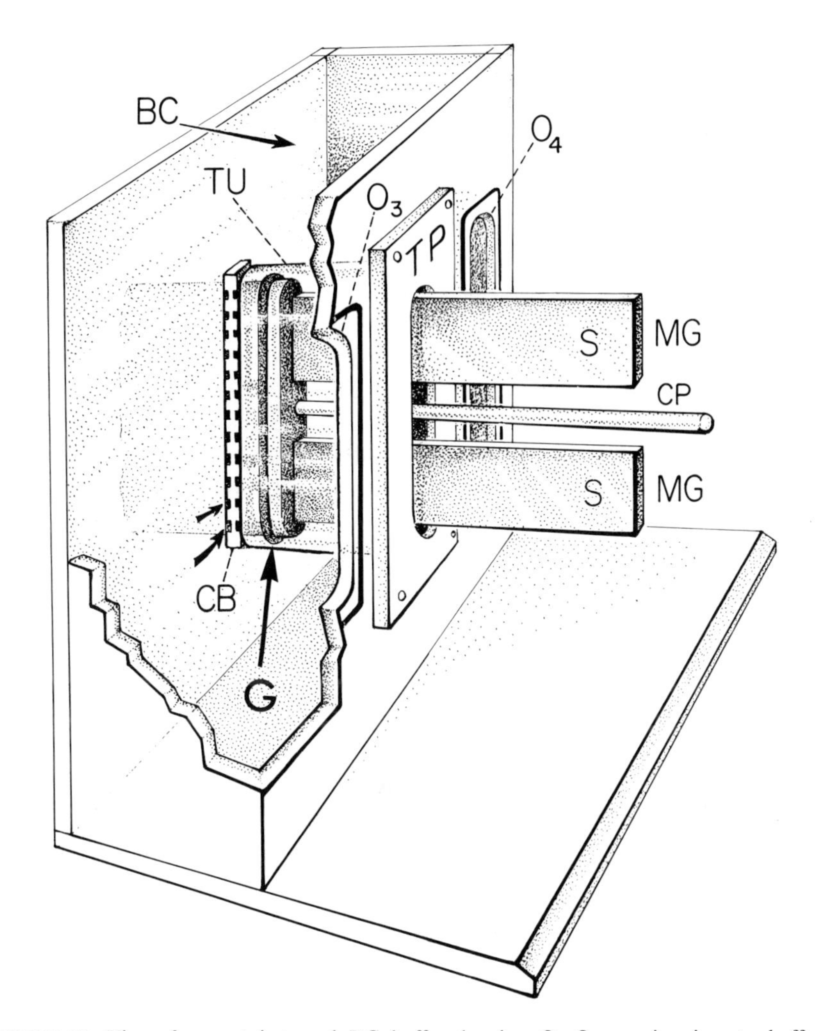

FIGURE 20. View of magnets in tunnel: BC, buffer chamber; O_3, O_4, openings in outer buffer chamber wall against which the perforated plates P of Fig. 18 are pressed; TU, plastic tunnel with inner gasket G with prevents buffer from leaking from buffer chamber BC into tunnel TU; CB, anticonvection baffle; CP, pipe conveying liquid coolant to iron core; C, iron core which fits snugly through gasket G; MG, magnets; S, south poles of magnets; TP, end plate of tunnel TU.

current between the right and left buffer compartments but inhibit thermal convection at the two extreme ends of the buffer belt surrounding the core C. These end points are sites of steep temperature gradients where the high-current-density region of the annular buffer belt contacts the low-current-density regions in the buffer compartments.

B. The Iron Core

The iron core C is hollow. Channels Ch are drilled into it, as shown in Fig. 21, for the purpose of cooling it by a circulation of cooled water through the tube CP and vent V (provided for flushing out air trapped inside the core lumen). The end plates E shown in Fig. 21 seal the hollow iron core.

As seen in Fig. 19, four cavities CC are milled out of the plastic mantle MA so as to create four external cooling compartments which contact the endless buffer belt through the thin membrane-like walls m (about 0.5 mm thick). Cooling water is supplied to and drained from the cooling chambers CC via connecting tubes CW shown in Fig. 18. The course of the cooling fluid is indicated by arrows in the diagram. The appearance of the cooling chambers is the same on the backside of the cell as seen frontally in Fig. 18. The circulating cooling fluid is refrigerated by a Neslab Instruments, Inc., cooling unit model HX-50.

C. The Injector System

The mixture of cells to be separated is injected by means of a motor-driven syringe SY of Fig. 22 via the capillary Cap (0.18 mm i.d., 0.66 mm

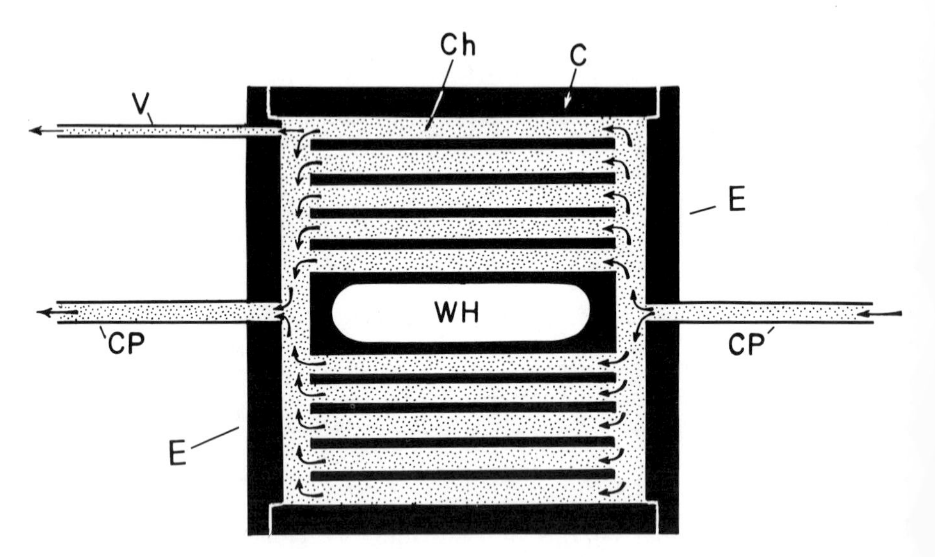

FIGURE 21. Section through iron core: C, core; WH, window openings; CP, tubes for entry and exit of coolant; V, vent for air escape; Ch, channels drilled into core for passage of coolant; E, end plates of core. The flow of coolant is indicated by arrows.

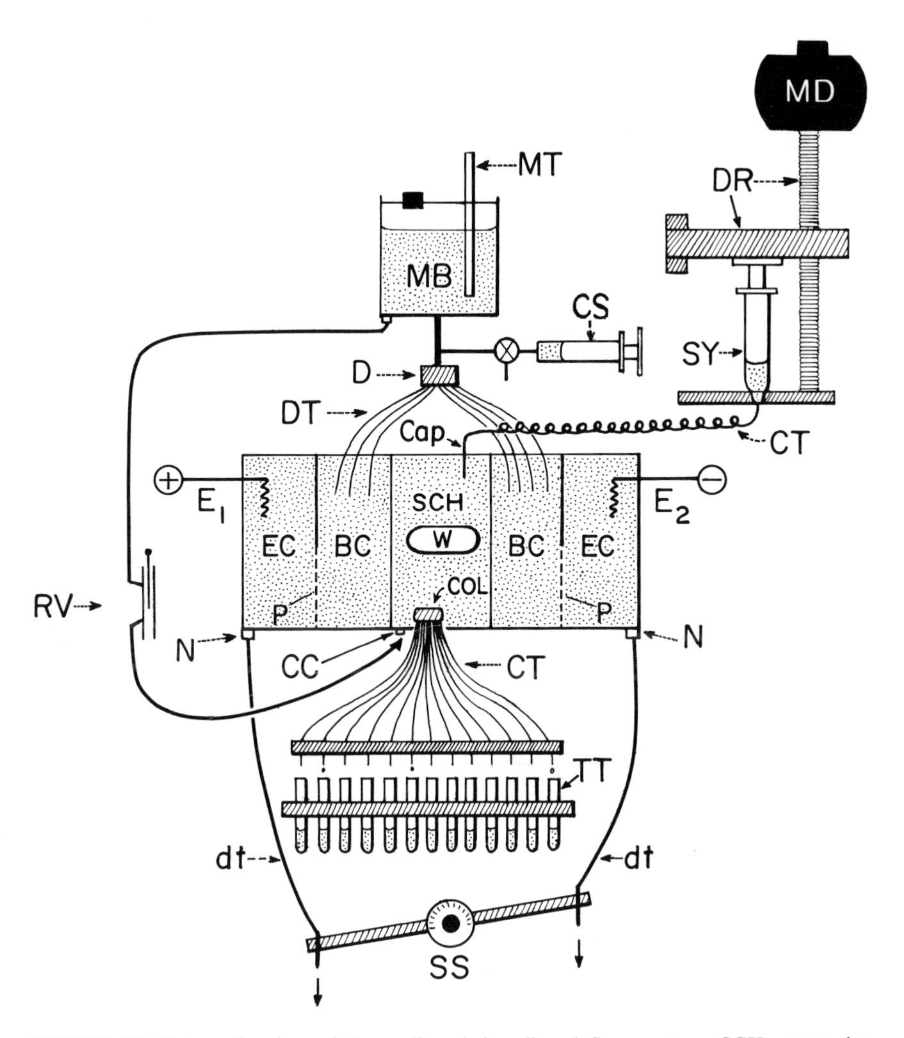

FIGURE 22. Schematic view of the endless belt cell and flow system: SCH, separation chamber; W, window; Cap, injector capillary; COL, collector; CT, collector tubing; CC, collector compensator nipple; TT, test tubes; BC, buffer compartments; EC, electrode compartments; E_1, E_2, electrodes; N, nipples of rigid drainage tubes (not shown); dt, narrow plastic drainage tubes; SS, "see-saw"; P, perforated plates; MB, Mariotte bottle; MT, tube of Mariotte bottle; CS, clean-out syringe; D, distributor; DT, distributor tubes; CT, coiled tubing linking capillary to sample syringe; SY, sample syringe; MD, motor drive; DR, screw and plate which drive the plunger of syringe SY; RV, regulator valve for control of collector compensator inflow.

o.d.) into the endless belt, as shown in Figs. 6B, 7, 18, and 19. The capillary passes through a plastic tube IN whose channel aligns and centers the capillary within the annulus. The "smokestack" S is a 13-gauge syringe needle to which a syringe can be attached to remove air bubbles which may be trapped at the top of the annulus during the process of filling the cell with buffer.

D. Plug-in Windows and Collector

Window openings WO (cf. Fig. 18) have been milled out in the front and back walls of the mantle MA. Plug-in windows Wm (made preferably of 2-cm-thick optically polished glass or quartz and enclosed in a plastic frame) fit snugly into these openings. The plastic window frame has a stop so that on full insertion the inner surface of the plug-in window is flush with the inner wall of the mantle MA, as shown in Fig. 19. A silicone rubber gasket insures a water-tight seal when the window frame is fastened to the mantle by means of four corner screws indicated in the frame of Wm in Fig. 18.

Because the windows are removable it is possible to clean them thoroughly after prolonged separation runs with cells. This is important for dark-field photography of the streaks of cells since deposition of even a few cells on the windows creates a disturbing background of light scattering which masks the visibility of faint streaks.

A similar plug-in system is used for the collector COL. A collector opening CO surrounded by a silicone rubber gasket shown in black outline in Fig. 18 provides a snug fit for the collector which abuts against the wall of the core C in the manner shown in Fig. 6C. The end portion actually has adjacent milled channels, rather than vertical holes shown for clarity in Fig. 6C. The circulating buffer intercepted by these channels is guided to fine PVC tubes t (about 0.6 mm i.d. and 70 cm long) from which it drips with the particles suspended in it into an array of test tubes T. The collector compensator (CC) openings shown in Fig. 6C are omitted in Fig. 18.

E. Centrifugal Buffer Flow

The central mantle section MA (cf. Figs. 7, 18, 19) is attached to identical lateral sections on the right and left sides. The two lateral sections BC (buffer compartments) and EC (electrode compartments) are shown screwed together as in actual use in Fig. 18 on the left-hand side and separated on the right-hand side to expose details which are hidden in the assembled sections.

The buffer compartments BC are separated from the electrode compartments EC by plastic plates which are perforated in the lower half by about 50 holes approximately 1.6 mm i.d. It is through these holes that the buffer compartments communicate with the electrode compartments electrically as well as hydraulically. Their function is to eliminate the use of membranes as described below.

In the fluid curtain apparatus (Hannig, 1961, 1964) as well as in the earlier version of the endless belt apparatus (Kolin, 1967a), the electrode compartments were partitioned from the electrophoretic separation space (fluid curtain or endless belt) by a membrane to keep the electrolysis products out of the separation zone. The presence of the membranes leads, however, to nonuniformities in pH and conductivity within the separation space which change in the course of time (Luner, 1969; Kolin and Luner, 1971; Hannig *et al.*, 1975; Zeiller *et al.*, 1975). This is undesirable not only in analytical work when a measurement of electrophoretic mobility at a well-defined pH and temperature is desirable, but also in preparative work where a shift of the components entering the test tubes as a well-defined particle distribution is to be avoided.

The replacement of the membranes by the perforated plates combined with a "centrifugal" buffer flow from the buffer compartments toward the electrodes via the perforations in the plates P (Figs. 18 and 22) can eliminate the above-mentioned drifts in pH and conductivity in the annulus. The centrifugal buffer flow through the perforations must be fast enough to prevent electromigration of ions of the electrolysis products formed in the electrode compartments EC into the buffer compartments (Kolin and Luner, 1969; Luner, 1969). It came to my attention after crediting this idea to Luner (Kolin, 1972) who implemented it in the endless belt system that the basic idea for such avoidance of changes in pH and conductivity by centrifugal buffer flow was first described by Bergrahm (1967) in connection with an electrophoretic separation column.

In order to generate the centrifugal buffer flow, buffer is supplied at a constant rate via tubes DT (Fig. 22) to the buffer compartments by a constant-pressure head delivery system, such as a Mariotte bottle MB (Kolin, 1966, 1967a). The flow velocity of the buffer which enters the compartments BC is greatly increased as it flows through the narrow perforations of the plates P toward the electrode chambers EC.

If not eliminated, the gas developed at the electrodes could present a problem, because it could get into the drainage tubes and thus affect the rate of axial buffer flow in the annulus. This is avoided by allowing the buffer to flow toward the drainage tubes D via the "balconies" B (Fig. 18). The latter are open channels through which the buffer flows outward slowly enough to allow the gas bubbles carried from the electrode compartments to escape into the air. Thus the buffer flows upward past the electrodes, horizontally across the balconies B, where the bubbles escape via the buffer surface, and downward in the drainage ducts D, and escapes via the PVC tubing dt attached to the nipples N as indicated schematically in Fig. 22.

F. Regulation of Buffer Flow

The maintenance of the centrifugal buffer flow can be accomplished by supplying buffer via the tubes DT in Fig. 22 at equal rate (i.e., equal numbers of tubes enter the compartments BC on both sides of the center section). If we wish to create lateral flow of buffer, say to the left, we increase the number of tubes entering the right buffer compartment, thus decreasing the number entering the left compartment BC. Conversely, we can generate a left-to-right buffer flow through the annulus, by transferring several tubes DT from the right to the left buffer compartment. Changes in lateral (axial) buffer flow by tube transfer are stepwise and thus represent a coarse flow adjustment. A fine-adjustment is accomplished by the "see-saw" SS shown schematically in Fig. 22. It is a horizontal bar pivoted at the center (controllable by a vernier dial) to the ends of which are attached the ends of the PVC drainage tubes dt of Fig. 22 (about 1.5 mm i.d., 30 cm long) which drain the buffer at both sides of the electrophoresis cell. Clockwise rotation of the see-saw, for instance, lowers the end point of the right drainage tube dt relative to the rising end point of the left drainage tube. This tends to increase the left-to-right buffer flow through the annulus or to decrease the rate of an existing right-to-left buffer flow (Kolin and Luner, 1969; Luner, 1969).

Changing the height of the pivot of the see-saw alters the rate of the buffer drainage from the electrophoresis cell. In this fashion, the rate of buffer outflow can be adjusted to equal the rate of inflow from the tubes DT to achieve a steady state.

The rate of buffer delivery to the cell from the Mariotte bottles can be changed most conveniently by changing the total number of delivery tubes DT. Thus, one can operate normally with some of these tubes closed. Opening some of them or closing more tubes will increase or decrease the rate of buffer delivery. A fine-control can be achieved by raising or lowering the tube MT of the Mariotte bottle.

The rate of buffer outflow from the collector can be changed by adjusting the height of the bottom openings of the collector drip-out tubes (CT of Figs. 18 and 22). The proper rate of collector drainage is determined as follows. By injection of dye through injector IN we can measure the linear velocity of the revolution of the buffer at the center of the annulus. Assuming a parabolic velocity profile, we can calculate the mean velocity.

If the lateral width of the collector intercepting the revolving buffer is, say, 2 cm, the area of the intercepted flow in the 1.5-mm-wide annulus will be 2 $\times$ 0.15=0.3 cm^2. The product of this area and the mean tangential flow velocity of the circulating buffer is the rate of volume flow through the cross-section occupied by the collector in the annulus. We must thus remove buffer via the collector at the same rate at which the buffer is supplied to it by the circulation in the endless belt. This is easy to adjust for since we know the volume of a drop and can count the number of drops leaving the collector tubes per minute. The total minute volume of the issuing drops must be made about equal to the volume flow entering the collector as calculated above.

G. Sample Injection

The cell suspension is injected via a capillary tubing Cap which passes through a channel in injector stub IN (Figs. 18 and 22). Figure 22 illustrates how the capillary is linked by a Teflon tube helix (28 gauge "microthin" Teflon tubing, Shamban & Co., Newbury Park, Cal.) which follows a mostly horizontal course until it reaches the injection syringe Sy which is driven by a motor MO and a screw drive DR. The turns of the coiled tubing CT guide the cell suspension in a circular–helical motion around a horizontal axis and thus inhibit sedimentation in the cell suspension delivered to the capillary injector (Kolin, 1954, 1960, 1964). An additional factor in the suppression of cell sedimentation is the small diameter of the tubing which leads to a high speed of the suspension flow through it.

One disadvantage of the above injection system is the waste of cell suspension which remains in the Teflon coil and syringe when the syringe piston reaches its terminal position. In dealing with small amounts of scarce materials, this is a serious drawback. To circumvent this, an alternative cell injector shown in Fig. 23 has been developed. Its capillary Cap fits directly into the injector stub IN of Fig. 18. The body of the injector consists of an upper half u and lower half L which can be screwed together. When assembled, they are separated by a silicone rubber membrane M which is sandwiched along the rim between two O-ring gaskets. The membrane thus creates a water-tight separation between the spaces above and below it. The upper space is filled with a colored driving solution (aqueous dye solution DS) which is linked by tubing T to the injector syringe Sy of Fig. 22. The space below the membrane is filled with the cell suspension (CS) to be fractionated electrophoretically. The syringe Sy makes the membrane M bulge downward as fluid is injected into the upper space. The pigment in the driving solution makes it easy to see what fraction of the original cell suspension has been expelled into the endless belt. When the membrane

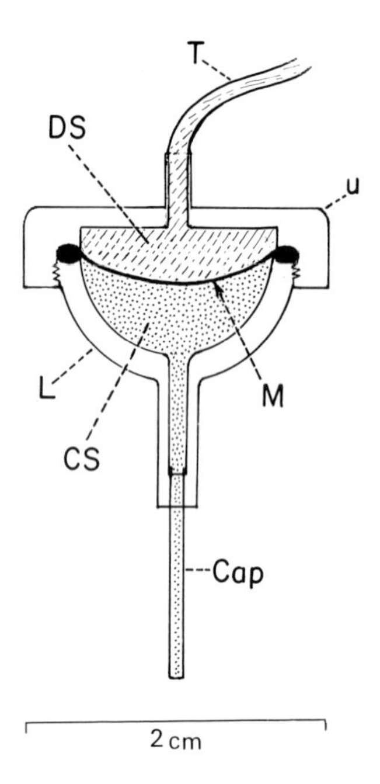

FIGURE 23. Cell injector: U, upper half of injector body with inner thread; L, lower half of injector body with outer thread; M, rubber membrane separating upper from lower half of injector; D, driving solution; T, tube conveying the driving solution; CS, cell suspension; Cap, capillary.

has expanded to make contact with the hemispheric wall of the lower space, all of the original cell suspension has been expelled, except for the negligible residue in the capillary.

The thickness of the injected streak is of great importance for the following reasons. In analytical cell separations, where high resolving power is essential and several components of a cell mixture are to be visualized, very thin streaks are advantageous. On the other hand, large-scale preparative separations are normally carried out with thicker streaks at a sacrifice in resolving power. It would be inconvenient to have to change capillaries to vary the streak thickness. Fortunately, the thickness of the injected streak can be varied for a given capillary quite simply so that the same capillary could expel a streak much narrower or wider than the internal capillary diameter.

According to the continuity equation applied to the flow of an incompressible fluid through a tube of varying diameter, the rate of volume flow remains constant: $v_1A_1 = v_2A_2$, where A_1A_2 are cross-sectional areas in two different tube sections and v_1v_2 the corresponding mean flow velocities. Thus, if A_2 is a narrower cross-section the velocity v_2 in it $v_2 = (A_1/A_2)v_1$ will be enlarged as compared to the wide-cross-section velocity v_1 by the factor A_1/A_2. Suppose now that the streaming velocity in the endless belt is faster than the suspension flow in the injector capillary Cap. The ejected suspension will be accelerated as it leaves the capillary and enters the faster buffer belt. Concurrently, the diameter of the injected streak contracts below the value of the capillary's inside diameter. Conversely, an increase in the rate of suspension flow inside the capillary above the buffer flow velocity in the endless belt will lead to expansion of the streak of cell suspensions as it enters the slower endless belt. Adjustment of the rate of buffer flow in the capillary to the value of the ambient flow rate in the endless belt avoids the above changes in the diameter of the injected streak.

H. Protection of the Buffer Delivery Line

Figure 22 shows a second syringe CS which has nothing to do with cell injection. Its purpose is to periodically clean out the distributor D and tubes DT. The distributor contains a perforated stainless steel plate (Millipore support screen #3002510) for removal of coarse dirt particles issuing from the Mariotte bottle which may enter the small-gauge distributor tubes DT and thus cause fluctuations in lateral flow in the annulus. The syringe CS permits one to rapidly aspirate fluid from the buffer compartments via the distributor tubes DT and thus to clean the perforated coarse filter plate.

I. Overall View of the Apparatus

Figures 24A and B depict the actual appearance of the cell and some of its accessories. In both photographs DI is the distributor linked by the tube T to the Mariotte bottle MB, the bottom surface of which is seen in Fig. 24B. MB is a lucite cube holding 60 liters of buffer and delivering it to the cell at a constant rate corresponding to a pressure head determined by the height of the bottom of tube MT (Fig. 22) above the buffer level in the electrophoresis cell. The Mariotte bottle is mounted at the top of a relay rack and the remainder of the instrument components at appropriate levels below it.

The PVC tubes DT issuing from the distributor DI are apportioned between the buffer compartments BC so as to obtain the desired rate of buffer flow from right to left in the annulus. The distributor DI consists of an upper and lower half which can be pulled apart. The lower part is larger than the upper part which "plugs" into an O-ring gasket. The stainless steel coarse filter plate is sandwiched between the two parts of DI. To insure against pulling air into the system when the syringe CS of Fig. 22 (not shown in Fig. 24) aspirates fluid from the buffer compartments via DI, the lower part of DI has a ring-shaped "bathtub" surrounding the upper (inner) compartment DI. The water filling this annular tub prevents air from leaking through the gasket when the fluid pressure in DI drops during aspiration of buffer into CS.

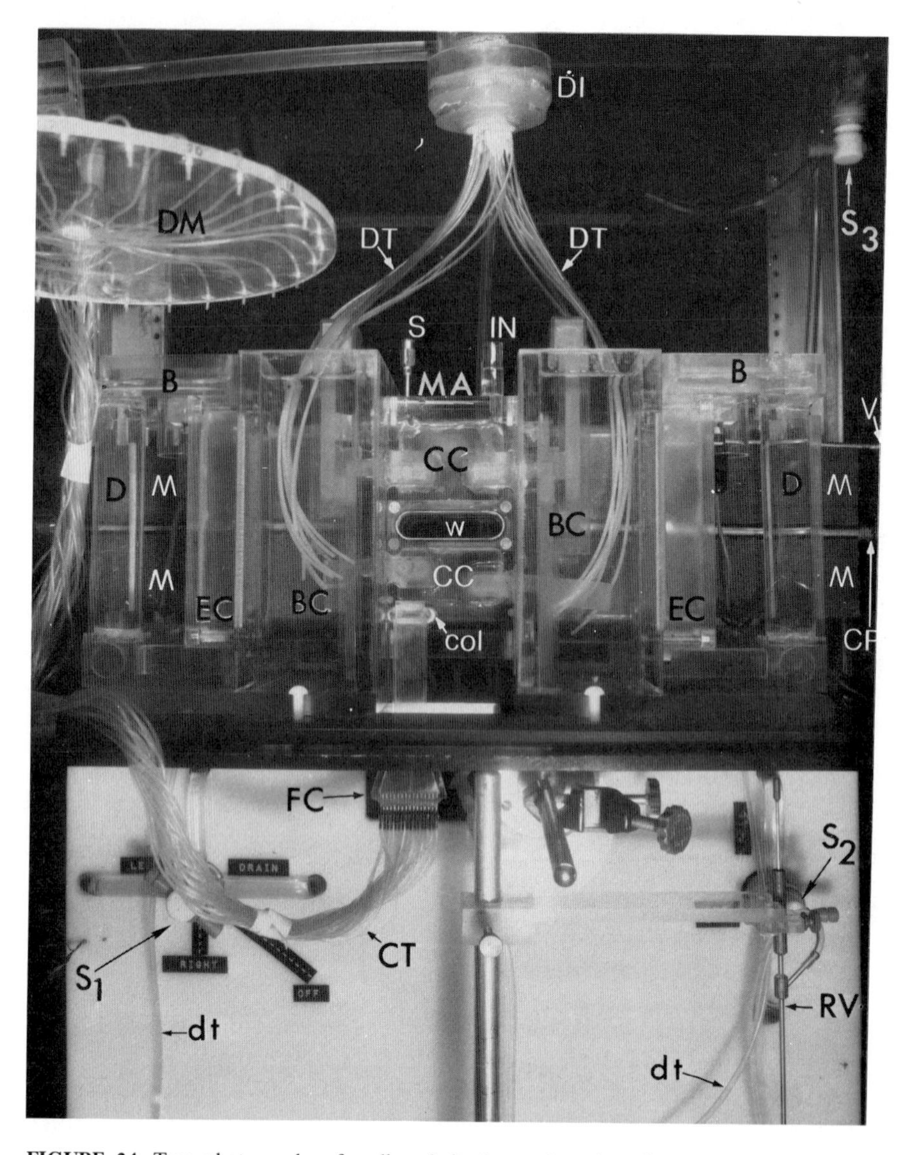

FIGURE 24. Two photographs of endless belt electrophoresis cell and accessories: MA, mantle; S, syringe needle for air bubble removal; IN, injector; CC, cooling chambers; W, window; col, collector; FC, fan collector exit; CT, collector tubes; DM, plate with terminals of tubes CT; dt, terminal drainage tubes; S_1, S_2, S_3, stopcocks; RV, collector compensator regulating valve; BC, buffer chambers; EC, electrode chambers; B, balconies; D, large drainage tubes; M, magnets; CP, cooling water pipe linked to iron core; DT, distributor tubes; DI, distributor; MB, Mariotte bottle; T, tubing linking distributor DI to Mariotte bottle; IT,

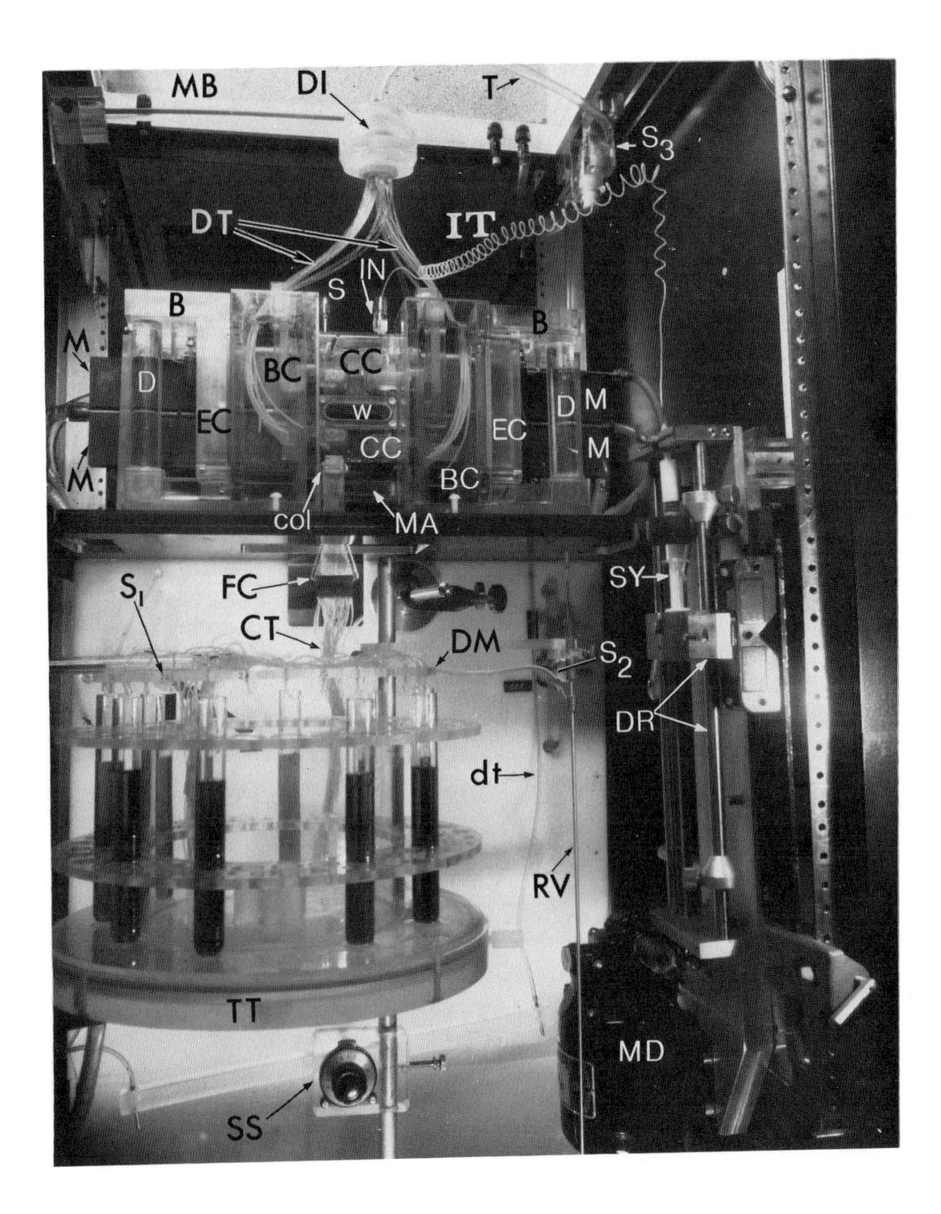

coiled injector tubing linking syringe SY to IN; SY, sample syringe; MD, motor drive; DR, syringe drive; TT, test tube stand. (*Left*) Cell prior to activation of collector. (Its exit tubes lifted with terminal plate DM.) (*Right*) Cell during collection. Collector end plate DM lowered and resting over test tube stand TT. The sample syringe and its driving mechanism are shown inverted to avoid obstructing other structures. In normal use the syringe and its drive is mounted so that the plunger descends as it ejects sample.

Tubing IT (labeled CT in Fig. 22) is the fine 28-gauge teflon tubing which delivers the cell suspension from syringe Sy (driven by the motor MD and drive DR) into the injector IN. This syringe orientation is opposite to the one shown in Fig. 22 which has been used normally. The inverted position shown in Fig. 24B was chosen for greater clarity of illustration. The most advantageous arrangement would be a horizontally mounted *rotating* syringe. The rotation about a horizontal axis would inhibit sedimentation of cells inside the syringe. The design of such a rotating reservoir is complicated. We used instead the membrane injector shown in Fig. 23.

Figure 24 shows the projecting ends of the magnets M, the "balconies" B, the electrode chambers EC, the cooling chambers CC located in the mantle MA of Figs. 18 and 19, and the drainage tubes D through which buffer escapes from the balconies B. This buffer drainage is completed by the passage of the buffer from the conduits D into the thin plastic tubes dt, the ends of which are attached to two short metal tubes fixed in openings at the ends of the see-saw SS from which the buffer drained from the balconies finally escapes.

W is the front window through which the cell streaks injected at point IN are observed. The gasketed insertion window col for the plug-in collector FC ("fan collector") will be described in section XI. The tubes leading from it terminate in a circular distribution mount DM which is elevated in Fig. 24A above the buffer level in the cell so as to avoid drainage of buffer from the collector. To activate the collector, DM is mounted at an appropriate depth below the buffer level in the cell as shown in Fig. 24B. The buffer is then drained by drops escaping at regular intervals from the ends of collector tubes CT into test tubes in a circular rack mounted below M. Both DM and test tubes TT can be moved simultaneously up and down to adjust the rate of buffer outflow from the collector. Stopcocks S_1 and S_2 control buffer drainage from the cell and buffer delivery from the Mariotte bottle. Stopcock S_3 permits the connection of distributor DI to the cleanout syringe CS of Fig. 22.

The inclination of the "see-saw" SS can be adjusted by the central vernier dial, thus fine-adjusting the right-to-left buffer flow through the annulus. Regulator valve RV (cf. Fig. 22) adjusts the rate of buffer flow to the collector compensator (shown to illustrate its principle in Fig. 6C but omitted in all subsequent figures). This regulator was built in the laboratory out of two hypodermic tubes as depicted in Fig. 25. Outer tube OT is about 50 cm long (1.6 mm i.d.) and terminates in a cast rigid plastic plug PL which centers and aligns a *closely fitting* inner rod IR (1.5 mm o.d.). A cast silicone rubber plug G acts as a water-tight gasket (with a "cup" above it for water to secure an air-tight seal, if necessary). The annular space between the two tubes is very narrow so that the main hydraulic resistance in this valve is in the space between IR and OT, while the flow resistance of

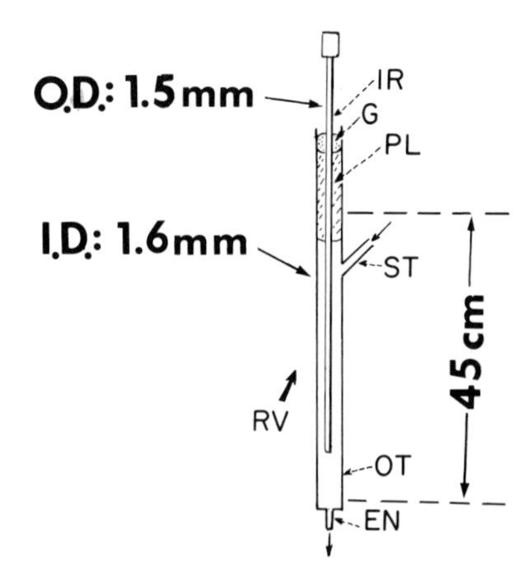

FIGURE 25. Collector compensator regulating valve: RV, regulator valve; OT, outer tube; IR, inner sliding rod; PL, rigid plastic plug; G, gasketing soft rubber plug; ST, side tube; EN, end tube. The arrows indicate direction of flow.

the outer tubing OT below the bottom of the inner rod IR is negligible. Thus, up-and-down motion of the inner rod IR permits nearly linear variation of the principal flow resistance in the buffer delivery line to the collector compensator. The buffer enters RV through the side tube ST and leaves it at the end EN. Adjustment of RV permits centering of ascending streaks behind the core window between the descending streaks in front of it.

Two important general-purpose commercially available accessories are not shown: (1) The cooling fluid was derived from a model HX-50, Neslab Instruments cooling unit which circulated a 12% aqueous solution of ethylene glycol with sodium chromate added (about 0.05% solution, to inhibit rust formation) through the iron core and the mantle cooling chambers CC connected in parallel. The temperature stability of the cooling unit is ±0.05°C. (2) The electrophoretic current is derived from a Sorensen DC Power Supply model #DCR3000-.5 (Sorensen Power Supplies, Raytheon Co., Norwalk, Conn.) 1500-W constant-current DC power supply.

X. PREPARATIVE INSTRUMENT WITH SUBMERGED MAGNETS

An instrument which has been put in operation relatively recently has certain advantages over the apparatus described in the preceding section and is still in the process of further development. It is depicted in perspective in Fig. 26, it is briefly described below. The parts which serve the same function as the corresponding parts of Fig. 18 are labeled by the same lettering.

The "heart" of the instrument is as before the endless buffer belt which is sandwiched between the iron core C and the mantle MA whose

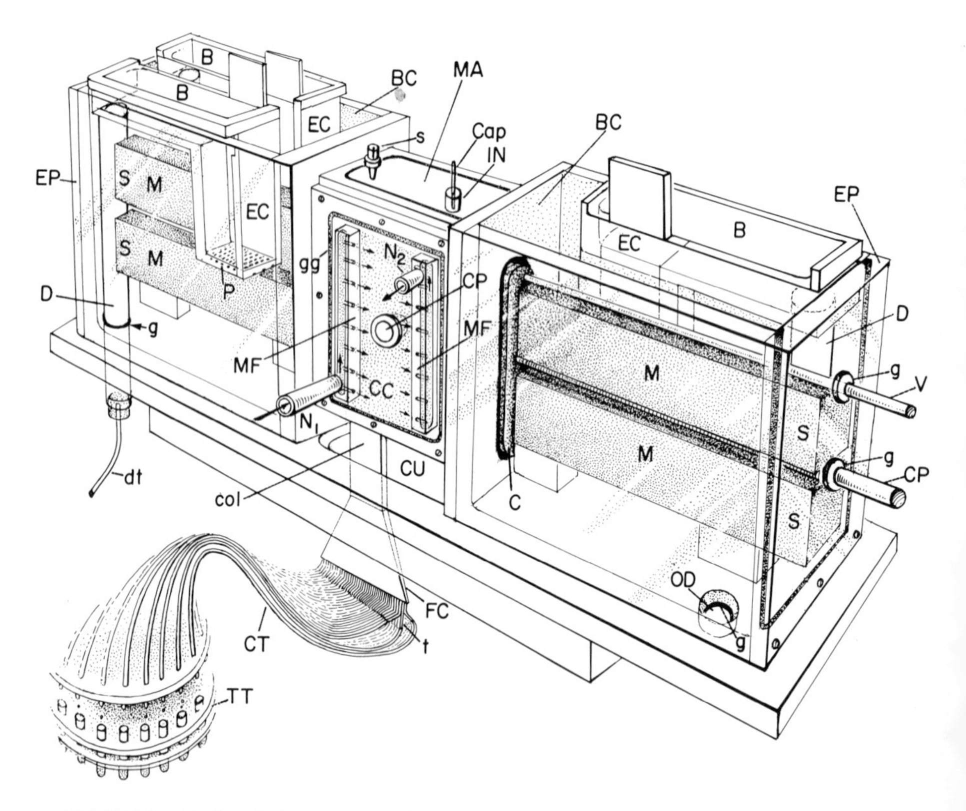

FIGURE 26. Endless belt apparatus with submerged magnets: MA, mantle; S, syringe needle for removal of air bubbles from annulus; IN, injector mount; Cap, capillary; CC, cooling chamber; CP, center post; N_1, N_2, coolant supply nipples; gg, gasket; MF, cooling manifolds (arrows indicate flow in the cooling chamber); CU, cutout in the base plate for passage of fan collector; col, collector; FC, fan of collector; t, terminal tubes of collector; CT, collector tubing; TT, test tubes; BC, buffer chambers; B, four balconies (one of them has been removed—front right—to avoid obstructing view of magnets); EC, electrode compartments; R, perforated plates separating electrode compartments from the buffer compartments; D, drainage tubes; dt, terminal drainage tubes; g, gasket; OD, opening for drainage tubes which act as support columns for balconies; C, iron core; CP, coolant pipe of iron core; V, vent pipe of iron core; EP, removable, gasketed end plates of buffer chambers; M, magnets; S, magnet south poles.

inside is of the same shape as the core C but larger in size so as to leave a 1.5-mm gap which is occupied by the endless buffer belt. As can be seen in Fig. 26, the design of the mantle and the lateral chambers is less complex than in the instrument of Fig. 18. The central mantle section MA and the buffer chambers BC form one piece and only the end plates EP can be removed by unscrewing. The electrode chambers EC, the "balconies" B, and large drain tubes D are in one piece, as can be best seen from the coherent unit D-B-EC shown in front in the left buffer chamber. The tube D fits snugly through an O-ring gasket g and acts as a column supporting the balcony B and the attached electrode chamber EC. The outer edge of the balcony rests on the upper edge of the buffer chamber wall and is thus aligned horizontally at a fixed level. The perforated plate P in EC serves the same function as in Fig. 18. There are two such units at each side of the cell supported by drainage tubes D passing through gasketed openings OD. The electrodes (which are not shown) reside in the chambers EC.

The iron core C is constructed as shown in Fig. 21, except that there is no opening WH for the window. Its absence yields the advantages of simple construction, of utilizing the full extent of the core and the surrounding mantle for cooling the buffer belt, and of obtaining a more uniform temperature and magnetic field distribution. The disadvantage is the inability to see the particle streaks until they reach the collector col.

The iron core C is centered in the mantle opening by spacers in similar fashion as indicated in Fig. 19. The two end plates EP are removed from the cell and the iron core C is inserted through the "tunnel" in the mantle. The magnets are then attached at both ends of the core C as shown in Fig. 26, relying on magnetic attraction to hold them. The end plates EP are then screwed back in place with the outer ends (S-poles) of the magnets fitted into supporting niches milled out for them in the end plates. The cell can now be filled with buffer if the collector opening is closed.

The magnets, being exposed to an electric field, must be well insulated. They are encased in a lucite case of 2 mm wall thickness, except for the N-poles which contact the core C. The wall thickness separating the magnet core from the magnet poles should be as thin as possible (preferably no more than 0.3 mm) to minimize losses in magnetic field intensity due to magnetic leakage.

The collector is plugged into the cell through a gasketed opening as in Fig. 18, except that in this cell the opening is located at the bottom of the annulus. The advantage of this arrangement is that it avoids a horizontal section of the collector in which cell sedimentation could occur. The collector has a transparent vertical rectangular section through which the separated streaks can be viewed by light scattering. The lower portion of the collector (FC) develops into a transparent "fan" in which the cell streaks can also be visualized by light scattering (see section XI). The front plate of FC can be made removable for cleaning. The collector compensator openings located behind the collector are not shown. The location and function of the injector IN and air removal vent S are as in Fig. 18.

The cooling chambers CC in this cell are different from and more effective than those of the Fig. 18 design. There is only one chamber on each side of the cell. The chambers plug into the mantle MA by insertion through a rectangular frame gasket gg. The cooling chamber CC is essentially a plastic frame with manifolds MF on the right and left sides. We see in the figure the cooling fluid enter the left manifold via nipple N_1 and direct a horizontal stream of coolant toward the right manifold, from which it is conveyed to the upper nipple N_2. The inner wall of the cooling chamber CC facing the iron core is made of a glass plate, 0.9 mm in thickness. This is more advantageous than the plastic membranes m of Fig. 19 separating the coolant from the buffer belt because of the much higher (about sevenfold) thermal conductivity of glass. The glass is cemented to the plastic frame with RTV silicone rubber cement. The pressure in the cooling chamber may range from 6 to 12 lb/in^2. As a result, a large force is exerted upon the glass window. To minimize its deformation and the danger of its breaking, a cylindrical metal post CP is cemented to the glass and allowed to protrude through a snugly fitting opening in the thick plastic outside wall of the chamber CC to which it is cemented with RTV silicone rubber cement. This post links the center of the thin glass plate almost rigidly to the thick outside plate thus minimizing variations in the thickness of the buffer belt by deformation of the glass plate from pressure in the cooling chamber. The ease of removing the cooling chambers is a great convenience in cleaning the electrophoretic separation space of the cell.

The ends of the buffer belt are separated from the buffer volume in the buffer chambers BC by anticonvection baffles similar to those shown in Fig. 20 (CB). Except for the design differences described above, this cell is operated exactly as the apparatus described in the preceding section.

XI. THE "FAN" COLLECTOR FOR INCREASED RESOLUTION

The device described in this section (Kolin, 1965) is not necessarily limited in its applicability to the endless belt apparatus. It is, however, of particular importance for the endless belt separator because the width of the collector COL (Fig. 18) is typically only 2 cm. Technical difficulties in milling collection channels normally limit their number to about ten channels per centimeter. The electrophoretic separation pattern would thus be collected at most in twenty fractions. The ideas described below made it possible to greatly increase both the total number of collection channels as well as the number of channels per centimeter.

Imagine the gap between Q_1 and W_1 in Fig. 27A to represent the width of the collector at the collector window CO in Fig. 18. Assume that instead of plugging in the collector COL at this point, we insert a fan-shaped flow channel consisting of two nearly parallel plates of the shape shown in Fig. 27A which fan out to a greater width Q_2–W_2 at the bottom end of this laterally enclosed flat flow channel. The streaks passing through the line Q_1–W_1 diverge as they move with the flow in the expanding channel and enter the collection openings (to which collection tubes CT are attached) located between Q_2 and W_2. Thus, two streaks (for instance S_3 and S_4) located so close to each other between Q_1 and Q_2 that they could have passed through a single collection tube will have diverged far enough by the time they reached the boundary Q_2–W_2 to pass through two separate exit tubes. Thus, we have achieved without electrophoresis an additional, purely kinematic, separation of streaks. At the same time as the distance between the streaks increases, their width is proportionally augmented, as indicated in the figure.

To maintain a constant linear mean flow velocity in the "fan" channel, the distance between the trapezoidal plates must diminish as their width increases so as to present a constant cross-sectional area to the flow. This configuration is shown in perspective in Fig. 27B. Thus, the product of the dimensions $d \times W$ in Fig. 27B remains constant: $W_1 \times d_1 = W \times d = W_2 \times d_2$.

If we assume that the channel density (i.e., number of exit tubes per centimeter) is fixed by technical limitations, we can increase the number of fractions by the ratio W_2/W_1 with the use of a fan collector.

We can increase the resolving power, however, even more by taking advantage of the fact that there is no electric current flowing within the "fan." The exit tubes CT of Fig. 27A can thus be made of thin metallic tubes (hypodermic tubing). It is quite easy to line up hypodermic tubing at a density of two tubes per millimeter and to cast them in denture material. By bending tube #1 backward, leaving tube #2 straight, and bending tube #3 forward, and so on in the same pattern, we separate the end points of these metal tubes sufficiently to attach flexible plastic tubing to them to convey the separated fractions to test tubes. Thus, using a ratio $W_2/W_1 = 3$ we could discharge the output of a 2-cm-width collector into 120 channels at a channel density of two exit tubes per millimeter.

The collector shown in Fig. 24 is of this "fan" type. The flow from the collector opening COL is bent 90° downward and continues between two vertical parallel plates before they begin to widen to form a fan at the bottom. The collector shown in these photographs has a ratio $W_1/W_2 = 1/2$ and terminates in 30 exit channels.

It must be pointed out that increasing the density of exit channels is advantageous only if the streak pattern is very stable. If there is a drift or a fluctuation in the positions of the streaks relative to the exit channels, an

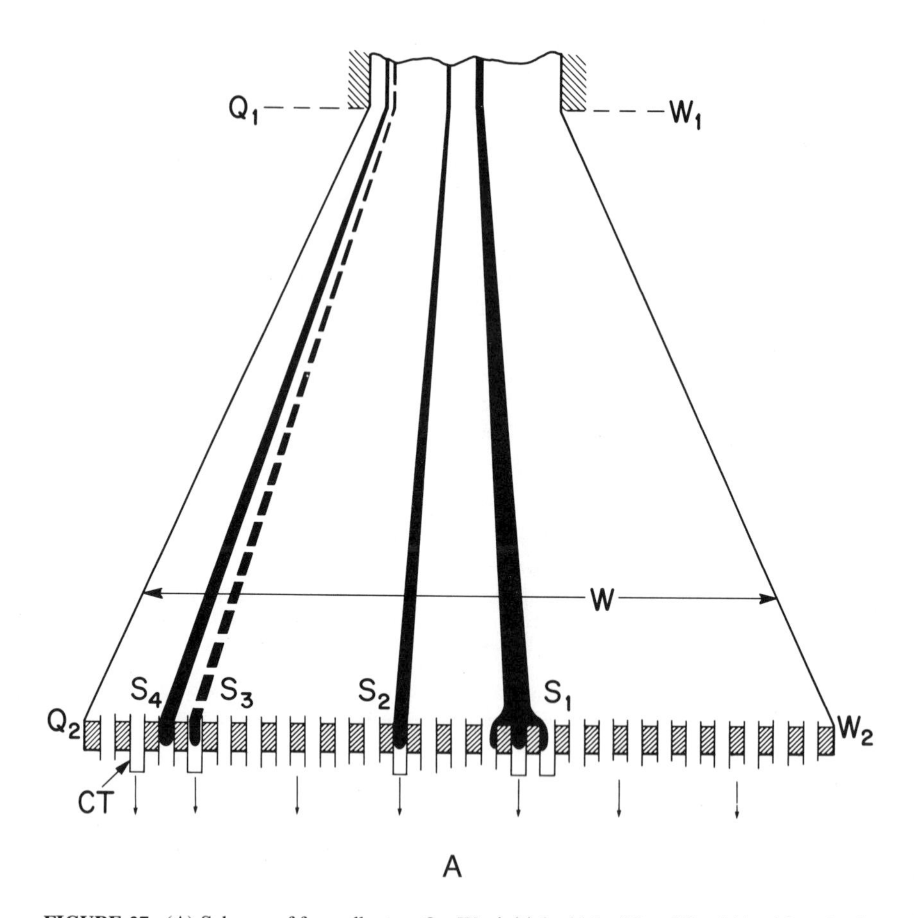

FIGURE 27. (A) Scheme of fan collector: Q_1–W_1, initial width of fan; W, width of fan; S_1–S_4, streaks of separated components; Q_2–W_2, exit width of fan; CT, collector exit tubes. (From Kolin, 1965.) (B) Perspective view of fan collector: FC, fan collector's rectangular input channel; W_1, initial width of fan; W_2, terminal width of fan; W, intermediate width of fan; d_1, d_2, d, the initial, final, and intermediate widths of the fan channel, respectively; CT, nipples for collector tube attachment; TT, test tubes. (Redrawn from Kolin, 1965.)

increase in channel density will accentuate the variations in the location of the streak components within the fraction collector. Addition of a tracer dye to the cell suspension to be fractionated permits confinement of the collection of this dye to a preselected test tube of the collection rack by appropriate rotary displacement of the circular test tube rack TT under the circular distributor DM of Fig. 24B. This ensures stable collection of the other components of the separation pattern.

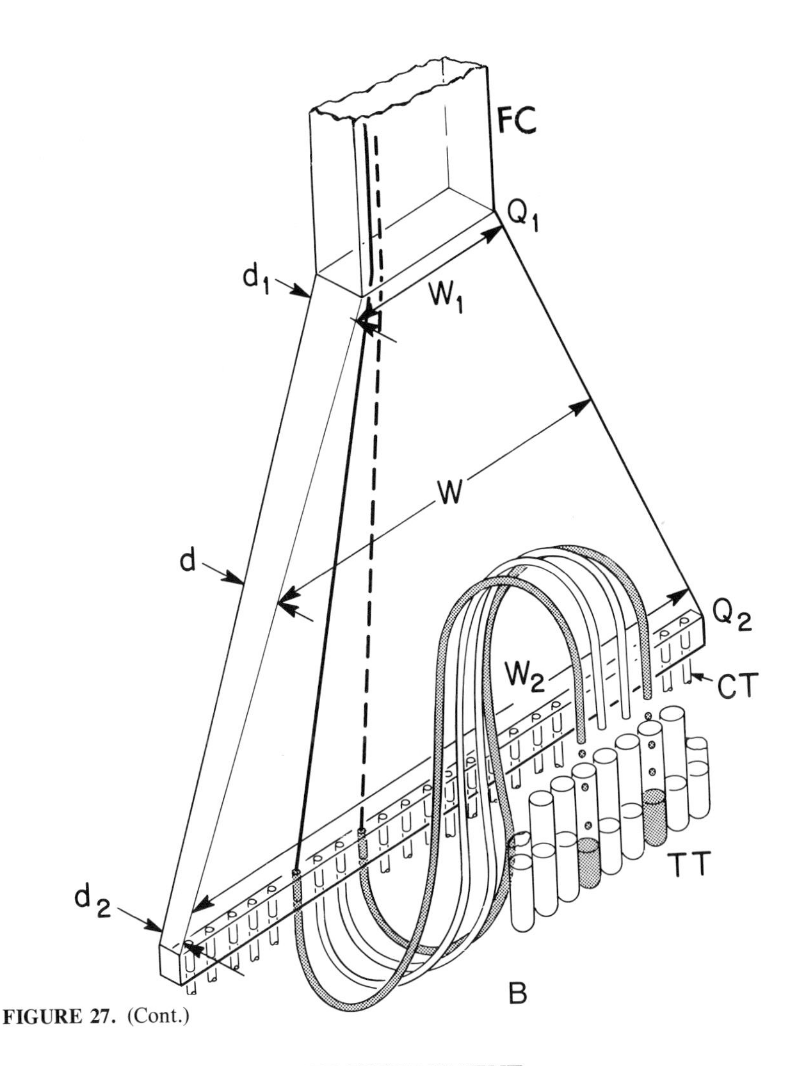

FIGURE 27. (Cont.)

XII. OPERATION OF THE INSTRUMENT

To give an idea of the operation of the instrument, we will briefly describe a typical preparation for a collection run. The description will be based on Figs. 18, 22, and 24.

First, the cell is filled with buffer solution by means of stopcocks S_1 and S_2 (Fig. 24B) which control the buffer inflow from the Mariotte bottle MB and the drainage of the cell through nipples located in the back of the bottom of the cell and which are not shown in any of the illustrations. The bubbles which may accumulate above the core C during the filling process are then withdrawn by a syringe plugged into the 13-gauge syringe needle S.

The accumulation of such bubbles can be avoided in filling the cell by raising the left side of the cell while allowing the buffer to enter the cell on the right-hand side. The air at the top of the iron core in the annulus is thus driven out into the left buffer compartment.

The buffer delivery tubes DT are then placed into the buffer chambers BC and filled with buffer solution by aspiration with a syringe (CS of Fig. 22, not shown in Fig. 24) attached to the distributor DI via the stopcock S_3. The same procedure is used to remove air bubbles from the tubes DT as well as from the distributor. The stopcock S_3 is then turned so as to connect DI to the Mariotte bottle MB, the bottom of which is seen in Fig. 24B. The buffer delivered to the right and left chambers BC via tubes DT is freed from coarse particles and mold fragments as it passes through the stainless steel grid (Millipore support screen #3002510) incorporated into the distributor DI. As the buffer level in the cell rises, the buffer flows over the "balconies" B into the large drainage tubes D and escapes via the thin drainage tubes dt whose exit points are fixed to the ends of the "see-saw" SS. The liquid level in the balconies rises until the rate of the buffer outflow through tubes dt becomes equal to the inflow rate via tubes DT. Raising or lowering the center see-saw raises or lowers the liquid surface in the balconies, thus permitting its adjustment to a desired level.

The aforementioned manipulations are performed with the plate DM harboring the terminals of the collector drip-out tubes CT in the elevated position (above the buffer level in the balconies) shown in Fig. 24A. To activate the collector, plate DM is lowered and placed over the test tubes TT in the circular rack shown in Fig. 24B. (Some of the test tubes have been removed from the rack.) The rate of buffer outflow is varied by raising or lowering the test tube rack with the plate DM resting on it. This is accomplished by sliding the rider to which the test tube rack is attached along the left perforated rail of the relay rack and fixing it in the desired position by the screws. The rate of collector drip-out flow is measured easily and accurately by timing the interval between two consecutive drops. The knowledge of the drop volume and of the number of tubes determines the rate of collector outflow. Section IX described how the optimal rate of collector outflow is determined.

The final step is turning on the cooler which circulates the cooling fluid through the core C and through the mantle chambers CC and simultaneously energizing the constant-current power supply which is set to the desired current value (normally about 250 mA). The collection of the separated fractions requires great stability. There must be no shift of any of the fractions to different tubes over a long period of time. For such a stable steady state to be established requires operation of the instrument for about 15 to 20 min. This waiting time is, however, not necessarily lost, since the following essential actions can be taken during this interval.

The injection syringe SY is filled with the cell suspension to be fractionated and fixed in the mechanical injection drive DR (driven by motor MD). It is helpful to add a small amount of tracer dye to the cell suspension. We ascertained that dilute brilliant blue did not perceptibly affect the electrophoretic mobilities of the lymphocytes in our experiments. The stabilization of the tracer dye location indicates the end of the initial drift and the establishment of the steady state where the dye accumulates in the same test tube. The dye also permits short collection runs *prior* to establishment of the steady state. The entry of the dye can be confined to the same test tube by angular displacement of the plate DM in case the dye entry tends to shift to a different test tube. This automatically insures that the cell fractions do not shift to other test tubes.

The cell suspension is conveyed to the injector opening IN by a "microthin" 28-gauge coiled Teflon tubing which fits snugly over a 30-gauge hypodermic needle attached to syringe SY. The other end of the Teflon tube is attached to the glass capillary Cap by means of a short piece of thin silicone rubber tubing which passes snugly through the bore in the injector opening IN. Cell sedimentation in this delivery line is inhibited by the rapid flow through the thin tubing and by the rotary motion about a horizontal axis via the coiled Teflon tube.

During this interval, the lighting (parallel light passing through the window W from the back of the cell toward the experimenter who is viewing the front of the cell) is adjusted so that it is possible to visualize the separated cell streaks by forward scattering of light without being blinded by the direct light beam (and keeping it from entering the lens of the camera). The descending streaks move to the left, forming an acute angle with the left–right axis. The ascending streaks in back of the core form an obtuse angle with the same axis so that it is easy to distinguish the descending from the ascending streaks seen through the core window. Nevertheless, there may be a problem in obtaining a clear view and photograph in cases where the ascending streak lies directly behind a descending streak. This situation can be easily corrected by the collector compensator (CC of Fig. 6C) using the regulating valve RV of Figs. 22, 24, and 25. Regulation of the flow through the collector compensator permits adjustment of the ascending streak so as to place it between the two descending streaks, thus making all of them visible without overlapping, as can be seen from subsequent photographs of cell separations (Figs. 31–40). After this adjustment, a photograph of the separation pattern can be taken without waiting for the establishment of the steady state.

The final step before collection consists of deciding after how many turns the streaks of separated cells can be collected with adequate resolution. The number of turns prior to reaching the collector is adjusted by variation of the lateral buffer flow. The coarse adjustment is made by transferring one or more tubes DT from the left to the right buffer compartment or vice versa. The fine adjustment is made by rotation of the see-saw

SS. Reduction in the rate of the right-to-left flow lowers the helical pitch and increases the number of turns the cells perform prior to reaching the collector.

Normally, we process in one run 0.5 cm^3 of a cell suspension of 5×10^7 to 10^8 cells/ml. The duration of the separation run varies from 30 45 min. In most cases the special cell injector shown in Fig. 23 has been used.

XIII. MEASUREMENT OF ELECTROPHORETIC MOBILITIES

The endless belt electrophoresis apparatus permits absolute as well as relative measurement of electrophoretic mobilities of biological particles. It is thus possible to characterize cells by their electrophoretic mobilities in a specified buffer system at a known temperature. The electrophoretic mobilities will be stated in this review in Tiselius units (TU) (Catsimpoolas *et al.*, 1976):

$$1\text{TU} = 10^{-5}\,\frac{\text{cm/s}}{V/\text{cm}}$$

The main experimental difficulty in measuring electrophoretic mobilities is electroosmotic streaming. As will be pointed out in greater detail in section XV, an electroosmotic convection is established in the annulus by the electric field. The buffer moves parallel to the electric current in the annulus. The direction of the horizontal electroosmotic flow *in the central plane* of the vertical straight section of the annulus is *opposite* to the flow *near the annulus walls* (i.e., near the surfaces of the core and the mantle). The velocity distribution is parabolic as depicted in Fig. 44. Thus, if a particle species of zero mobility were injected through the injector capillary, it would be deviated by the electroosmotic streaming and appear to have a finite mobility.

The electroosmotic streaming is demonstrated in Fig. 28. Figure 28A defines the baseline of zero deviation (under arrow). A fine straight hypodermic tubing has been inserted through the capillary channel of the injector at zero current. Its photograph indicates the path of a zero-mobility particle in the absence of electroosmosis. The neutral yellow dye "Apollon" (Microchemical Specialties Co., Berkeley, Cal.) can be used as an electrophoretic component of zero mobility. Since it is difficult to visualize we preferred to use as an approximation for demonstration purposes a 1% Ficoll solution. Its streaks can be easily photographed by illumination with a point source, such as a zirconium arc (Burton Mfg. Co., Los Angeles, Cal. model #2020) as suggested by Dr. Benedict Cassen. Figure 28B shows the helical path of the Ficoll streak in the absence of imposed lateral flow injected from the capillary in the direction of the vertical wire seen under the arrow in Fig. 28A. The Ficoll streak is injected at the center of the

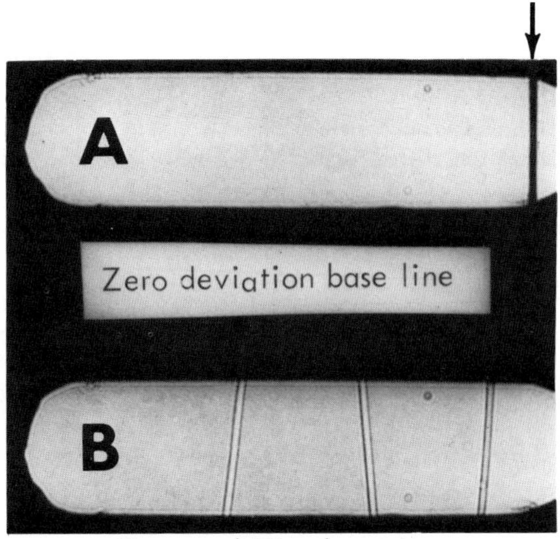

FIGURE 28. Demonstration of electroosmotic streaming: (A) Under the arrow, a wire emerging from the injector capillary indicates the "baseline" of zero deviation, i.e., the course of a streak of electrically neutral particles in complete absence of lateral streaming. (B) From right to left: the first descending, the first ascending, and the second descending streak of a particle of zero mobility (approximated by Ficoll). Due primarily to electroosmotic streaming at the annulus center, the streak is carried to the left along a helical path in the circulating endless buffer belt.

annular gap and thus depicts the horizontal electroosmotic flow in the central region between the core and mantle. The measurement of the pitch of a zero-mobility helix (approximated by the Ficoll helix) of the period of revolution of the buffer at the center of the annulus and of the electric field intensity in the annulus permits the measurement of the electroosmotic velocity and of the cell wall zeta potential (cf. section XV). The helical path of a neutral substance (such as Apollon dye) can serve as a baseline of zero mobility in measurements of electrophoretic mobilities. Such a zero-mobility reference retains its validity in the presence of imposed lateral flow in the annulus.

To make an *absolute* measurement of the electrophoretic mobility of a particle species, proceed as follows:

1. Determine the electrical field intensity in the annulus. This can be done most simply by measuring the potential difference between two horizontally spaced points in the annulus; for instance, between the "smokestack" S of Fig. 18 and a metal wire inserted through the injector capillary channel IN. The ratio of the measured voltage and the distance between the points of measurement gives the field intensity dV/dy in volts per centimeter.

2. Measure the period of revolution in the central region of the annulus by injecting a fine streak of a dye through the injector capillary and measuring the time from the moment when the leading point of the first descending streak passes the lower edge of the window W till the moment when the second descending streak reaches the same window edge.
3. The particle whose mobility is being measured is injected together with Apollon dye or another zero-mobility reference. The distance between the particle streak and the reference streak after one revolution, divided by the revolution time, measures the electrophoretic velocity of the particle. Dividing this value by the electric field intensity dV/dy from No. 1 yields the electrophoretic mobility. Figure 29 shows how such a mobility measurement can be performed by injecting a mixture of a dye (brilliant blue in this case) with a reference substance (Ficoll). The reference streak need not be a component of zero mobility. It may be a substance of known mobility relative to which the mobility of the unknown component is measured.

It is more convenient to make *relative* mobility measurements by establishing a mobility standard. The diazo dyes brilliant blue and amaranth (Werum *et al.*, 1960) appear to be suitable mobility standards (K and K Labs, Hollywood, Cal.). They maintain a constant ionic charge in the pH range of 3.3 to 9.3. We used brilliant blue as mobility standard in our laboratory. Its mobility has been determined and is known as a function of temperature (Luner, 1969). Brilliant blue is thus useful not only as a primary standard in relative measurements of mobilities of other materials but also for determination of the temperature at the center of the annulus.

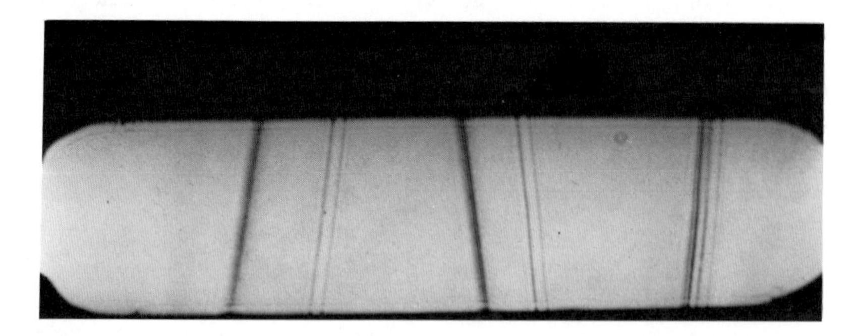

FIGURE 29. Electrophoresis of brilliant blue relative to a Ficoll "baseline." Brilliant blue is the faster component. Migration is from right to left. The first ascending streaks of Ficoll and brilliant blue are between the first and second descending streaks.

Such temperature measurements are based on the fact that electrophoretic mobility μ is inversely porportional to viscosity μ and on the availability of tables listing the viscosity as a function of temperature. Knowing the brilliant blue mobility $\mu_{18°}$ at 18°C and the viscosity $\mu_{18°}$ at the same temperature, we can find the viscosity η_t at an unknown temperature in the annulus from the relation

$$\eta_t/\eta_{18°} = \mu_{18}\ /\mu_t \tag{1}$$

if we measure the mobility at the unknown temperature t in the endless belt as described above (Luner, 1969). By consulting the tables in the *Handbook of Chemistry and Physics,* we infer the temperature t which corresponds to the calculated viscosity η_t. We have thus in effect a "brilliant blue thermometer" which permits to sharply localize temperature measurements in the endless belt annulus within a central buffer layer about 100 μm in thickness.

The relative measurement of electrophoretic mobilities with respect to the brilliant blue standard is extremely simple, as shown in Fig. 30. We photograph, after an arbitrary number of helical turns, a zero-mobility streak F (Ficoll, instead of Apollon, has been used for sharper visibility) along with a streak of brilliant blue B and of the component U of unknown

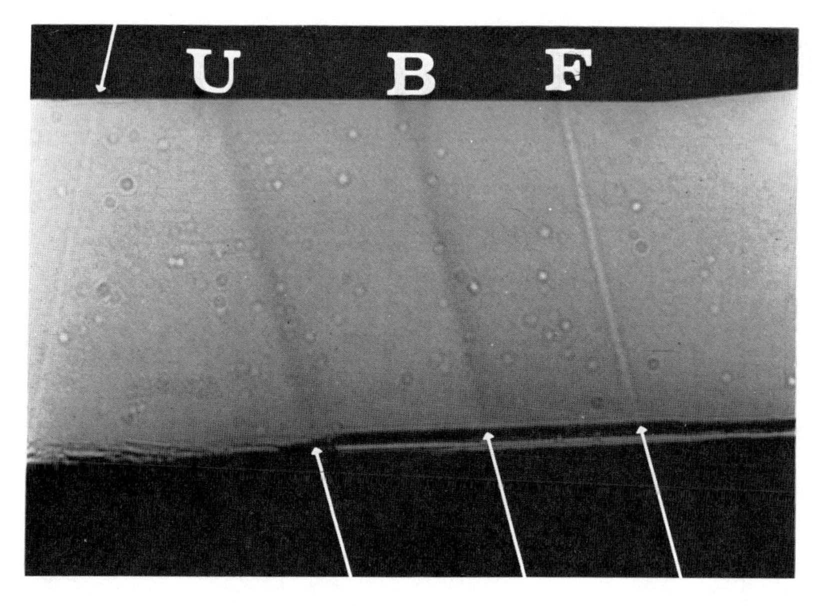

FIGURE 30. Scheme of relative mobility measurement. The three bottom arrows point at the first ascending streaks of three electrophoretic components: F, the baseline of zero mobility; B, component of known mobility (The top arrow points at second descending streak of component F.); U, component of unknown mobility.

TABLE 1
Examples of Typical Operating Parameters[a,b]

i, μA	E, V/cm	σ, μmho/cm	η, cP	t, °C	τ, s	$-\mu_B$ TU
220	97.7	692	0.91	24	31.0	29
180	87.2	633	1.00	20	40.7	26
120	71.4	517	1.23	12	76.0	21

[a]These operating conditions apply to a cell similar to the one shown in Fig. 18. i, current in the annulus; E, electric field intensity in the annulus; σ, buffer conductivity (from current and voltage measurements); η, average viscosity in buffer belt; t, average temperature in buffer belt (η and t calculated from average electrical conductivity); τ, period of circulation of buffer belt around the core; μ_B, mobility of brilliant blue (by absolute measurement).
[b]Excerpted from Luner, 1969.

mobility. The ratio of the distance between the streaks U and F and B and F is the ratio of the mobilities of the unknown component. Thus,

$$\mu_U = (UF/BF)\mu_B \qquad (2)$$

This gives us the Evans blue mobility at an unknown temperature. Measuring the absolute value of μ_B gives us the temperature at which the mobility μ_U has been measured relative to μ_B.

The abbreviated Table 1 (Luner, 1969; Kolin and Luner, 1971) exemplifies changes in the electrophoretic mobility of brilliant blue in a tris–acetic acid buffer at different temperatures.

XIV. EXAMPLES OF ELECTROPHORETIC SEPARATION OF LIVING CELLS BY ENDLESS BELT ELECTROPHORESIS

A. Buffers

This section presents examples of analytical and preparative modes of using endless belt electrophoresis as it can be applied to studies of living cells. Although the composition of the buffer is immaterial for the physical performance of the instrument, the requirement for biological compatibility between the cells and the suspension medium limits the selection of usable buffers. A thorough discussion and review of buffer solutions suitable for free-flow electrophoresis has been published recently by Zeiller *et al.* (1975). We shall refer to their paper for details. These workers examined the cytotoxicity of a variety of buffers and found four buffering solutions acceptable for cell separations: HEPES (Fisk and Pathak, 1969), triethanolamine (Hannig and Zeiller, 1969), ampholine (Haglund, 1967), and phosphate. In most of our separations of living cells, phosphate buffer has been used. For mammalian cells sucrose has been added to the buffer for osmotic compatibility. The composition of the pH 7.1 sodium phosphate buffer which we normally used for electrophoresis of mammalian cells was as follows (per liter of solution):

$Na_3PO_4 \cdot 12H_2O$	1.31	g
Sucrose	95.0	g
Glucose	2.0	g
EDTA	0.5	g

Sucrose was used to make the solution isotonic with the suspended cells, glucose was added to support cell metabolism, and the function of EDTA was inhibition of cell aggregation. The conductivity of the buffer usually was adjusted to be within the range of 600 to 800 μmhos/cm. This value is a compromise which avoids overheating the buffer at the high electric field intensity needed for rapid electrophoretic separation while permitting a high enough current density to secure rapid electromagnetic circulation of the fluid belt for inhibition of thermal convection.

Electrophoresis of erythrocytes was also carried out in tris–acetic acid buffers which proved convenient in the range between pH 3.5 and 9.3 (Kolin and Luner, 1971); 1.74 g tris per liter and 0.73 ml glacial acetic acid provided a suitable buffer near pH 7.0 and ionic strength of 1.3×10^{-2}. Sucrose in the amount of 30 g/liter suffices to inhibit osmotic hemolysis of erythrocytes (Sturgeon *et al.*, 1972).

B. Yeasts and Bacteria

In separations of bacteria and yeasts no sucrose was used in the buffer solutions. The aforementioned buffers will be referred to below for brevity as "tris buffer" and "phosphate buffer." Figure 12, obtained with the circular endless belt apparatus (Kolin, 1960, 1967a), and Fig. 31A, obtained with a noncircular vertical endless belt apparatus (Kolin, 1966, 1971; Kolin and Luner, 1969), illustrate the appearance of the streaks of microorganisms visualized by light scattering and the order of magnitude of separations obtained in less than a minute in a pH 7 sodium phosphate buffer. The time of descent of the particles from the capillary to the window (first descending streak) was of the order of five seconds. The time for reappearance of the microorganisms in the window moving upward behind the core (first ascending streak) was about 25 s, and the time for the second downward passage in front of the core window was about 45 s. Thus, the particles remaining in the endless buffer belt for a minimum of one and a half revolutions dwell in it for a little less than a minute before reaching the collector.

Figure 31B shows that the separation between the two particle streaks (the yeast *Rhodotorula* and the bacteria *Escherichia coli*) increases in proportion to the distance which they cover in circulating around the iron core (Kolin and Luner, 1969).

A

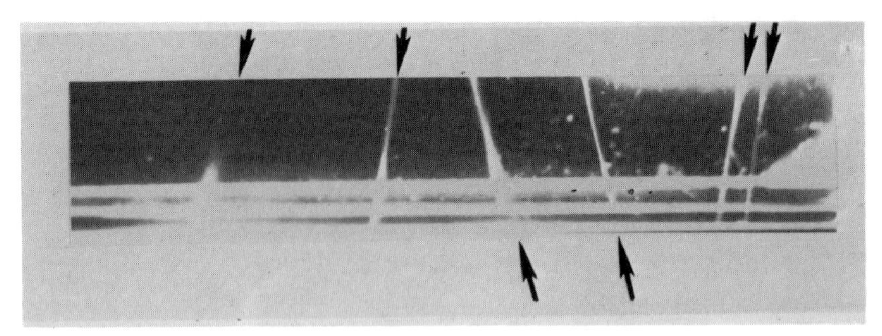

B

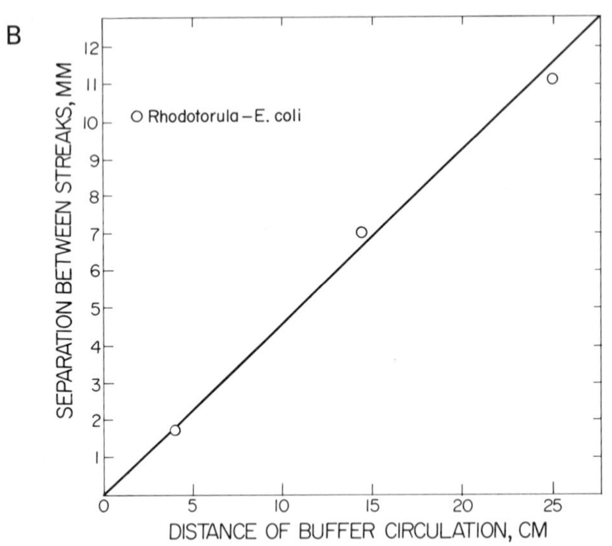

SEPARATION BETWEEN STREAKS, MM
O Rhodotorula – E. coli
DISTANCE OF BUFFER CIRCULATION, CM

C

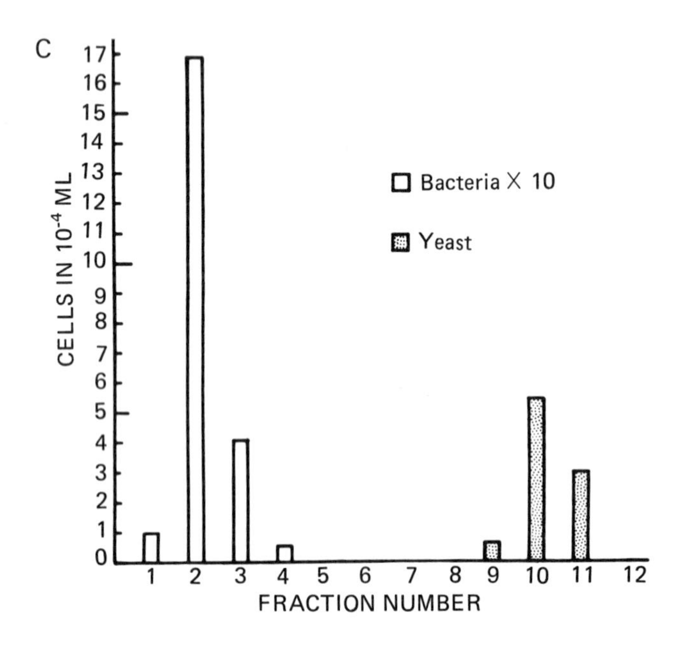

CELLS IN 10⁻⁴ ML
Bacteria X 10
Yeast
FRACTION NUMBER

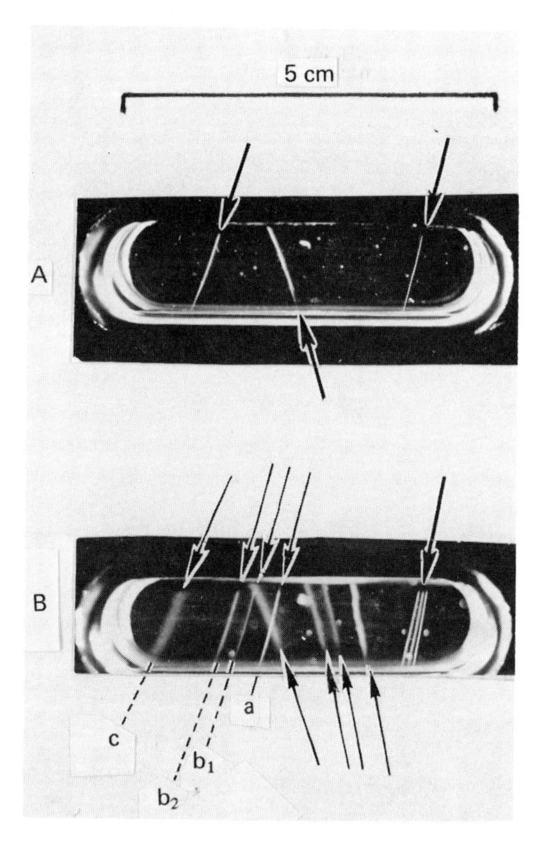

FIGURE 32. Separation of bacteria in suspension. (A) Single bacterial component: *E. coli* ML 35. (B) Separation of a mixture of three bacteria (two strains of *E. coli* and *Proteus vulgaris*) into four components (labeled in the second descending streak): a, *E. coli* ML 35; b_1 and b_2, two streaks into which the component *Proteus vulgaris* is split; c, E coli BE 30.

Figure 31C shows a histogram for the collection pattern corresponding to the separation pattern of *E. coli* and *Rhodotorula* shown in Fig. 31A. The microorganisms are well separated by four blank tubes in the fraction collector. Nevertheless, it is surprising to see that, in spite of the great sharpness and narrowness of the streaks, the bacterium is collected in four test tubes and the yeast in three. The resolution in the collection pattern is thus clearly inferior to that seen in the separation pattern of Fig. 31A. The reasons for such discrepancies will be considered in section XV.

Figure 32 illustrates the separation of a mixture of three bacteria:

←

FIGURE 31. Separation of *Rhodotorula* from *E. coli:* (A) separation pattern; (B) streak separation as a function of migration path; (C) histogram for collection pattern. (From Kolin and Luner, 1969.)

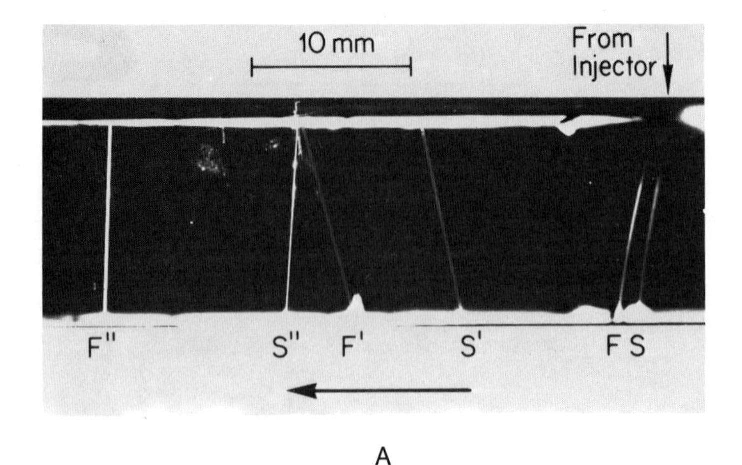

A

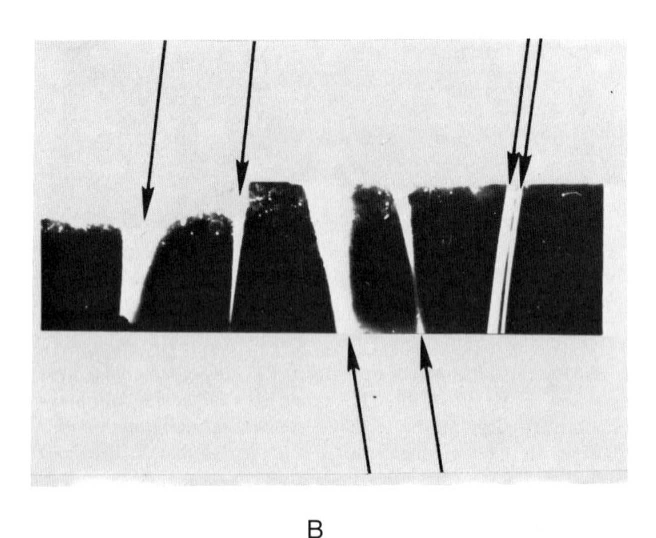

B

FIGURE 33. Splitting of streaks of one bacterial strain into two components. (A) Splitting of *Escherichia freundii* into a fast (F) and a slow (S) electrophoretic component. (From Kolin, 1971.) (B) Splitting of *E. coli* strain C600 $(P_1)^+$ into two electrophoretically distinct components. (C) Histogram for the separation shown in (B). (From Owen, 1972.)

Proteus vulgaris and two strains of *E. coli* (BE 30 and ML 35) in pH 7.1 phosphate buffer. Figure 32A obtained with *E. coli* ML 35 shows the degree of electrophoretic homogeneity which can be exhibited by a single bacterial component. Fig. 32B shows a sharper streak for the slowest component (a), *E. coli* ML 35 (presumably indicating greater electrophoretic homogeneity), than for the fastest (c), *E. coli* BE 30. *P. vulgaris* is

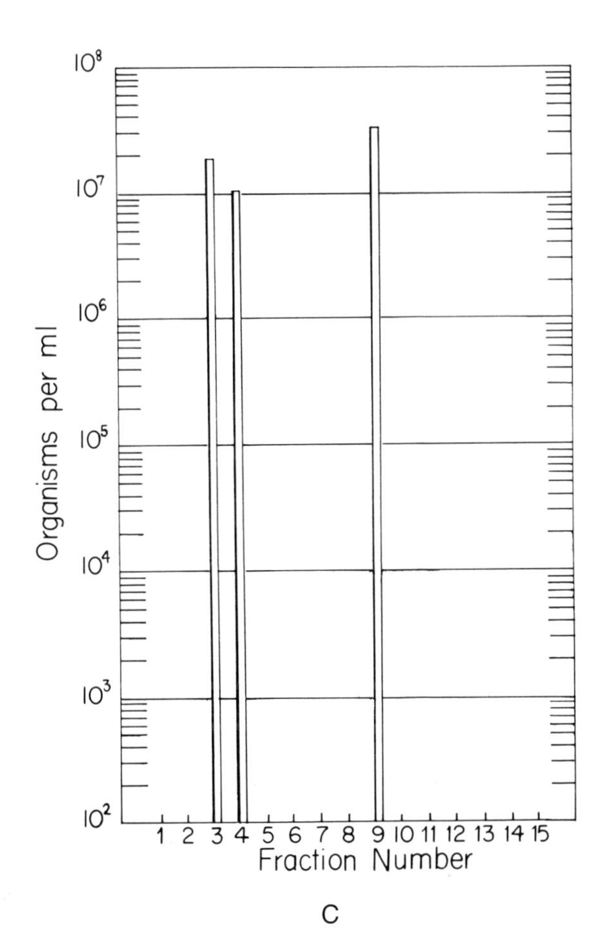

FIGURE 33. (Cont.)

seen to split into two well resolved components (b_1 and b_2). This does not necessarily indicate a contamination of the *P. vulgaris* culture, which was pure. We observed many instances of pure bacterial strains which yielded two sharp, widely separated streaks in the endless belt apparatus, as illustrated below.

Figure 33A shows the separation pattern of *Escherichia freundii* (Kolin, 1971) whose components are exceptionally sharp and widely separated. Figure 33B shows a similar splitting of a bacterium, *E. coli* strain C600 $(P_1)^+$ (Owen, 1972). The faster component is clearly more abundant, as can be seen in the photograph and the histogram of Fig. 33C.

Experiments suggest that the two streaks seen for *E. coli* C600 $(P_1)^+$ are due to separation of the suspension into piliated and nonpiliated bacte-

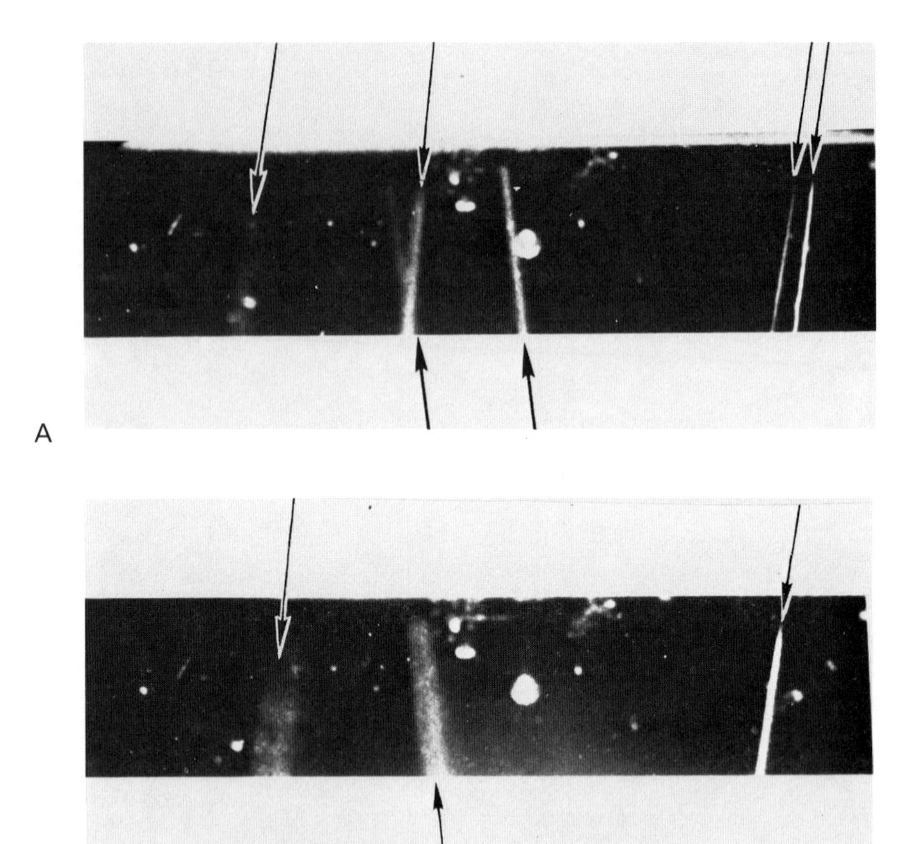

FIGURE 34. Effect of removal of pili on the splitting of *E. coli* C600 $(P_1)^+$ strain into two components. (A) The top arrows indicate the first (on the right) and second (on the left) descending streaks of the components into which the injected streak splits. The bottom arrows point at the first ascending streak. (B) After removal of pili, the bacterial suspension does not split into two electrophoretically distinct components. (From Owen, 1972.)

ria (Owen, 1972). Figure 34A shows the separation pattern of a suspension of *E. coli* C600 $(P_1)^+$ at the outset of the experiment. Figure 34B shows the drastic change in the separation pattern after removal of the pili from the bacterial surface by blending. The slower fraction has been removed and one no longer sees two sharp widely separated fractions, but rather one wide diverging streak exhibiting considerable electrophoretic inhomogeneity. [The removal of the pili was accomplished by a method which, according to Brinton (1967) does not appreciably affect the viability of the bacteria.] According to Brinton (1967) the electrophoretic mobility of piliated bacteria is proportional to the number of pili per cell. If this is true, the electrophoretic inhomogeneity observed in Fig. 34B may be due to variations in piliation among the bacteria following the blending process.

In the above study (Owen, 1972), 13 strains of *E. coli* have been studied and it was found the 69% of the examined cultures consisted of two subpopulations differing in their electrophoretic mobility. A mobility difference of 0.2 TU (cf. section XII) was sufficient for separation of the bacteria. Samples of 15 μl were sufficient for an endless belt electrophoretic analysis.

C. Mammalian Cells

Among mammalian cells, human erythrocytes have been subjected to more endless belt electrophoresis studies than have other types of cells. The mean electrophoretic mobility of human erythrocytes was determined with the endless belt apparatus from blood specimens obtained from 106 healthy medical students (Sturgeon *et al.*, 1972). The value found was 24.6 TU. The standard error of the mean was ± 0.073, the standard deviation was ± 0.75, and the coefficient of variation was $\pm 3.05\%$. Figure 35 shows the frequency distribution of the electrophoretic mobility of erythrocytes for the aforementioned student sample. The abscissa indicates the mobility in Tiselius Units (TU) and the ordinate indicates the percent of the sample. The mobility distribution was found to be bimodal (Sturgeon *et al.*, 1972).

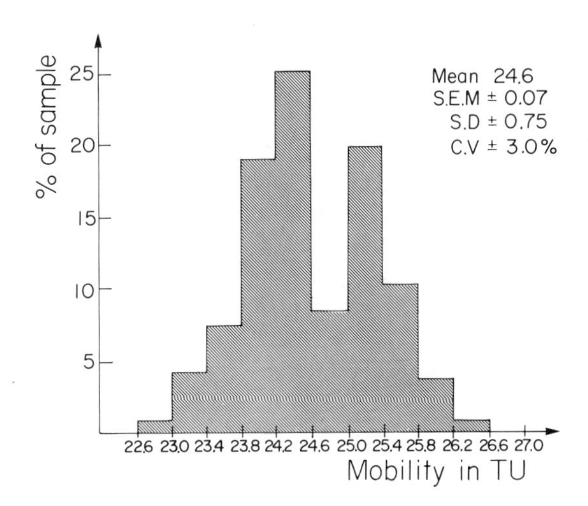

FIGURE 35. Frequency distribution of electrophoretic mobility of red blood cells from 106 human subjects. The mobility is measured in Tiselius units (TU). (Redrawn from Sturgeon *et al.*, 1972.)

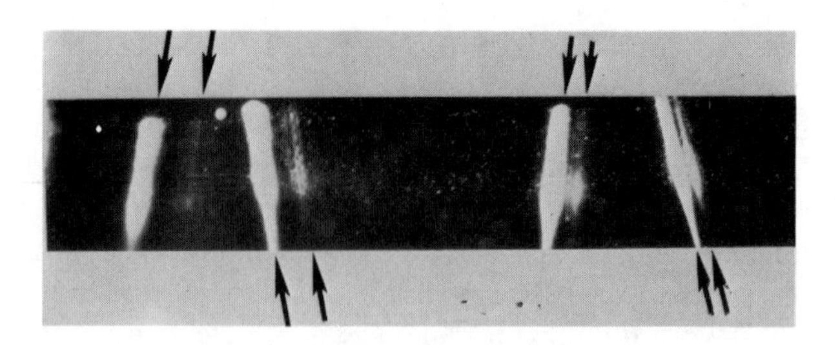

A

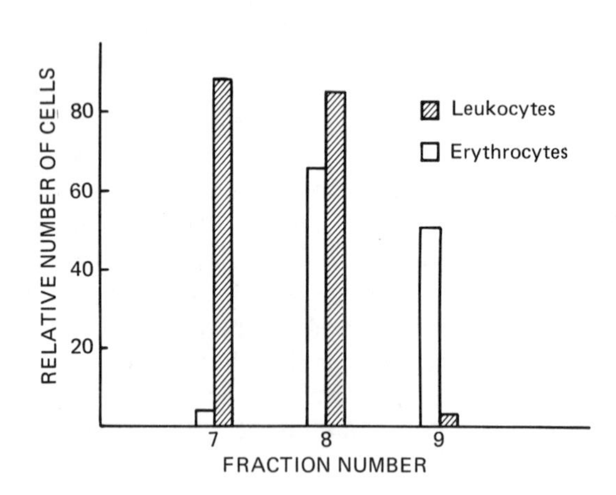
RELATIVE NUMBER OF CELLS
80
60
40
20
Leukocytes
Erythrocytes
7
8
9
FRACTION NUMBER

B

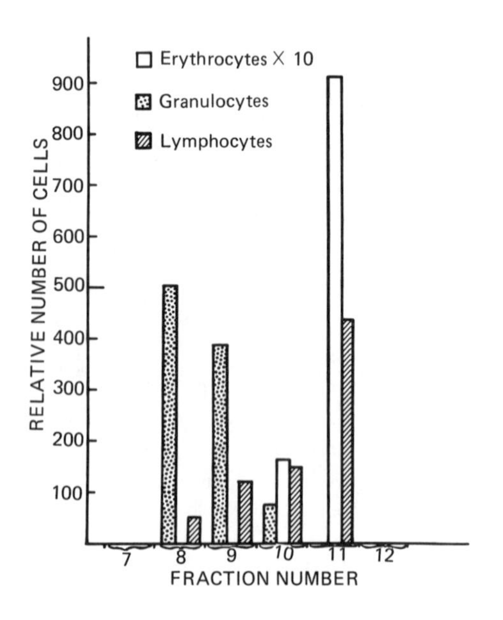
Erythrocytes × 10
Granulocytes
Lymphocytes
RELATIVE NUMBER OF CELLS
900
800
700
600
500
400
300
200
100
7
8
9
10
11
12
FRACTION NUMBER

C

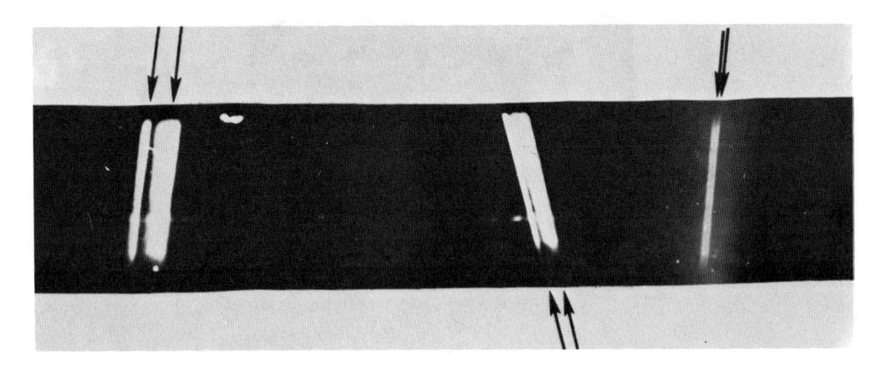

FIGURE 37. Splitting of erythrocytes of a donor into two electrophoretically distinct components. The donor's blood exhibited partial polyagglutinability. (From Sturgeon *et al.*, 1972.)

Figure 36A shows the separation pattern of human erythrocytes (fast component on the left) and granulocytes (slow component). Figure 36B and C show histograms for collection patterns of blood cells from two different hospital patients fractionated by endless belt electrophoresis (Kolin and Luner, 1969).

Figure 37 presents an unusual case. The erythrocytes of a blood donor, whose cells exhibited partial polyagglutinability, split into two discrete subpopulations of different electrophoretic mobility (Sturgeon *et al.*, 1972).

Electrophoresis of human lymphocyte suspensions prepared from blood samples by the Isopaque–Ficoll interface centrifugation method (Davidson and Parish, 1975) yielded a separation pattern shown in Fig. 38A. This procedure removes about 99% of the red cells, and dead cells are removed by forming clumps and precipitating in the centrifuge with the red cells below the Isopaque–Ficoll interface. The lymphocytes which remain at the Isopaque–Ficoll interface are 95–100% viable. There is thus some contamination by red cells to be expected. An additional potential contaminant is blood platelets as can be seen in Fig. 38B, which shows an evaluation of a collection pattern obtained by electrophoresis of a lymphocyte suspension prepared by the above method. In addition to a bimodal distribution curve for the lymphocytes, we see a sharp peak indicating the distribution of the blood platelets in the fraction collector and a small peak locating the erythrocytes.

The practical utilization of the method's ability to separate B and T lymphocytes is at the moment somewhat impeded by the low recovery rate

←

FIGURE 36. Separation of human erythrocytes from leukocytes. (A) Photograph of the separation pattern. The erythrocytes are the faster component (on the left). (B) Histogram for collection pattern of separated blood cells of a hospital patient. (C) Histogram for collection pattern of separated blood cells of a different hospital patient. (From Kolin and Luner, 1969.)

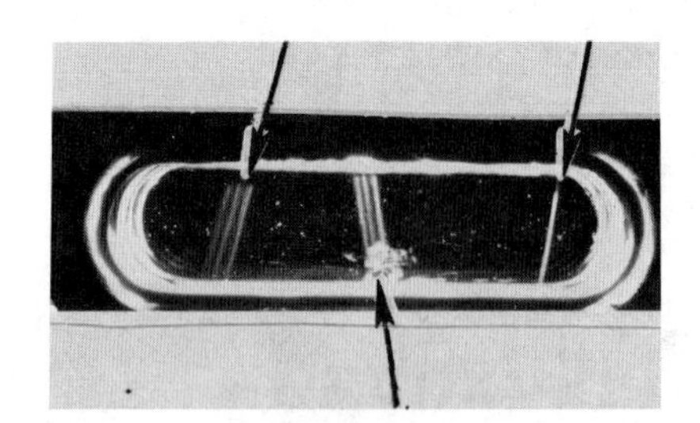

A

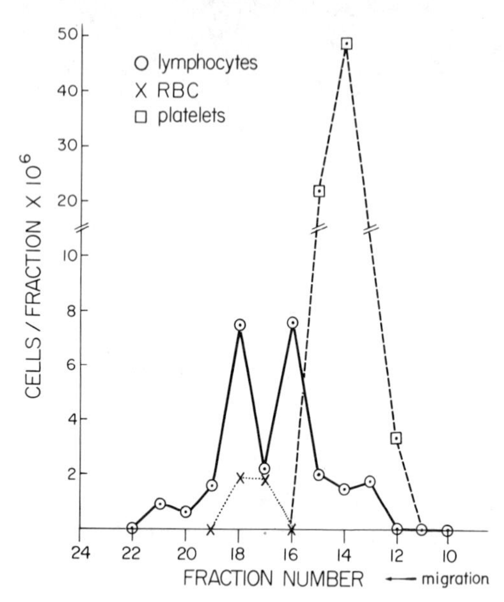

O lymphocytes
X RBC
□ platelets
CELLS / FRACTION X 10^6
50
40
30
20
10
8
6
4
2
24
22
20
18
16
14
12
10
FRACTION NUMBER
migration

B

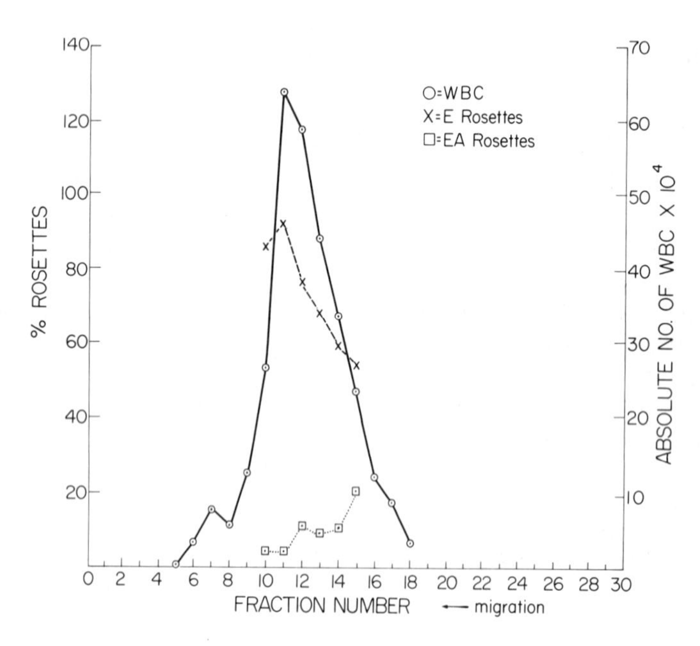

O=WBC
X=E Rosettes
□=EA Rosettes
% ROSETTES
ABSOLUTE NO. OF WBC X 10^4
140
120
100
80
60
40
20
70
60
50
40
30
20
10
0 2 4 6 8 10 12 14 16 18 20 22 24 26 28 30
FRACTION NUMBER
migration

C

of the lymphoid cells in the centrifugation and resuspension procedures which follow the electrophoretic separation and collection. While the recovery of cells after traversing the endless belt electrophoresis apparatus is between 85 and 100%, as determined with erythrocyte suspensions, the final recovery of lymphocytes after electrophoresis, centrifugation, and resuspension can vary between about 25 and 60%. The following reasons contribute to the low recovery. Cell aggregation can lead to large cell clumps which are eliminated from the electrophoretic process by rapid sedimentation. Cell aggregation may be due to release of DNA by damaged cells and may be reversed by treatment with deoxyribonuclease. This treatment may, however, lead in itself to some cell damage. Adhesion of cells to the centrifuge tubes represents another potential source of cell losses. Cell damage may also occur when cells are transferred from their original suspension medium to the electrophoretic buffer and from it to the media in which they are subjected to subsequent processing. Cell recovery problems of this kind are common to Hannig's free-flow electrophoresis apparatus and to endless belt electrophoresis. They have been extensively reviewed by Zeiller *et al.* (1975).

A representative test shown in Fig. 38C, performed in collaboration with Dr. Robert Seeger, clearly indicates substantial enrichment of E-rosette-forming cells and depletion of EA-rosette-forming cells in the collection pattern. While the E rosettes are a unique characterization for T lymphocytes, the formation of EA rosettes is not limited to B lymphocytes; it could also be due to binding of EA to monocytes, K cells (which are non-T, non-B, $F_c^{(+)}$ cells), or T cells with F_c receptors (Jondal *et al.*, 1972; Elhilali *et al.*, 1976).

Prior to electrophoretic separation, the blood sample contained 69% T cells and 20% EA-rosette-forming cells in the cell population. We recognize thus a substantial enrichment of T cells to 92% in fraction No. 10 whereas fraction No. 16 shows a depletion of T cells to 56%. In addition, EA-rosette-forming cells are depleted in fractions 10–14.

Much of the work with lymphocytes has been carried out with cells obtained from mesenteric lymph nodes of mice, as a rule in phosphate–sucrose buffer at neutral pH. Figure 39A shows a photograph of a separation pattern obtained with a suspension of mesenteric lymph node lymphocytes of a Swiss white mouse. Fig. 39B shows two plots of collection patterns. The dashed plot corresponds to a low injection rate of the cell

←

FIGURE 38. Separation of suspensions of human lymphocytes with contaminants. The lymphocytes were prepared by the Ficoll–Isopaque interface centrifugation method. (A) Photograph of separation pattern. (B) Collection patterns of lymphocytes and contaminants. (C) Distribution of E-rosette- and EA-rosette-forming cells in a lymphocyte collection pattern. The vertical scale on the right applies to the curve drawn through the circles. The percent scale on the left applies to the curves drawn through the crosses (×) and squares (□).

suspension and the solid plot corresponds to a high injection rate. Both graphs show two peaks corresponding to the two streaks appearing in the photograph. The resolution of the two cell components is, however, clearly higher at the slow injection rate (dashed plot). Similar photographs and plots have been obtained with murine lymphocytes prepared from spleens of SJL/J mice.

Electrophoretic analysis of cells and their characterization by their electrophoretic mobilities can be combined with biochemical or immunological alterations of the cell surface which may modify the electrophoretic mobility in characteristic fashion. Such alterations could be, for instance, produced by interactions of the cell surfaces with enzymes or antibodies. Figure 40 shows a comparison between the effects of treatment with neuraminidase and trypsin on the electrophoretic mobility of erythrocytes (Sturgeon *et al.*, 1972). After washing with saline, the suspensions containing the enzyme at suitable concentration were incubated at 37°C in several

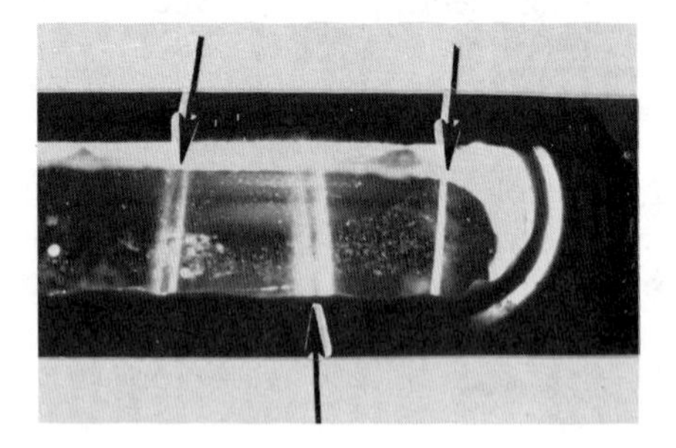

A

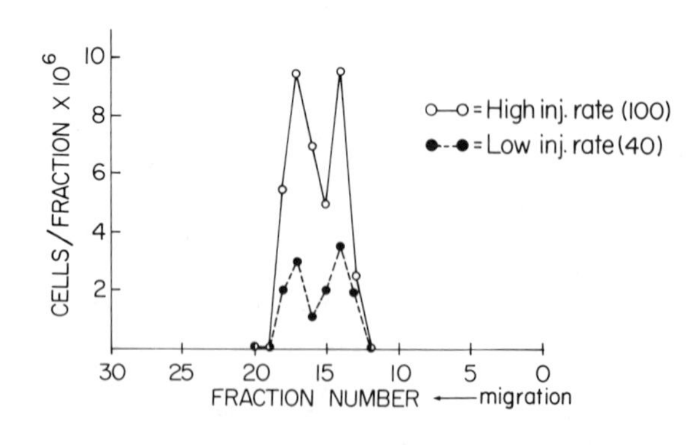

B

FIGURE 39. Separation of murine mesenteric lymph node cells. (A) Photograph of separation pattern. (B) Collection patterns. The solid graph of lower resolution represents a collection at high injection rate, whereas the dashed graph a better-resolved collection at a low injection rate.

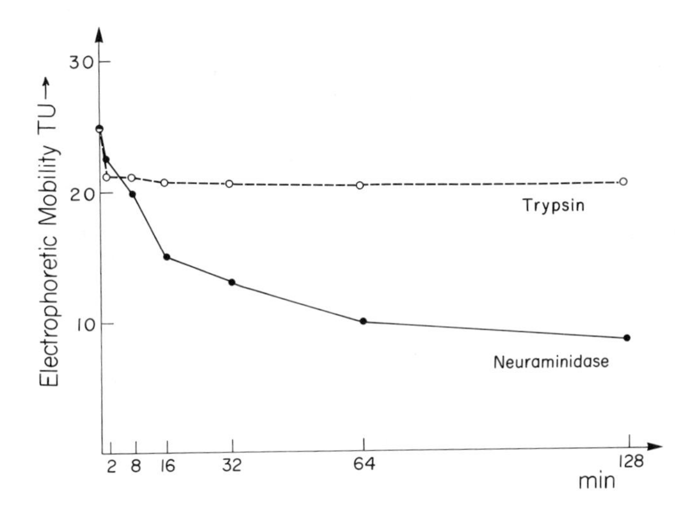

FIGURE 40. Effect of enzyme treatment on electrophoretic mobility of erythrocytes. The duration of treatment is indicated along the abscissa. The electrophoretic mobility in Tiselius units (TU) is indicated along the ordinate. Neuraminidase is more effective than trypsin in changing the mobility. (Redrawn from Sturgeon *et al.*, 1972.)

tubes at different periods of time for each tube (2, 8, 16, 32, 64, and 128 min). At the end of each selected time interval the reaction was stopped by addition of cold saline and immersion of the test tube in crushed ice for 10 min. The cells were then washed in saline and suspended in a 3% sucrose–tris buffer for electrophoretic analysis. While the effect of neuraminidase after a period of about two hours results in a drop of the electrophoretic mobility to about 40% of the initial value, the trypsin-treated cells retain a mobility of about 83% of the initial magnitude.

It is not inappropriate to mention electrophoresis of viruses in connection with cell electrophoresis since electrophoresis could be used to purify viruses by isolating them from fine subcellular fragments. Figure 41 shows two sharp streaks obtained with a mixture of two strains (U_1 and U_2) of tobacco mosaic virus photographed by ultraviolet light (Kolin and Luner, 1969). The faster component (U_1) is on the left and the slower on (U_2) on the right. The second (ascending) streak corresponds to electromigration in the endless belt of less than half a minute. This method is thus quite suitable for rapid purification and electrophoretic characterization of viruses.

XV. THEORETICAL CONSIDERATIONS

In the preceding descriptions, we disregarded the velocity distributions in the vertical and horizontal flow patterns encountered in the annular

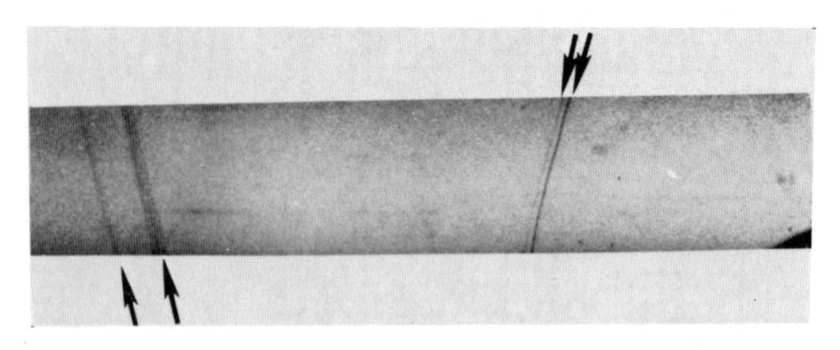

FIGURE 41. Separation of subcellular particles: two strains of a virus. The top arrows point at the first descending streaks of the U1 and U2 strains of tobacco mosaic virus which have been visually separated about five seconds after leaving the injector. The bottom arrows point at the first ascending streaks. U1 is the faster component. (From Kolin and Luner, 1969.)

buffer belt of the endless belt electrophoresis separator. We shall now consider the conditions which actually prevail.

A. Tangential Buffer Flow

Figure 42 illustrates in perspective the tangential flow of the buffer solution which circulates around the iron core C in the annulus of the endless belt separator. Only the front portion of the annulus is drawn. The curved arrow indicates the flow of the circulating buffer caused by electromagnetic forces. The width of the annulus is h. We center our attention on the vertical portion of the fluid sheet of thickness h in the front section of the buffer belt and choose the X axis in the midplane of this fluid sheet as shown in the figure. The Y axis of our coordinate system designates the plane of the lateral buffer flow (which is parallel to the direction of the electric current density vector **J**) and the Z axis coincides with the direction of the magnetic field vector **B**.

The fluid in the annulus is driven by the electromagnetic force density

$$\mathbf{f}_x = {}^1\!/_{10}\,(\mathbf{J} \times \mathbf{B}) \tag{3}$$

where **J** is in A/cm², **B** in gauss, and $\mathbf{f}_x$ in dynes/cm³. This force gives rise to viscous flow in which the velocity distribution $u = f(z)$ is such that the force per unit volume is

$$f_x = \eta(\partial^2 u/\partial_z^2) \tag{4}$$

where η is the fluid viscosity in poise (Lamb, 1945). After two integrations and consideration of the vanishing of the velocity u at the walls ($z = \pm h/2$),

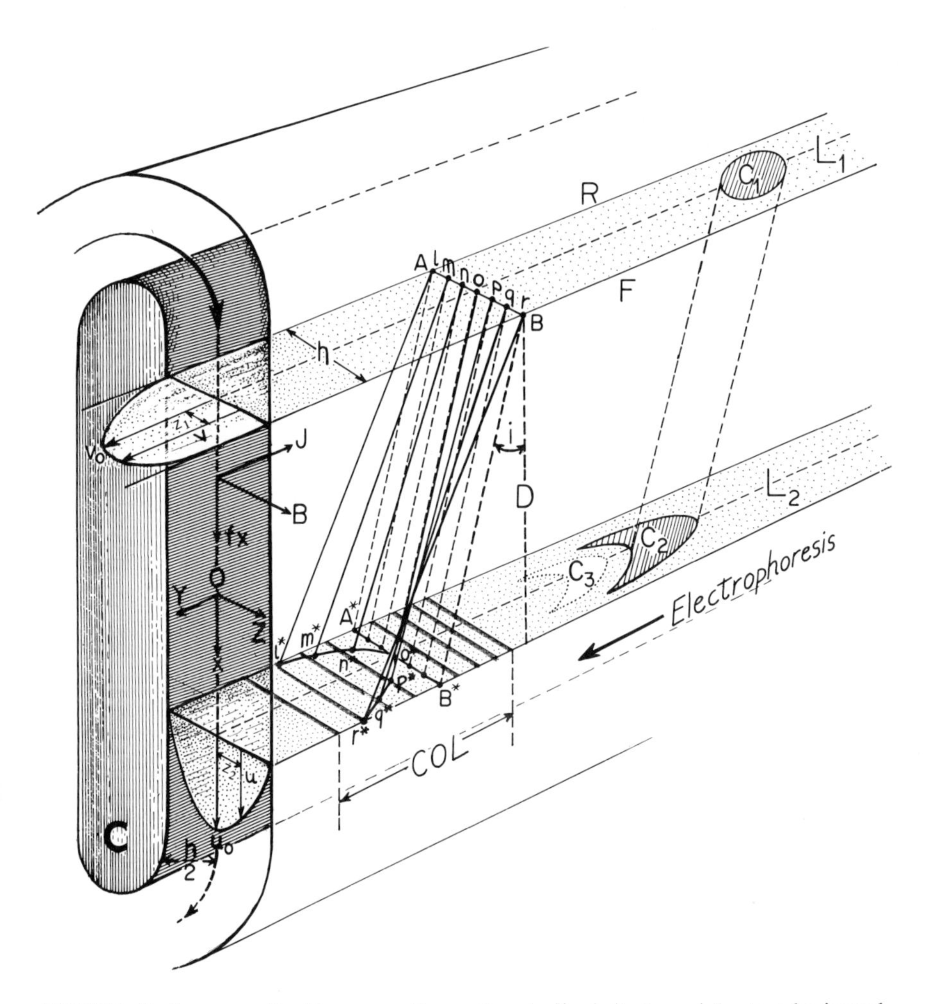

FIGURE 42. Iron core C with surrounding endless buffer belt: L_1 and L_2, two horizontal sections through the buffer belt; R, rear boundary of buffer belt; F, front boundary of buffer belt. [Parabola on the left in plane L_1 shows laminar velocity distribution of lateral flow (maximum velocity v_0). The parabola perpendicular to plane L_2 on the left (maximum velocity u_0) depicts the parabolic velocity profile of the tangential buffer flow in endless belt.]; h, thickness of fluid curtain (endless belt); **B**, magnetic field vector; **J**, current density vector; $\mathbf{f}_x$, electromagnetic force density vector; C_1, circular cross-section of streak entering the buffer at level L_1 from above; C_2, distorted shape of the streak cross-section by the time the particles in it reach level L_2; C_3, distorted cross-section of a streak of electrophoretically faster particles entering the buffer belt through C_1; BD, perpendicular to the planes of L_1 and L_2; D, distance between the planes L_1 and L_2; A–B, a narrow slit on level L_1 through which a band of particles enters the buffer belt; A*–B*, one of the slots of collector COL on level L_2. The other parallel collector slots are shown on either side of A*–B*. The particles entering slot A–B are shown to proceed in a band toward slot A*–B* in the collector through which they exit. Such a band can exist only under exceptional circumstances discussed in the text. Normally the band is distorted as shown by curve l* m* n* o* p* q* r* on level L_2.

we obtain the familiar expression for the velocity distribution (Dryden *et al.*, 1956):*

$$u = (f_x/2\eta)[z^2 - (h/2)^2] \tag{5}$$

Introducing in above expression the maximum fluid velocity u_0 at the center of the annulus ($z = 0$)

$$u_0 = -(f_x/2\eta)(h/2)^2 \tag{6}$$

we obtain

$$u = u_0[1 - 4(z/h)^2] \tag{7}$$

The mean flow velocity is (Dryden *et al.*, 1956):

$$\bar{u} = \tfrac{2}{3}\, u_0 \tag{8}$$

The parabolic tangential circulation velocity distribution which is magnetohydrodynamically engendered in the annulus is depicted in Fig. 42 near the bottom of the annulus. We can easily calculate the velocity of fluid flow in the annulus. From equations (3) and (6) we get

$$|u_0| = (h^2/80\eta)(\mathrm{J} \times \mathrm{B}). \tag{9}$$

Assuming typical values for experimental parameters we can estimate the value of u_0. For $h = 0.15$ cm, the viscosity at 16°C: $\eta = 1.11 \times 10^{-2}$ poise, $i = 200$ mA, J = 0.061 A/cm², B = 340 G, we obtain: $u_0 = 0.53$ cm/s (and $\bar{u} = \frac{2}{3}u_0 = 0.35$ cm/s). For an annulus L of 22 cm circumference, the circulation time for a well-centered streak will thus be

$$\tau_0 = L/u_0 = 41.5 \text{ s} \tag{10}$$

which is in good agreement with observations.

B. Lateral Buffer Flow

Unlike the free-flow curtain electrophoresis instrument (Hannig, 1972), the endless belt apparatus utilizes a horizontal lateral flow, in addition to the buffer circulation in the endless buffer belt. Both of these laminar flows have a parabolic velocity profile like the one shown in Fig. 42 for the circulation in the annulus. The parabolic distribution of the imposed lateral velocity v is depicted at the extreme left in the plane of the upper horizontal section L_1 through the annulus in Fig. 42. Both instruments,

*This equation is identical with the expression which I gave in my first paper (Kolin, 1960) except that the origin of the coordinate system is at the center of the annulus in equation (5), whereas it is placed at the boundary of the buffer belt in the above publication.

however, have in common an *unintentional* lateral fluid motion due to electroosmosis (Kolin, 1960). As a result of charge separation at the cell wall–electrolyte interface (ionic double layer), the charged electrolyte layer near the cell wall is set in motion toward the electrode of opposite polarity. In a closed system, this flow must be balanced by an opposite flow in the central region of the cell cross-section so that the net fluid transfer through the cell cross-section is zero. This phenomenon has been studied by Smoluchowski (1921) who showed that the electroosmotic streaming has a parabolic velocity profile with *nonzero velocity* at the cell walls.

Figure 43 shows an electroosmotic velocity profile between two parallel plates P_1 and P_2, which are perpendicular to the plane of the paper and are separated by a small distance h that is negligible as compared to the plate dimensions. The vector **J** indicates the direction of the electric current and the vectors $\mathbf{v}_0$ and $\mathbf{v}_W$ the directions of the electroosmotic streaming in the central plane and at the plate surfaces, respectively. We see that the streaming velocity is zero in two parallel zones Z_1 and Z_2 (Smoluchowski zones) which are located at the distance 0.21 h from the plate surfaces. The streaming velocity distribution is parabolic and the streaming direction is opposite on the left and right sides of O axis. This axis passes through the intersection of the velocity profile curve with the Smoluchowski zones of

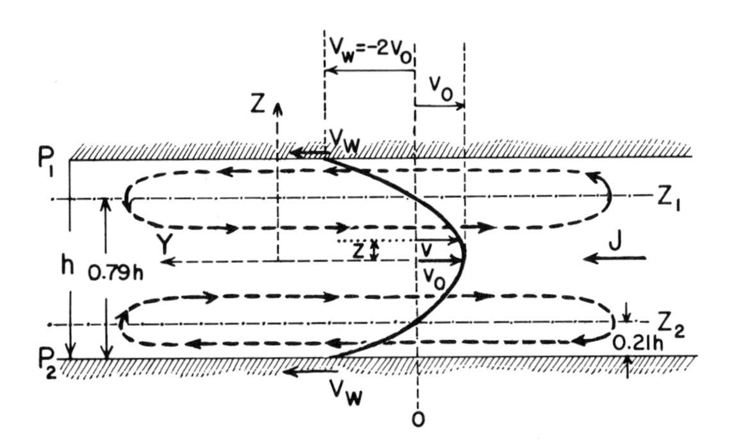

FIGURE 43. Electroosmotic convection: P_1, P_2, two parallel plates of infinite extent as compared to their separation distance h; **J**, electrical current density vector; z_1, z_2, Smoluchowski zones of zero velocity (The closed dashed lines depict qualitatively electroosmotic convection. The parabola shows the electroosmotic velocity distribution.); v_0, central velocity between the plates; v_w: velocity at the walls ($v_w = -2v_0$).

zero velocity; i.e., the streaming at the center between the plates is opposite to the streaming at the two plate walls P_1 and P_2.

To obtain the velocity distribution for the electroosmotic flow, we begin with a differential equation similar to equation (4) (Brinton and Lauffer, 1959):

$$f_y = \eta \, \partial^2 v / \partial z^2 \tag{11}$$

where f_y is the horizontal force density component responsible for the electroosmotic flow. Integration of equation (11) yields

$$v = (f_y/2\eta)(z + h/2)^2 + A(z + h/2) + B \tag{12}$$

The integration constants A and B are evaluated from the condition that the velocity becomes v_w at the walls ($z = \pm h/2$). We obtain thus

$$v = (f_y/2\eta)[z^2 - (h/2)^2] + v_w \tag{13}$$

which is the velocity distribution shown in Fig. 43 (Kolin, 1960). It is similar to the vertical and horizontal parabolic velocity profiles shown in Fig. 42 for the endless belt flow, except for the velocity value v_w at the walls, which is zero in Fig. 42 and

$$v_w = -2v_o \tag{13a}$$

in Fig. 43 (Brinton and Lauffer, 1959).

In addition to the electroosmotic flow, there will be, in general, a lateral laminar flow through the annulus due to a difference in buffer levels in the right and left buffer compartments maintained by unequal rates of inflow and drainage of buffer from the lateral buffer chambers. The equation representing this flow is analogous to equation (5):

$$v' = [(dp/dy)/(2\eta)][z^2 - (h/2)^2] \tag{14}$$

where $(dp/dy) = f_y$ is the horizontal force per unit volume which maintains this flow (dp/dy being the lateral pressure gradient). In analogy to equation (7):

$$v' = v'_0[1 - 4(z/h)^2] \tag{15}$$

where v'_0 is the maximum horizontal central velocity of the flow maintained by the pressure gradient and

$$v'_0 = -[f_x/(2\eta)](h/2)^2 \tag{15a}$$

C. Idealized Particle Motion in the Endless Belt

Figure 42 illustrates what the motion of negatively charged particles would be in the endless belt in the absence of lateral streaming and electroosmosis under the unrealistic assumption that the tangential circulation velocity u, instead of being parabolic (as shown at the lower left of the annulus) is uniform. The injector in this example is not a capillary, but rather a slit A–B through which negatively charged particles are continuously injected into the revolving buffer belt across its entire width. The electrophoretic velocity of the particles is actually uniform throughout the annulus as the particles electromigrate toward the anode on the left. The superposition of the two uniform, mutually perpendicular migrations moves the particles along a sloping path as a wide band joining the lines A–B and A*–B*. The collector COL is symbolized by parallel slots on the lower level L_2. The band of particles enters a particular collector slot A*–B* from which it is guided further by a channel not shown in the figure. Components of different mobilities in the particle band would be deviated to different degrees and would enter other slots in the collector. Such a perfect collection for all components over a great width within the annulus never occurs in practice in the endless belt electrophoretic separator nor in the liquid curtain free-flow electrophoresis apparatus for reasons discussed below.

D. Impairment of Preparative Resolving Power by Mismatching of Horizontal and Vertical Velocity Profiles

The angle i of inclination of the deviated particle streak against the vertical (line BD) is measured by the ratio of the horizontal particle velocity v to the vertical velocity u of the buffer belt, as illustrated in Fig. 42:

$$\tan i = v/u \tag{16}$$

It has been pointed out (Kolin, 1967b) that the angle i can be the same over the entire width h of the annulus independently of the value of the particle coordinate z, not solely for the case of the ideal uniform velocity distributions assumed in the preceding section C and illustrated by the dashed lines joining the points l, m, n, o, p, q, r between A and B in section L_1 (Fig. 42) to the corresponding points between A* and B* in section L_2. This uniformity of streak deviation will in fact occur for any arbitrary velocity distribution $v = f(z)$, provided the velocity distribution function is the same for the horizontal $[v = f(z)]$ as well as the vertical flow $[u = F(z)]$, where $f(z)/F(z) = \text{const}$. Thus, for instance, if we inject particles (in the absence of an electric field) into a vertical parabolic flow described by equation (5) and superimpose a lateral flow with a parabolic velocity profile given by equation (14), we will obtain an inclination for the particle path which will be independent of the value of z, i.e., will be the same at the center of the annulus as at its walls:

$$\tan i = \frac{v'}{u} = \frac{[(dp/dy)/(2\eta)][z^2 - (h/2)^2]}{[f_x/(2\eta)][z^2 - (h/2)^2]} = \frac{dp/dy}{f_x} = \text{const.} \tag{17}$$

Under these conditions a band of particles entering the superposition of the two parabolic flows through the slit A–B located in section L_1 (Fig. 42) will proceed without distortion to its exit through the slit A*–B* in section L_2.

This situation is, however, drastically changed if the vertical and horizontal velocity profiles are mismatched. Let us consider again the simplest case of a vertical parabolic velocity profile (from which we cannot escape) combined with a perfectly uniform horizontal velocity profile. The latter is obtainable, in principle, in the absence of imposed lateral streaming and of electroosmosis (which can be arranged by a suitable matching of buffer solution with the materials covering the walls of the annulus). The horizontal particle velocity is thus due only to electrophoresis and is independent of the particle position (z) between the annulus walls. The lateral displacement of an ion which passes through the slit A–B into the electrophoretic curtain, is then equal to its electrophoretic velocity ($E \times \mu$) times travel time τ (where μ is the electrophoretic mobility and E the electric field intensity in the annulus). The travel time is given by

$$\tau = D/u \tag{18}$$

where D is the distance between the levels L_1 and L_2 in Fig. 42 (injector and collector levels) and u is the vertical curtain velocity for the coordinate z value corresponding to the particle position between the annulus walls.

Since the curtain velocity u is given by equation (7) and is represented by the vertical parabolic velocity profile shown near the bottom of the annulus in Fig. 42, we see that the particles entering the injector slit A–B centrally (i.e., at point o where $z = 0$) will have the highest downward speed u_0 and, hence, will reside in the electric field, which displaces them toward the left, a shorter time than particles entering at points l, m, n, p, q, r ($z \neq 0$). Particles entering at n and p will travel longer than the central particle from level L_1 to level L_2 and will thus be exposed for a longer time to the horizontal electric field and will therefore reach the collector plane L_2 displaced to the left of the point o* where the particles originating from point o arrive with a minimum lateral displacement. Particles which travel closer to the wall (originating at l, m, q, r for instance) will require an even longer time (depending on their wall distance) to reach the level L_2 and will thus be displaced even further to the left, namely to points l*, m*, q*, r*. By joining the corresponding points (l–l*, m–m*, n–n*, o–o*, p–p*, q–q*, r–r*), we see that the angles of deviation of the particle paths increase with the particle distance from the central plane of the annulus. As a result, the "image" in the plane of section L_2 of the slot A–B formed by the charged particles which passed through it is no longer the straight line A*–B*, but rather, the curved line l*, m*, n*, o*, p*, q*, r*. The centrally located particles will be the only ones to enter the collector slot A*–B*. Particles located off-center will enter other collector slots, so that an initially sharp band will end up in many collector tubes. This is an obvious degradation of collection resolving power, since particles entering collector slot s at points l* and q*, for instance, would find themselves in the company of particles of a different (faster) electrophoretic mobility which enter the same slot at its center. To avoid infinite horizontal displacements of particles to the left, we must imagine that the end points of the slits A–B and A*–B* are some distance removed from the annulus walls, where the vertical downward velocity $u_w = 0$.

Actually, the injectors commonly used are not slots but tubes of circular cross-section. The initial particle distribution will thus be a circle C_1 as particles enter at level L_1. We can imagine lines drawn within this circle parallel to line A–B in Fig. 42. The configuration of particles lying on such lines will be distorted as just described for particles entering along the line A–B. The result is a "crescent" deformation C_2 of the circular cross-section C_1. Actually, the term "crescent," used for lack of a better term, is a misnomer (Luner, 1969; Strickler and Sacks, 1973) since the shaded area C_2 is not formed by intersection of eccentric circles. In my earlier papers, I referred to this distortion as "parabolic divergence" because of the divergence between the directions of the central edge of the streak and its lateral edges caused by superposition of the vertical parabolic velocity profile with a horizontal uniform velocity distribution. The "crescent" distortion is easy to observe in the endless belt apparatus by looking at the streaks end-on toward the origin of the light beam L as illustrated in Fig. 7. Figure 9 shows a photograph of the streak cross-section thus obtained (Luner, 1969; Kolin and Luner, 1971). Such photographs can also be taken with a free-flow curtain apparatus (Strickler and Sacks, 1973).

Such degradation of resolution can be avoided by making the circular injector aperture very small (about 0.2 mm or less) (Kolin, 1960). For mobility measurements, a thin streak is not required, as the "parabolic divergence" is no problem, since the edge of the streak located in the central plane is sharp and gives the streak deviation undistorted by the "crescent" deformation. However, for preparative work, a thin streak is undesirable despite the higher resolution which it offers because of reduced throughput of particles. Thus, in practice, one must make a compromise between high resolution and high throughput in preparative work.

E. Superposition of Electroosmotic Streaming

Contrary to a possible intuitive anticipation of further deterioration of resolution by superposition of the complex electroosmotic streaming pattern upon the combination of velocity profiles considered above, one actually can make use of electroosmosis to eliminate the "crescent" distortion ("parabolic divergence"), as has been shown in the first paper describing this method (Kolin, 1960).

In the absence of imposed lateral streaming, the horizontal velocity of particles, such as negatively charged cells, will be due to superposition of their electrophoretic velocity $v_e = -\mu E$ and the electroosmotic velocity given by equation (13), in which we will set $v_w = E \times W$ (where W is the "electroosmotic mobility," i.e., $W = v_w/E$). We obtain thus for the resultant velocity of the cells (Kolin, 1960):

$$v^* = [f_y/(2\eta)][z^2 - (h/2)^2] + E(W - \mu) \tag{19}$$

The slope of the streak will thus be, according to equations (5) and (19):

$$\tan i = \frac{v^*}{u} = \frac{f_y[z^2 - (h/2)^2]}{f_x[z^2 - (h/2)^2]} + \frac{E(W - \mu)}{z^2 - (h/2)^2} \tag{20}$$

$$\tan i = \frac{f_y}{f_x} + \frac{E(W - \mu)}{z^2 - (h/2)^2} \tag{20a}$$

This is in essence equation (14a) of the original publication (Kolin, 1960) which stated that the helical pitch of the injected ions (and thus the slope of the injected particle streak) will in general depend on z, the wall distance of the ion streak, because of the z-dependence of the second term of equation (20a). The paper pointed out, however, that there is one condition under which the pitch of the helix (and, hence the slope of the streak) becomes independent of z [condition for vanishing "parabolic divergence" (Kolin, 1967b)]. That happens when the second term of equation (20a) vanishes; i.e., when $W = \mu$. In this case, the electrophoretic particle velocity ($E\mu$) becomes equal and opposite to the electroosmotic velocity (EW) near the walls of the annulus or the liquid curtain apparatus.*

The consequences of equation (19) can be understood and visualized as follows. We have seen [equation (17)] that the combination of a parabolic vertical curtain flow along the X axis (velocity profile $u = f(z)$ shown near the bottom of the annulus in Fig. 42) with a horizontal parabolic velocity distribution (velocity profile $v = f(z)$ shown at the left end of section L_1 in Fig. 42) produces a slope of particle paths which is independent of their wall distance z. In other words, the cross-section of the injected streak (or band) remains undistorted! Figure 44 shows how such a horizontal parabolic velocity profile matching the vertical parabolic veloc-

*Despite the clarity of the statement in Kolin's publication (1960), one reads in a more recent paper (Strickler and Sacks, 1973), referring to a sequel to the above article (Kolin, 1967b) the following curious statement in which the authors appear to take credit for this insight: "Though prior studies accorded a role in band broadening to velocity profiles, an important relationship was not recognized, that is, that for any band, broadening due to these profiles disappears at a particular value of cell wall zeta potential (ZP) such that the electroosmotic velocity adjacent to the cell walls is equal and opposite to the electrophoretic band velocity."

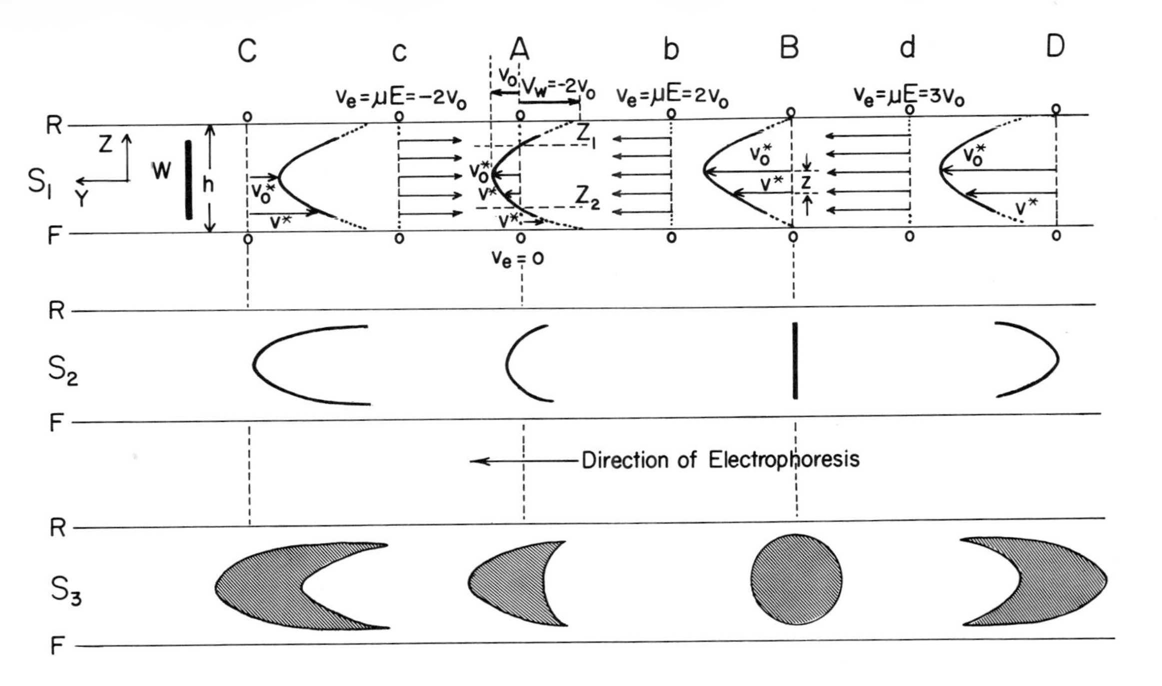

FIGURE 44. Analysis of the distortion of the streak profile: S_1, S_2, S_3, perpendicular sections through the fluid curtain; R, rear boundary of the fluid curtain; F, its front boundary (The fluid curtain is perpendicular to the page and the flow is away from the reader.); W, slit through which particles enter the fluid curtain; *h*, curtain width; o–o: reference axis of velocity distribution; Z_1, Z_2, Smoluchowski zones of zero velocity. (A) Electroosmotic velocity profile. (The dotted line in all velocity distributions is an extrapolation beyond the width of entry slot W.) (B) Velocity distribution of (A) with a superimposed uniform velocity $2v_0$ to the left. (C) Superposition of a uniform velocity $v = -2v_0$ upon the velocity profile of (A). (D) Superposition of a uniform velocity $v = 3v_0$ upon the velocity profile of (A). *Curves shown in section* S_2 under corresponding velocity profiles: shapes into which the originally straight particle band is distorted in the presence of the horizontal velocity distribution shown above it. *Areas shown in section* S_3: shapes ("crescents") into which an originally circular streak cross-section is distorted in transit through the fluid curtain in the presence of a horizontal velocity profile shown above it. In all cases the vertical velocity profile in the buffer belt (or curtain) is assumed to be parabolic with vanishing velocity at the walls.

ity distribution can be obtained. Imagine S_1 to be a horizontal section through the vertical fluid curtain in our annulus of width h, such that lines F and R represent the rear and the front wall of the buffer curtain, respectively. The particles are introduced through a slot of width $W < h$. W indicates the relative width and thickness of the slot but not its location, which is to be imagined to be along the o–o axes of the diagrams A, B, C, D and b, c, d in section S_1. The electromagnetically engendered flow of buffer through the section S_1 is perpendicular to the page away from the reader and particle electrophoresis proceeds from right to left.

Imagine now that we introduce a row of particles of electrophoretic mobility zero along the line o–o in diagram A of section S_1 in Fig. 44. If we turn on the current for one second the particles will be displaced from their original linear array by electroosmotic streaming everywhere except at the intersections of the o–o axis with the lines Z_1, Z_2 which mark the Smoluchowski zones of zero electroosmotic movement. The particle displacement in one second will be equal to the electroosmotic velocity and the deformed row of particles will represent the electroosmotic velocity distribution. As shown in the diagram, the displacement will be to the left between the zones Z_1, Z_2 and to the right beyond them. This electroosmotic velocity distribution, although parabolic, does not match the transverse parabolic curtain flow profile because the electroosmotic velocity near the wall is $v_w = -2v_o \neq 0$. We can, however, achieve a matching velocity distribution for horizontal particle motion by replacing our particles of zero electrophoretic mobility by particles of mobility μ for which the electrophoretic velocity v_e becomes $v_e = 2v_o$. Superimposing this *uniform* velocity, shown in diagram b, section S_1, upon the electroosmotic velocity profile of diagram A which the particles share with the streaming fluid, we obtain the distribution of the resultant particle velocity shown in diagram B. A row of cells of the chosen mobility distributed initially along the o–o axis of diagram B will be distorted after one second by combined motions of electrophoresis and electroosmosis so as to form a parabola intersecting the walls F and R at the o–o axis of zero displacement. This horizontal parabolic velocity distribution with a vanishing velocity at the walls of the curtain matches the vertical curtain velocity, thus yielding a particle streak of undistorted cross-section as in Fig. 42 for the particles emanating from slit A–B on level L_1 and terminating along the line A*–B* on level L_2. This freedom from distortion is also illustrated by the straight line under diagram B in section S_2 of Fig. 44. S_2 is to be imagined as a horizontal section through the vertical buffer curtain some distance below the section S_1. Due to horizontal streaming, the particles will be deviated laterally from the positions which they occupy in section S_1. The lateral deviation from the o–o axis has, however, been disregarded in Fig. 44 for purposes of space conservation and clarity of correlation. The shapes of the originally linear particle bands altered by electrophoresis, electroosmosis, and parabolic streaming while the particles move from level S_1 to level S_2 are shown in section S_2. They appear below the diagrams A, B, C, and D which depict the particle velocity distributions produced in the electric field by electrophoresis and electroosmosis. We see in section S_2 below diagram A that the linear particle band of zero mobility is distorted by electroosmosis with a concavity matching that of the electroosmotic velocity profile.

We will now choose particles of an electrophoretic mobility equal and opposite to that of particles used in diagram b. Their electrophoretic velocity distribution ($v_e = -2v_o$) is shown in diagram c. The superposition of this uniform velocity upon the electroosmotic velocity profile of diagram A results in the velocity distribution shown in diagram C. The corresponding distortion of the streak is shown below the diagram in section S_2. Its concavity matches that for the zero-mobility particles of diagram A.

Finally, we choose particles of higher electrophoretic mobility than was necessary in diagrams b and B to achieve an undistorted linear streak. In diagram d the mobility is such that $v_e = 3v_o$ and diagram D shows the corresponding velocity profile for superposition of electrophoresis upon the electroosmotic displacement. The streak is distorted as shown under the diagram D in section S_2, but now the concavity of the curve is opposite to the previous cases.

Section S_2 shows qualitatively the distortions electrokinetically imposed upon streaks which have originally the shape of linear bands and relative cross-sectional dimensions indicated by W in section S_1. Section S_3 shows in a very rough *qualitative* manner the distortions corresponding to the reviewed cases, for a streak of originally circular cross-sections are "crescents" similar to that photographed in Fig. 9, concave to the right or to the left, depending on the ratio of the electrophoretic particle velocity to the electroosmotic velocity near the annulus wall.

In addition to the above-mentioned horizontal motions, a laminar lateral flow can be superimposed in endless belt electrophoresis. Since the velocity distribution of this flow is parabolic with zero velocity at the walls, its combination with the vertical tangential buffer flow of matching velocity profile does not introduce further streak distortion.

XVI. RESOLVING POWER

A. Flow Fluctuations

The final aspect of the endless belt apparatus to be considered is its resolving power. Some of these considerations will be equally applicable to liquid curtain free-flow electrophoresis. All previous discussions presupposed ideal constancy of the buffer inflow from the Mariotte bottle and outflow through the collector. Neither assumption is realistic, because of surface tension forces. As atmospheric air enters the Mariotte bottle MB of Fig. 22 via tube MT, which may have a lumen about ⅓ cm in diameter, a backpressure due to surface tension is opposing the entry of air which eventually rises as a bubble to the top of the buffer solution. This backpressure is given for a spherical bubble (with one surface) of radius r by the following expression

$$p = 2\alpha/r \qquad \text{dynes/cm}^2 \tag{21}$$

where α is the surface tension in dynes/cm and r the radius of curvature of the liquid surface in centimeters. As we see, this backpressure varies from 0 when the liquid surface at the bottom of tube MT is flat to a maximum at about $r \simeq 1$cm when the air bubble is ready to detach itself. The magnitude of $p_{\max}$ is of the order of 500 dynes/cm², which is about 2% of the pressure head driving the buffer from the Mariotte bottle into the electrophoresis cell (which may range from 10 to 20 cm of water). The fluctuation of the buffer delivery rate may cause a slight lateral fluctuation of the streak separation pattern as it enters the collector. Thus, even though an instantaneous photographic exposure may yield a sharp well resolved streak pattern, the slow fluctuation of the pattern at the collector entry may cause overlap of the components in the collector. The resolution of collection patterns presented with the photographs of separation patterns (cf. Figs. 36, 37, and 39) indeed shows that the resolution in collections is, as a rule, inferior to the resolution in the visible separation pattern.

The effect of this source of fluctuation could be minimized by separating the delivery of the centrifugal buffer flow past the electrodes (which consumes by far the major fluid volume) from the supply of buffer for the lateral flow (which requires about 10% of the centrifugal buffer flow rate). The centrifugal buffer inflow, being perfectly symmetrical, is less likely to have a noticeable effect on the slopes of the streaks and could be supplied by the Mariotte bottle in its present low-level mounting. A separate small Mariotte bottle could be mounted as close to the ceiling as possible to deliver buffer for lateral flow through a thin high-resistance tube. The pressure fluctuation due to the variable backpressure of the bubbles would have a much smaller effect on the lateral buffer flow in view of the much higher pressure head.

A much greater surface tension effect on the collection pattern is to be expected from the droplets which detach themselves from the ends of the collector tubes and carry the separated components into test tubes. These drops may be as small as 1 mm in diameter, giving rise to an appreciable fluctuation in backpressure resisting buffer outflow. Since the pressure head accounting for the collector outflow may be as low as 10 cm of water or less and the maximum backpressure due to surface tension may be as high as 1200 dynes/cm^2, it may cause more than a 10% fluctuation in the pressure difference across a collector outflow tube. This may actually be the major cause of the present inferiority of the collection pattern as compared to the visual separation pattern. The elimination of this drawback, which is not peculiar to endless belt electrophoresis, requires redesign of the collection system so as to avoid an air–water interface at the exits of the collector tubes.

B. Distortion of Streak Profile

The resolution in analytical observations of the visual separation pattern may be impaired by the "parabolic divergence" ("crescent" distortion) as follows. Let us consider in Fig. 42 the circle C_1 as the entrance point at level L_1 of a circular streak of particles which are undergoing electrophoresis in the concomitant streaming field. The streak profile will be distorted to the shape of "crescent" C_2 when the particles reach level L_2. Let us further assume that there is a second (electrophoretically faster) particle component entering the curtain at level L_1 through entry port C_1 in the same streak. The faster particles will form at level L_2 the "crescent" C_3 somewhat to the left of C_2. If the right *(central)* edge of C_3 is close to the left (also *central*) edge of "crescent" C_2, the trailing edge of C_3 may be hidden from view by the slower streak terminating in crescent C_2. The right, trailing edge of the faster streak which terminates in crescent C_3 is harbored in the horseshoe-shaped "niche" of the hollow slower streak so that when viewed from the side, (i.e., along the Z axis) the two streaks will appear to fuse in projection into a single broad streak.

For further clarification, it is helpful to consider a linear band entering through the slit A–B on level L_1 of Fig. 42. We draw the central line o–o* representing the right *central* edge of the band-shaped streak. Similarly we join two points of the slit A–B which are located off center (r and l) to the points where the particles originating at r and l cross the level L_2 in proximity to the rear wall R and front wall F of the buffer curtain. These points, r* and l*, are located on the curve into which the originally straight band A–B is distorted at level L_2. When projected upon the rear wall, the lines o–o* and r–r* will enclose an angle α.* Thus the streak, will appear in projection to be enclosed between two diverging lines and will thus appear to broaden in proportion to the distance from the injection point.

The points l, r, l, r* are to be imagined fairly close to the annulus walls R and F but not in their planes as roughly drawn in Fig. 42.

A faster electrophoretic particle component emanating from the same slit A–B will terminate in points l′, m′, n′, o′, p′, q′, r′ of a curve in plane L_2 similar to curve l* m* n* o* p* q* r*, but displaced somewhat to the left of it in the same plane, and its *(central)* right edge will enclose an angle α_2 with the projection of the line joining point r of line A–B to point r′. This will be a second diverging streak located to the left of the first slower streak. For the two streaks to appear as separate in projection, the *trailing edge* of o–o′ of the faster streak must be slightly to the left of the *leading edge* r–r* of the streak of the slower component.

C. Definition of Resolving Power

Adopting this as a criterion of resolution (Kolin, 1967b) and defining the resolving power R as the ratio of the mean mobility $\bar{\mu}$ of the two components to be resolved and $\Delta\mu$ as the difference between their electrophoretic mobilities:

$$R = \bar{\mu}/\Delta\mu \tag{22}$$

It has been shown (Kolin, 1967b) that the resolution of the endless belt apparatus (or of a free-flow electrophoretic curtain apparatus) is determined by the ratio of the diameter d of the circular injector and h, the width of the annulus (or fluid curtain), as follows:

$$R = \bar{\mu}/\Delta\mu = (h/d)^2 \tag{23}$$

Very high resolution can thus be obtained by suitably diminishing the diameter of the injected streak. It is also clear that the resolving power deteriorates rapidly as one increases the streak diameter in order to achieve a high throughput of cells in preparative work. In practice, one must make a compromise between requirements of high resolution and high throughput.

A numerical example of achievable resolution may be helpful. Suppose we want to resolve two components differing by 1% in their mobilities: $\Delta\mu = 10^{-2}\ \bar{\mu}$ How narrow an injector capillary must we choose in an instrument with a 1.5-mm annulus? From equation (23) we obtain $d = 0.15$ mm. It is quite easy to use narrower capillaries (if necessary, with microscopic streak observation) and thus achieve much higher resolution.

D. Resolution in Collection

The problem of resolution in collection is somewhat different. As a glance on level L_2 of Fig. 42 shows, the problem lies in the mismatching between the normally linear slots of the collector COL which are to receive the separated fractions and the distorted shape of the streak (or band) (for instance, curve l* m* n* o* p* q* r*) when it arrives at level L_2, depositing the contents of a homogeneous streak population in several adjacent collector slots instead of in one. In principle, one could curve the collector slots to coincide with the cross-section of the streaks at level L_2 so that only one collector slot would receive the contents of the curved streak. But this is impractical! It is much more reasonable to attempt to rectify the shape of the streak to match the straight collector slots.

E. Band Rectification by Matching Electrophoretic and Electroosmotic Velocities

A paper entitled ''Focusing in Continuous Flow Electrophoresis Systems'' (Stickler and Sacks, 1973) actually aimed at streak (or band) rectification rather than focusing. Focusing implies an increase in particle concentration (e.g., increase in photon concentration at the focus of a lens or of ions in a condensation zone in isoelectric focusing). The basic idea for such rectification is contained in equation (17) (Kolin, 1967b) and equation (20a) (Kolin, 1960) and it was pointed out in the first paper on endless belt electrophoresis that the helical pitch (and hence the shape of the streak) becomes independent of z for particles whose electrophoretic velocity is equal and opposite to the electroosmotic velocity at the cell wall; i.e., the boundaries of a streak of such particles will not diverge, regardless of diameter d of the streak as compared to the width of the annulus h (Kolin, 1960). Stickler and Sachs (1973) had an interesting idea for modifying the zeta potential of the walls of a free-flow curtain apparatus so that a rectification of the shape of the slot in the L_2 plane (cf. Fig. 42) could be obtained for *one* particle species in the electrophoretic spectrum. This component could be collected efficiently but the streaks of the remaining components still remained afflicted by the ''crescent'' distortion. The above rectification idea is based on transforming a parabolic velocity distribution with finite velocity at the curtain wall into one with vanishing velocity at the wall (Kolin, 1960). This approach is different from the rectification idea described below.

The final question we shall ask is, whether it might be possible, in principle, to achieve rectification of the band for *all* electrophoretic components *at the same time,* which would be the ideal solution of the problem of preparative collection of wide bands filling out nearly the entire annulus width without distortion of their profile.

F. On the Possibility of Universal Band Rectification

As we have shown in equation (17), rectification of the band (avoidance of streak profile distortion) is possible if the velocity distribution of the migrating particles is represented by the same function in the vertical and horizontal directions. In the previous discussion we achieved rectification for one particular particle component whose electrophoretic velocity was equal and opposite to the electroosmotic wall velocity. The rectification came about by addition of the uniform electrophoretic particle velocity at all z values to the electroosmotic streaming velocity. This shifted the resultant particle velocity to zero at the wall and yielded a parabolic particle profile which matched the parabolic profile of the vertical curtain flow.

Such rectification is obviously possible for only one of the many components of an electrophoretic separation spectrum covering a wide mobility range. The only way one could, in principle, achieve a mobility-independent separation would be by rectification of the vertical and horizontal velocity profiles; i.e., one would have to distort the parabolic profiles of the vertical curtain flow on one hand as well as the horizontal laminar flow with the superimposed electroosmotic velocity distribution on the other hand in such a way that both flows would proceed with constant velocity independent of coordinate z (i.e., neither flow should vanish at the curtain walls). Superposition of the uniform electrophoretic velocity upon the established uniform horizontal flow would then result in a horizontal velocity distribution matching the uniform vertical velocity profile *and this would hold for particles of any arbitrary electrophoretic mobility!*

Inspection of Fig. 44 shows how such a rectification of a parabolic velocity profile could be accomplished. Diagrams A, B, and c of section S_1 show that the electroosmotic velocity profile of A may be conceived as a superposition of the uniform velocity distribution of c ($v = -2v_0$) upon the parabolic velocity distribution of B. Instead of adding a uniform velocity distribution to the parabolic one shown in A, we could have added the parabolic profile shown in diagram B, but with a negative sign. This superposition of a parabolic profile of a flow to the right upon the electroosmotic profile of A would cancel the parabolic component of this velocity distribution, leaving only the uniform motion to the right of velocity—$2v_0$. The superposition of the uniform electrophoretic motion upon this uniform flow will not perturb the rectification of the *horizontal* motion which we have thus achieved. All that remains to be done is rectification of the *vertical* motion. The method for doing it is described in a recent publication (Kolin, 1979).

ACKNOWLEDGMENTS

The development of endless belt electrophoresis was supported originally by the Office of Naval Research and subsequently by Medical Testing Systems, Inc. (MTS) and the American Cancer Society. I am particularly indebted to MTS for an indefinite loan of an endless belt apparatus (illustrated in Figs. 18 and 24) constructed at UCLA under their support and placed at our disposal with accessories.

In the conduct of cell separations, the advice and cooperation of several colleagues proved most helpful. I am particularly indebted to Dr. C. W. Boone, Head of the Cell Biology Laboratory of the National Cancer Institute for his highly stimulating advice, loan of a cytocentrifuge, supply of special breeds of normal and tumor-bearing mice, and most effective cooperation. The cooperation of Dr. Robert Seeger of the UCLA Department of Pediatrics and his staff, notably Mr. Joseph Rosenblatt, proved most helpful in work on separation of human B and T lymphocytes (cf. Fig. 38C). Similar cooperation of Dr. Benjamin Bonavida of the UCLA Department of Medical Microbiology and Immunology in efforts to separate murine B and T lymphocytes is equally appreciated. The assistants who performed in my laboratory cell separations such as those illustrated in Fig. 32, 38, and 39 included J. Murai and S. Peak. Nancy Muleady performed helpful preparatory work. I am grateful to Miss Alice Wing of the Clinical Laboratories of UCLA for excellent work in analyzing slides of cell fractions processed by the cytocentrifuge. I am also indebted to Mrs. Hermine Kavanau for excellent cooperation in preparing the drawings for this chapter, to Mrs. Nancy Ellerbroek for proofreading this manuscript and helpful comments, and to Mrs. Jane B. Walker for typing the manuscript.

Thanks are expressed to the following copyright owners for permission to reproduce illustrations from their journals: Elsevier Publishing Company, Academic Press, Akademiai Kiado, National Academy of Sciences (USA), California State College of Long Beach, UCLA. I am indebted to Mr. R. M. Owen for permission to reproduce from his thesis photographs and cytograms shown in Figs. 33 and 34.

REFERENCES

Barrolier, J., Watzke, E., and Gibian, H., 1958, Einfache Apparatur für die trägerfreie präparative Durchlauf-Elektrophorese, *Z. Naturforsch.* **136**:754.

Bergrahm, B., 1967, Apparatus for zone electrophoresis in vertical column, *Sci. Tools* **14**:34.

Brinton, C. C., 1967, Contributions of pili to the specificity of the bacterial surface, and a unitary hypothesis of conjugal infectious heredity, in *Specificity of Cell Surfaces* (B. D. David and L. Warren, eds.), pp. 37–70, Prentice-Hall, New Jersey.

Brinton, C. C., and Lauffer, M. A., 1959, Electrophoresis of viruses, bacteria, and cells and the microscopic method of electrophoresis, in *Electrophoresis* (M. Bier, ed.), Vol. 1, pp. 428–487, Academic Press, New York.

Catsimpoolas, N., Hjertén, S., Kolin, A., and Porath, J., 1976, Unit proposal: Tiselius unit of electrophoretic mobility, *Nature* **259**:264.

Davidson, W. F., and Parish, C. R., 1975, A procedure for removing red cells and dead cells from lymphoid cell suspensions, *J. Immunol. Methods* **7**:291.

Dryden, H. L., Murnaghan, F. D., and Bateman, H., 1956, *Hydrodynamics*, p. 184, Dover, New York.

Elhilali, M. M., Britton, S., Brosman, S., and Fahey, J. C., 1976, Critical evaluation of lymphocyte functions in urological cancer patient, *Cancer Res.* **36**:132.

Fisk, A., and Pathak, S., 1969. HEPES-buffered medium for organ culture, *Nature* **224**:1030.

Grassmann, W., and Hannig, K., 1950, Ein einfaches Verfahren zur kontinuierlichen Trennung von Stoffgemischen auf Filterpapier durch Elecktrophorese, *Naturwissenschaften* **37**:397.

Haglund, H., 1967, Isoelectric focusing in natural pH gradients: A technique of growing importance for fractionation and characterization of proteins, *Science Tools* **14**:17.

Handbook of Chemistry and Physics, 1975, Chemical Rubber Publishing.

Hannig, K., 1961, IV. Trennmethoden zur Analyse organischer Verbindungen. 1. Trennung durch kinetische Effekte, *Z. Anal. Chem.* **181**:244.

Hannig, K., 1964, Eine Neuentwicklung der trägerfreien kontinuierlichen Elektrophorese, zur Trennung hochmolekularer und grobdisperser Teilchen, *Z. Physiol. Chem.* **338**:211.

Hannig, K., 1972, Separation of cells and particles by continuous free-flow electrophoresis, in *Techniques of Biochemical and Biophysical Morphology*, Vol. 1 (D. Glick and R. M. Rosenbaum, eds.), Wiley-Interscience, New York.

Hannig, K., and Zeiller, K., 1969, Zur Auftrennung und Charakterisierung immunkompetenter Zellen mit Hilfe der trägerfreien Ablenkungselektrophorese, *Z. Physiol. Chem.* **350**:467.

Hannig, K., Wirth, H., Meyer, B. H., and Zeiller, K., 1975, Free-flow electrophoresis. I. Theoretical and experimental investigations of the influence of mechanical and electrokinetic variables on the efficiency of the method, *Z. Physiol. Chem.* **356**:1209.

Jondal, M., Holm, G., and Wigzel, H., 1972, Surface markers on human T and B lymphocytes. I. A large population of lymphocytes forming immune rosettes with sheep red blood cells, *J. Exp. Med.* **136**:207.

Kolin, A., 1954, A method for elimination of thermal convection. *J. Appl. Phys.* **25**:1442.

Kolin, A., 1960, Continuous electrophoretic fractionation stabilized by electromagnetic rotation. *Proc. Natl. Acad. Sci. USA* **46**:509.

Kolin, A., 1964, Kinematic stabilization of continuous-flow electrophoresis against thermal convection. *Proc. Natl. Acad. Sci. USA* **51**:1110.

Kolin, A., 1965, Magnification of resolving power of collectors in free flow electrophoresis, *J. Chromatogr.* **17**:532.

Kolin, A., 1966, Helical path electrophoresis in vertical fluid sheaths, *Proc. Natl. Acad. Sci. USA* **56**:1051.

Kolin, A., 1967a, Preparative electrophoresis in liquid columns stabilized by electromagnetic rotation. Part I: The apparatus, *J. Chromatogr.* **26**:164.

Kolin, A., 1967b, Preparative electrophoresis in liquid columns stabilized by electromagnetic rotation. Part II: Artifacts, stability and resolution, *J. Chromatogr.* **26**:180.

Kolin, A., 1971, Fractionation and characterization of cells and microbiological particles by means of endless fluid belt electrophoresis, *Proc. 1st. European Biophysics Congress,* Baden, Austria, pp. 481–485.

Kolin, A., 1972, Letter to the Editor, *Chem. Eng. News* Sept. 4:32.

Kolin, A., 1979. Endless belt continuous flow deviation electrophoresis, in *Electrokinetic Separation Methods* (P. G. Righetti, C. J. van Oss, and C. J. Vanderhoff, eds.), Elsevier, Amsterdam.

Kolin, A., and Luner, S. J., 1969, Continuous electrophoresis in fluid endless belts, *Analyt. Biochem.* **30**:111.

Kolin, A., and Luner, S. J., 1971, Endless belt electrophoresis, in *Progress in Separation and Purification,* Vol. IV (E. S. Perry and C. J. van Oss, eds.), pp. 93–132, John Wiley & Sons, New York.

Lamb, H., 1945, *Hydrodynamics,* p. 582, Dover, New York.

Luner, S. J., 1969, Electrophoretic studies of isolated mammalian metaphase chromosomes, UCLA Thesis.

Owen, R. M., 1972, Microbiological evaluation of endless belt electrophoresis, Cal. State College Thesis.

Smoluchowski, M. von, 1921, in *Handbuch der Elektrizität und Magnetismus,* Vol. 2 (L. Graetz, ed.), p. 366, Barth, Leipzig.

Strickler, A., and Sacks, T., 1973, Focusing in continuous-flow electrophoresis systems by electrical control of effective wall zeta potentials, in *Isoelectric Focusing and Isotachophoresis* (N. Catsimpoolas, ed.), pp. 497–514, New York Academy Sciences.

Sturgeon, P., Kolin, A., Kwak, K. S., and Luner, S. J., 1972, Studies of human erythrocytes by endless belt electrophoresis: I. A comparison of electrophoretic mobility with serological reactivity, *Haematologia* **6**:93.

Werum, L. N., Gordon, H. T., and Thornburg, W., 1960, Rapid paper ionophoresis using organic buffers in water–fromamide and water–urea, *J. Chromatogr.* **3**:125.

Zeiller, K. R. Löser, Pascher, G., and Hannig, K., 1975. Free-flow electrophoresis. II. Analysis of the method with respect to preparative cell separation, *Z. Physiol. Chem.* **356**:1225.

4

Buoyant Density Separation with Linear Gradients of Bovine Serum Albumin and Analysis by Centrifugal Cytology and Flow Techniques

ROBERT C. LEIF

I. INTRODUCTION

The last review of the work of my laboratory (Leif, 1970a) described the technique for buoyant density separation of cells in isotonic gradients of bovine serum albumin (BSA) and the application of that technique to the separation of human and rabbit erythrocytes. The various gradient media, BSA, Ficoll, iodothalamate, and colloidal silica, were reviewed. The method of preparation of the BSA, including deionization, filtration, and addition of salts and tissue culture media, were described in detail. The biological studies presented in that review were limited to the first class of cells studied, erythrocytes (human and rabbit). Briefly, reproducible buoyant density distributions of human erythrocytes were obtained, and individual fractions were shown to be capable of being rebanded. The average buoyant density of the erythrocytes from four individuals was 1.0808 ± 0.0004 g cm^{-3}. The average density from a fifth individual was 0.0028 g cm^{-3} greater. The entire buoyant density distribution shifts with salt content; the erythrocytes were shown to behave as "perfect" osmometers. Salt gradients were shown to spread or narrow the distribution predictably, and it was suggested that these gradients might be used to increase the resolving power of the density separations.

ROBERT C. LEIF • Papanicolaou Cancer Research Institute, Miami, Florida 33123.

Rabbit erythrocytes pulse-labeled with ^{59}Fe first appeared at the light edge of the distribution, and the mean of the radioactivity distribution progressed linearly through the red cell distribution. The width of the distribution of labeled cells also increased with time.

A study employing the Coulter Counter model B for cell volume distributions of the density fractions demonstrated that the mean cell volumes on the lighter side remained constant, while on the dense side the mean cell volume decreased. This decrease, if regarded as a water loss, does not quantitatively account for the increase in density. Recent studies with the AMAC II laminar flow electronic cell volume spectrometer indicate that the differences in mean cell volume of the density fractions are even less than were originally found. In short, we have established that buoyant density and cell volume are independent parameters in human erythrocytes.

Microscopic examination of the individual fractions of the buoyant density distribution demonstrated that the cells do not appear to be damaged by these manipulations, and that the cells in the denser fractions are significantly less biconcave than the average cell. The reticulocytes concentrated in the lighter fractions, but did not clearly separate from the erythrocytes. It was proposed that the buoyant density could be regarded as an index of the physiological state of the erythrocytes. A discussion of the aging of the erythrocyte was given.

Since this review is part of a multivolume series where the work of the other laboratories is described, it will be limited to the work of my laboratory and provide a detailed account of the methodology developed since my last review (Leif, 1970a).

Isopycnic buoyant density gradient centrifugation produces a final distribution of cells that is independent of the initial distribution in the gradient. Each cell either sediments or floats to a position in the gradient where the density of the solution is identical with that of the cell. Therefore the distribution of cells will not be affected by changes in either time or the gravitational field after the product of the time and the field exceeds a certain value, e.g., 2500*g*-hours for medium to large cells. At large *g* fields, however, effects due to differences in the compressibility of the cells and the medium should alter the distributions (Hearst and Vinograd, 1961a,b,c; Vinograd and Hearst, 1962). Since all gradient solutions are nonphysiological to at least some extent, the separation process produces a pseudoequilibrium in which exposure to the gradient medium will eventually result in a change in buoyant density. Centrifugation artifacts can also significantly distort the distribution, as will be described below.

Buoyant density centrifugation has the distinct advantage over all other methods of cell separation that as many as 10^9 cells can be separated in small fluid volumes of 25–60 ml. Since buoyant density is evidently related to the degree of maturation of a given cell type, this technique is particularly useful for studying the differentiation of normal and tumor cells, especially in conjunction with other physical separation techniques such as sedimentation velocity, electrophoretic mobility, or countercurrent distribution, which tend to produce separations based on cell type.

This chapter will give an introduction to the technique of isopycnic density gradient centrifugation and describe the ancillary techniques necessary to monitor the separations. After the first author's initial success in separating erythrocytes (Leif and Vinograd, 1964; Leif, 1970a), it became obvious that apart from improving the technology of cell separation, there was also an absolute necessity for developing techniques and equipment for monitoring the gradients. Just as the chemical separation techniques of liquid and gas chromatography have spawned a multitude of detectors, cell separation also requires (1) a technique for morphological analysis of cells, (2) flow analysis techniques which will permit counting and analysis of the various functions of separated cells, and (3) computer programs to analyze the data. The solution to the problem of morphological analysis was centrifugal cytology (Leif *et al.*, 1971), a technique which permits up to twelve gradient fractions to be prepared on the same microscope slide; this technique and its application to density gradient centrifugation will be described at length. Flow analysis requires in addition that the number of cells in individual fractions be counted and analyzed simultaneously, and that the data and calculations based on them be promptly available for subsequent dilution of the cells for centrifugal cytology or biological assays.

II. GRADIENT SEPARATION METHOD

Gradient methodology poses two basic questions: which type of gradient—linear or step—to use; and which gradient materials.

Two major arguments exist against step gradients. The first is that the cells are all concentrated at the density step interface, the volume of which is small compared to that of the total gradient. The presence of these high concentrations of cells at the interface impedes the redistribution of the cells in the gradient. This was best demonstrated in attempts to isolate Sendai virus agglutinates of chicken erythrocytes and Ehrlich ascites cells, which will be described later in this chapter.

The second problem is the choice of density steps, which is usually made on the basis of previous reports of procedures with *other* cells. Since the size of the cuts determines the total number of cells in the individual fractions, one should always be able to develop esthetically pleasing histograms with a little trial and error. However, unless there is some overriding preparative reason and the system has already been well-studied with linear gradients, the results obtained with step gradients are *not* suitable for publication in reputable journals. Pretlow *et al.* (1975) have gone so far as to state, "It is our opinion that the use of discontinuous gradients is rarely justified and, in fact, most often results in the production of artifacts." As a personal note—after the invention and fruitful development of a technique, it has been most disappointing to observe in the literature that the desire for facility appears to outweigh the desire for accuracy.

A. Density Gradient Media

The criteria for a density-increasing solute are the following: absence of cellular agglutinability, high molecular weight, exclusion by the cells (particularly if the material is nonphysiological), ease of sterilization, stability, and cost. If exposure to the gradient material results in agglutination, the cells will not be distributed according to their individual buoyant densities. Since a significant mass of solute is required to increase the density, the osmotic contribution of the solute must be minimized. It should be noted that the osmotic behavior of a polydisperse polymer such as Ficoll is proportional to the number average, not the weight average, molecular weight. In the case of low-molecular-weight solutes such as sucrose, Isopaque (*N*-methyl-3,5-diacetamide-2,4,6-triiodobenzoic acid sodium salt), or other X-ray contrast medium, the osmotic contribution is significant. A molecule of 650 molecular weight and density of 2.00, for example, would produce a concentration of 0.231 M at a density of 1.075 g cm^{-3}. In the case of a sodium salt such as Isopaque, both the cation and anion are excluded, thus doubling the net ionic effect to an osmolarity of 0.462. It has recently become fashionable to determine the osmolarity of concentrated polymers by freezing point depression and vapor pressure osmometry, but at the concentrations employed for gradient separation of cells, neither procedure would be expected to produce meaningful results. The physical chemistry of polymer solutions is only ideal at very low concentrations, and a 10 to 33% solute is a distinctly nonideal situation. The solute molecules obviously interact with each other and are present in sufficient concentrations to affect the hydrogen bonding of a substantial amount of the water present. In freezing point depression studies there is also the problem of supercooling, and in the case of vapor pressure osmolarity, the effect of heat of hydration may be significant. In short, these osmotic measurements may serve as a sensitive assay for the reproducibility of a solution but until a great deal more work is performed, the absolute osmotic pressure or water activity will remain undetermined and it is doubtful, even assuming a true value could be determined, whether it would provide sufficient information to permit extrapolation to a physiological solution which is plasma, not saline. All the same, this does *not* preclude accurate comparative studies, as will be described below. If the solute is not excluded totally by the cells, then either the absorbed or surface-bound solute will increase the density of the cells, which will in turn require an increase in the solute concentration and osmotic pressure, especially of low-molecular-weight solutes. In this way, obviously, absorption or binding of the solute can increase the density to the point where the solubility of the solute is exceeded or its nonphysiological effects become apparent.

The problem of sterilization has been solved by Millipore or Nucleopore filtration. There is no real advantage to autoclavability since the separated fractions are analyzed with a Coulter-type electronic cell volume instrument or an optical analyzer based on fluorescence or light scattering, or both, all of which are sensitive to background noise due to particulates in the gradient medium. Except for colloidal silica, which is unstable in physiological saline, all of the other gradient media are either stable after sterilization or, like BSA, can be stored indefinitely in a −70°C freezer. Iodothalamate and other X-ray contrast media must be shielded from light but this is not a significant objection to its use.

The cost of the gradient media, except for colloidal silica, probably has more to do with marketing practices than with intrinsic manufacturing costs; except for zonal gradient experiments, these are not significant when compared with labor and other costs. Large-scale utilization of any one medium should decrease the price. Even in the case of BSA the starting material, bovine blood, is very inexpensive.

Future Gradient Materials. In summary, although each of the gradient materials discussed here has its advantages and disadvantages, in my own admittedly prejudiced view, BSA is still the best at present. However, it is surprising to me that the polymer chemists and chemical supply houses have not made available high-molecular-weight dense hydrophilic polymers containing covalently bound iodine or other high-atomic-number elements.

B. Preparation of BSA and Salt Solutions

The composition of all the solutions and the BSA media utilized in these studies is shown in Table 1. The salt concentrations were derived by Leif (1970a) from the published values found in blood and plasma which were determined by use of either specific ion electrodes or standard chemical analyses. The solution nomenclature is as follows: If the solution is a gradient medium then BSA is applied as a prefix. The next group of characters specifies the type of tissue culture medium, CMRL (Parker *et*

TABLE 1
Composition of Salt Solutions and BSA Media

Substance	Mol. wt.	BSA-199L(CO_2)		199(B)		LP–0.2% BSA[b]		Counting medium		
		MCO[a] / kg H_2O	g / kg BSA	MCO / liter	g / liter	MCO / liter	g / liter	MCO / liter	g / liter	g / 20 liters
Medium 199 with glutamine but without salts or glucose			0.546		.820					
$NaHCO_3$	84.00			26.20	2.200					
Na_2CO_3		94.80	3.350							
$NaH_2PO_4 \cdot H_2O$	137.99	2.00	0.184	2.00	0.276	2.00	0.276	0.29	.040	.80
$Na_2HPO_4 \cdot 7H_2O$	268.07					13.10	1.755	1.68	.225	4.50
NaCl	58.44	49.50	1.929	118.10	6.903	118.10	6.903	129.8	7.586	151.71
NaF	41.99							11.9	.500	10.00
KCl	74.56	4.52	0.225	4.52	0.337	4.52	0.337	4.52	0.337	6.74
$MgSO_4 \cdot 7H_2O$	246.48	0.86	0.142	0.86	0.213	0.86	0.213			
$CaCl_2$	110.99	1.11	0.082	1.11	0.123	1.11	0.123			
Glucose	180.16	5.55	0.667	5.55	1.000	5.55	1.000			
BSA (33% deionized)							6.06			
Neomycin sulfate			0.089				0.100			
Total MCO Na^+		146.30		146.30		146.30		146.30		
Total MCO K^+		4.52		4.52		4.52		4.52		
Total Meq Cl^-		56.24		124.84		124.80		134.3		
Total Meq HCO_3^-		47.40		26.20						
Total MCO		152.79		152.79		152.79		150.82		
Total milliosmolality anions		106.50		153.90		140.80		149.96		
K^+/Na^+ Ratio		0.031		0.031		0.031				
HCO_2^-/Cl^- ratio		0.843		0.210						

[a]Millication osmolality.
[b]This saline is no longer used because of its high phosphate content. The counting medium is now used as the basis for all phosphate formulations.

al., 1957), as was used formerly, or 199 (Morgan *et al.*, 1950), which is presently used. The remaining part specifies the composition of the salts with (CO_3) representing carbonate, (P) phosphate, (B) bicarbonate, and (Cl) chloride. If for any reason the anion content is changed from the amounts previously specified (Leif, 1970a; Kneece and Leif, 1971), that is, 47.40 mmol of carbonate per kilogram of H_2O or 26.20 mmol of bicarbonate per kilogram of H_2O, that number is enclosed in the same parenthesis. For instance BSA-CMRL(CO_3, 50.35) was a 33% ρ_4^4 = 1.100 g cm^{-3}, BSA gradient medium containing CMRL tissue culture medium with Leif's salt formulation but with the carbonate increased at the expense of the Cl from 47.40 mmol to 50.35 mmol to produce a gradient medium of pH 7.2 (Kneece and Leif, 1971).

In the case of tissue culture media or saline the term BSA is of course not present at the front of the designation; however, if the solution contains a small amount of BSA to stabilize the cells, then this is added as a final suffix, for instance 199(B)–1% BSA for a bicarbonate-buffered tissue culture 199 medium containing 1% BSA. Parenthetically it should be noted that this nomenclature system can be made universal by specifying the source of the salt formation with the type of anion. Thus 199(L,P)–1% BSA would be Medium 199 with Leif's salt formation with phosphate as the buffer and 1% BSA added.

The compositions of four solutions are given in Table I. The first is the conventional 33% BSA ρ_4^4 = 1.100 g cm^{-3} employed as the dense medium. The second is the bicarbonate solution used to dilute it to form the less dense "light" gradient medium. The third is a phosphate-buffered saline employed for diluting the gradient fractions for subsequent centrifugal cytology and flow analysis.

The fourth is the medium presently used as the sheath flow for our flow analyzers, the AMAC II electronic cell volume analyzer and the AMAC III combined electrooptical cell multiparameter spectrometer. This saline can also be employed for centrifugal cytology of exfoliated cells.

The preparation of the BSA is as follows:

1. Into a 500-ml wide mouth plastic bottle is weighed in the following order: 800 g of water, 200 g mixed bed resin AG 5 01-X8(D) 20-50 mesh (BIORAD, Richmond, Cal.), and 432 g Bovine Serum Albumin Fraction V (Reheis Chemical Co., Div. Armour Pharm., Kankakee, Ill.). The BSA is placed on top of the water, which contains the resin.
2. The lid is sealed with tape, PVC household warp, or Parafilm, placed on a modified Cell Production Roller Apparatus (Bellco Glass, Vineland, N.J.) and rotated at 5 rpm at 2°C for 24–48 h.
3. The BSA solution is decanted from most of the resin into a 400-ml

Diaflow Model 401 filter with a 3-in. Millipore prefilter pad, and 10 lb of N_2 pressure is applied. The resin-free BSA is recovered in another large mouth plastic bottle.

4. New mixed bed resin (50 gms) is added. The lid is sealed and the container rolled in the cold an additional 24 h.
5. The BSA solution is decanted from most of the resin into the 400-ml Diaflow apparatus with a 5 μ Millipore or Nucleopore filter and about 10 lb of N_2 pressure is again applied. The liquid is recovered in a preweighed bottle. The amount of BSA is determined by the increase in weight. The refractive index is adjusted to 1.3986 by the addition of H_2O.
6. Powdered tissue culture medium and salts are added (Table 1).
7. The lid is sealed and the container rolled in the cold 12–24 h until the salts are dissolved.
8. The BSA is poured into the 400-ml Diaflow apparatus with a 0.22 μ Nucleopore filter and about 10 lb of N_2 pressure is applied.

In the event that the mixed resin in step 2 changes color strongly, the amount of resin in step 4 should be doubled to 100 g. Step 4 can be omitted if the resistivity of the BSA solution is greater than one million ohms or if the sodium content as determined by flame photometry is less than 1 mM.

C. The Effect of pH on Buoyant Density

There is a controversy between Leif and Shortman (Legge and Shortman, 1968) over the optimum pH for gradient separations. Leif prefers neutrality, Shortman prefers slightly acid conditions. Kneece and Leif (1971) have demonstrated that as long as the cation concentration is kept constant, the effect of pH on human erythrocytes is essentially minimal. The effect of the pH change on the buoyant density distributions, as measured by the ρ_{tmed} (the truncated median of the buoyant denstity distribution) value, of human erythrocytes from one donor (W.C.K.) with hemoglobulin was studied. Figure 1 shows the average curves calculated from several experiments at each pH value. For these studies, the anion concentration was reduced as the pH was increased. If the total osmolarity is kept constant (Williams and Shortman, 1972), then the erythrocytes increase in density as the pH is increased (Fig. 2) because the Na ion concentration must be increased as the pH is increased. In contradistinction to these results Kneece and Leif (1971) found (Fig. 2) that the buoyant density maximum was at 1.0836 g cm^{-3} at pH 6.8 and actually decreased to 1.0774 g cm^{-3} at pH 7.2. This density change is explained as the result of erythrocytes acting as cation osmometers. Shortman believes that the cells are responding to the Donnan equilibrium and binding anions, principally chloride ion, as the intracellular hemoglobin becomes positively charged. As Shortman states, "These two alternative explanations cannot be experimentally separated by studies in albumin media, since the albumin itself must be neutralized and the Na^{+} level altered to change pH at constant osmolarity." He then quotes Coulter Counter data on RBC volumes and Ficoll and nonaqueous density measurements (Williams and Shortman, 1972). None of these data are definitive. pH-induced shape as well as volume effects would easily explain the Coulter data. The Ficoll was hypertonic to begin with and nonaqueous media do not really separate single cells due to the surface tension effects. Most importantly, in all cases where the density of cells is measured in our laboratory under slightly acid

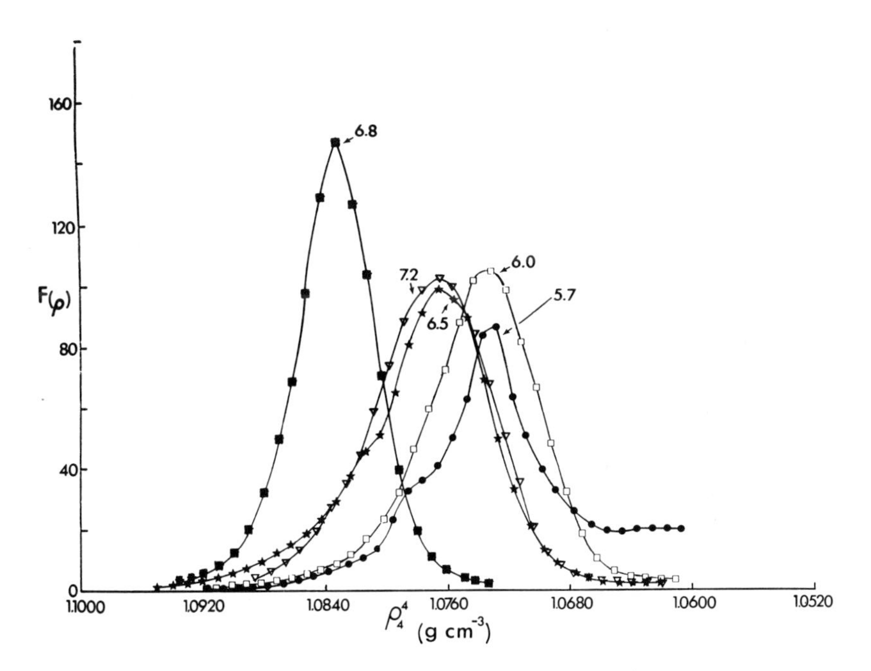

FIGURE 1. Buoyant density distributions of human erythrocytes at the pHs given in the figure from one donor (W. C. K.). The ordinate represents values of $F(\rho)$, a normalized distribution function which is described in section II. F. Briefly, this function gives the relative concentration of cells in each fraction but is independent of the absolute number of cells applied to the gradient and the density range of the individual gradient fractions. The average curves for each set of replicate experiments at a given pH pass through values of $F(\rho)$ determined by averaging the interpolated values from the individual experiments. The ρ_{tmed} value (the truncated median of the buoyant density distribution) of each individual experimental curve served as the fiducial point and values of $F(\rho)$ were read at increments and decrements of 0.00100 g cm^{-3} from the individual curves connecting the individual experimental points. The average value of ρ_{tmed} served as the initial point for plotting the average curves.

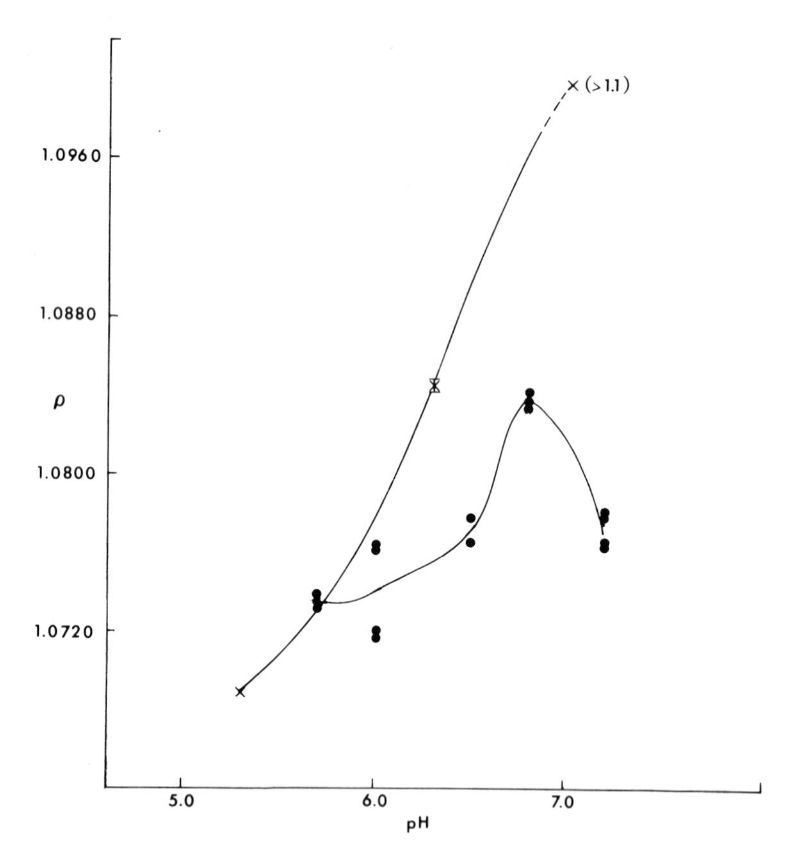

FIGURE 2. Variation of the buoyant density of human erythrocytes with pH. The filled circles represent the ρ_{tmed} of the individual experiments in the studies presented in Fig. 1. The ×s are taken from Table 2 of Legge and Shortman (1968). The cause of the large scatter of the values of ρ_{tmed} at pH 6.0 is presently unknown.

conditions, the results are not significantly different. When small agglutinates are found in the density fractions, these are similar cells which probably do not differ very much in density. In addition, it is significant that no one performs sedimentation studies, which are far more sensitive to agglutination, at acid pH.

The results of preliminary attempts at isolating heterokaryocytes revealed that the behavior of the fusion product of two different cells is relevant to this question. Sendai-virus-induced agglutinates of hen erythrocytes and Ehrlich ascites cells were pulled apart when the usual centrifugal force of about 10,000*g* was applied (Warters, 1972). These previously unpublished studies will be described below because they illustrate the methodology, show the difficulties in isolating aggregates, and compare the results obtained with step gradients as opposed to linear gradients. The isolation of heterokaryocytes from any type of cell rather than from specific mutants will permit studies of the induction of vegetative growth of defective viruses and of genetic complementation in general by this process.

D. The Gradient System

The gradient system now used is an updated version of the one reported earlier (Leif, 1968a,b, 1970a). It consists of special centrifuge tubes, a gradient mixing chamber, a double-sided undulating diaphragm peristaltic pump, a digital controller, a small fraction collector, and a cold bench. In addition to the 18-hole special gradient-forming tubes, new six-hole tubes (Fig. 3) have been fabricated for small gradients of less than 10 ml (Leif *et al.*, 1972). The tube shell is molded of crystal clear epoxide and an engraved Kel-F plate is pressed into it. The capillary in the side of the tube is formed by embedding a glass capillary which is later etched out with hydrofluoric acid. Since the Kel-F plate is denser than the gradient media, the centrifuge force shapes it to the bottom of the centrifuge tube. The mixing chamber (Fig. 4) consists of a synchronous 150-rpm Bodine motor (Bodine Motor Co., Chicago, Ill.) driving a glass driveshaft which in turn passes through a Teflon gland and a glass outer shell to which assorted Teflon paddles are attached. The gradient chambers are attached to the outer shell by an O-ring joint. In order to produce gradients of from 5 to 200 ml, the gradient chambers have been produced in three sizes: 15, 25, and 100 ml (Fig. 5). The volume of the gradient is twice the volume of the dilute gradient material placed in the chamber.

As shown in Fig. 6, the body of the peristaltic pump (PB) was cast from aluminum and then machined. The precision ramps (Ra) (Leif, 1968a), which eliminate pulsations in flow, are machined out of stainless steel and pinned to each side of the casting. A Slo-syn stepping motor (M) (Fig. 7), Model SS250-1027 (Superior Electric Co., Bristol, Conn.), is attached by a coupling (Co) (Fig. 6) to the driveshaft. Sprockets (Sp) on this shaft drive a hollow-pin chain (Ch) which holds the rollers (Ro) which in turn ride on the ramps and are supported by two ball bearings (BB) apiece. The pumping tubes (PT) are mounted in stainless steel tube holders (TH) (Fig. 8) resting on a mechanism which consists of a pair of tube stretchers (TS) (Fig. 7) mounted on captive lead screws (LS) connected at the center of the pump by a common driveshaft, which is driven by a crank (Cr). The tubes are compressed by pressure plates (PP) (Fig. 9) fabricated out of polycarbonate, and stiffened by an aluminum plate (AP) whose weight has been reduced by boring holes in a regular pattern. The pressure plates are

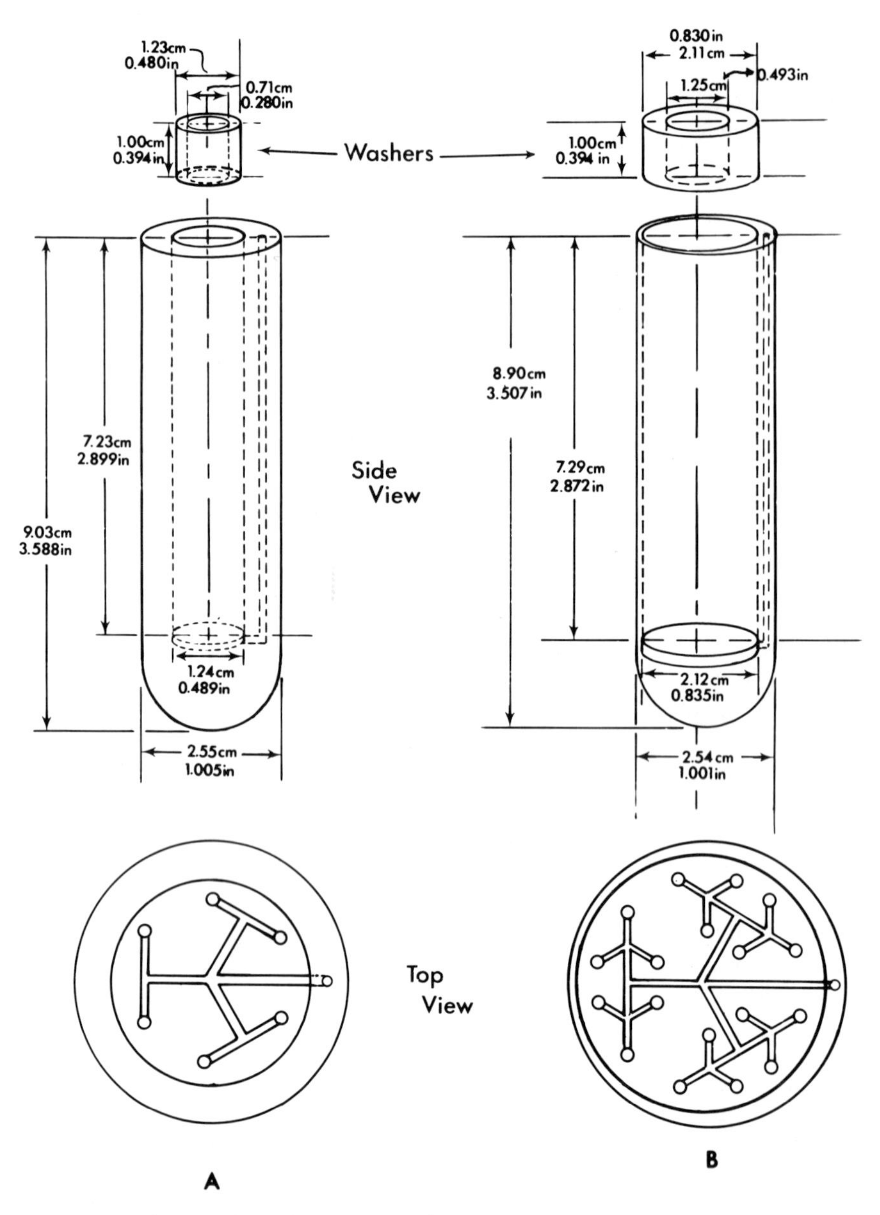

FIGURE 3. Diagram of special centrifuge tubes and polyethylene washers (not drawn to scale). Side view of centrifuge tubes shows capillary in the wall through which gradient is pumped into and out of the centrifuge tube. Placement of orifices and channels in the diffusing plate is shown in a top view. (A) 8-ml centrifuge tube and (B) 20-ml centrifuge tube. Both centrifuge tubes fit the International Equipment Company SB-110 and the prototype XYZ-40 swinging-bucket rotors.

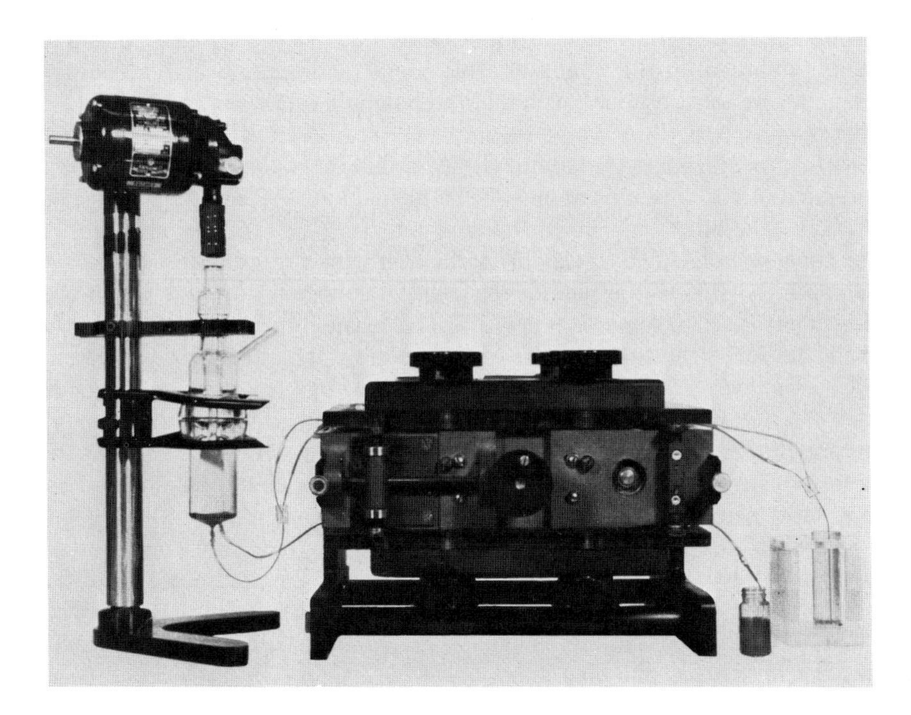

FIGURE 4. Photograph of the density gradient system. On the left are shown the mixer and 85-ml gradient-forming chamber. The Teflon paddle inside the chamber is rotated by a 150-rpm synchronous motor, which is attached to the top of the glass shaft of the mixer. The peristaltic pump is located in the center of the photograph. The dense solution is removed from its container, which is located at the right of the pump, and conveyed to the inlet at the periphery of the mixing chamber by a pumping tube stretched across the bottom of the pump. A pair of tubes stretched across the top of the pump are joined at both ends by plastic Ys and convey the gradient from the outlet at the base of the mixing chamber to the capillary in the wall of the special centrifuge tube. The location of the inlet and outlet pumping tubes on opposite sides of the pump permits them to pump in both directions.

tightened by eight screws (Sc) (Figs. 4, 9), four on top and four on the bottom, connected in pairs to four sliders (Sl) mounted in the walls of the pump. The pump itself is mounted in back by a pivot (Pi) attached to its base (B) (Fig. 7). A pair of retractable flat pins (obtained from an electrical chassis slide) allow for locking the pump in three positions; horizontal (the normal way), diagonal (45°), or vertical. The latter two positions make it easier to attach the bottom pressure plate which is always put on first and held by about three turns of the screws. When the top plate is removed, the bottom pressure plate (PP) then clears the tube holders (Fig. 9).

The undulating diaphragms are sheets of Teflon-coated Kapton (DuPont Inc., Wilmington, Pa.) secured to the body of the pump by two clamping plates (CP) (Fig. 6). Cloth tape is stuck to the top and bottom of each diaphragm at the points of attachment to the pump body. The diaphragms are set loosely enough that the pumping tubes can conform to the rollers.

In order to start the pump, the two stationary tube holders are first mounted on the pair of fixed pins (FP) attached to the side of the pump (Fig. 7). Next, the other pair of tube holders is mounted on the movable pins of the tube stretcher (TS) assembly, which are then retracted just past the ramp on the side of the pump. The crank (Cr) which turns their common driveshaft is set to top center (Fig. 7). The tension due to the stretching of the tubes locks the tube holders onto their pins. The top pressure plate is then mounted and screwed down tight. If the pump is not started immediately at this point, the plastic of the pumping tubes will be irreversibly deformed. After the pump is stopped, the top plate is removed, allowing the bottom plate to slide down and release the pressure on the pumping tubes. For short periods (one or two hours) the tubes can be left stretched but unpressurized, but for longer periods, the movable pins should be brought back as far as possible toward the center of the pump and one side of the tube stretcher then dismounted at top and bottom from its movable pin. Alternatively, the pump can be left assembled for one or two hours without any harm to the pumping tubes *providing it is not allowed to stop completely*.

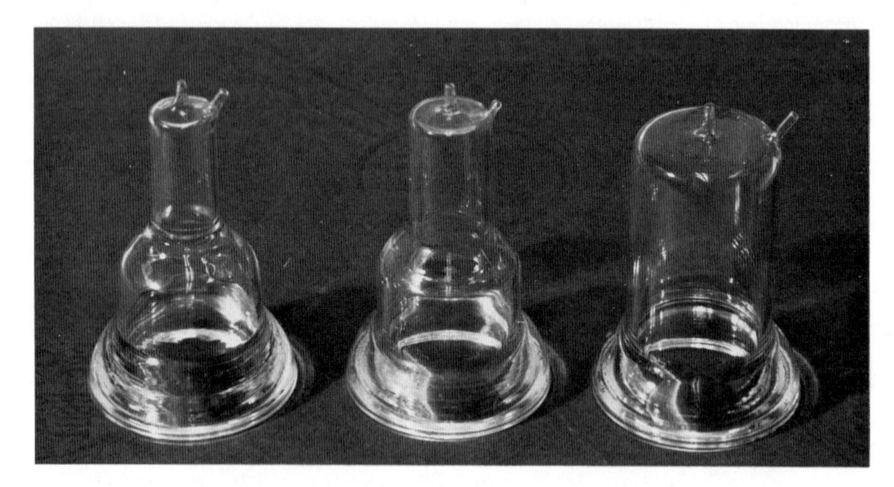

FIGURE 5. Photograph of three glass gradient chambers: 15-, 25-, and 100-ml volume. The total volume of gradient produced is twice the volume of these chambers. They all attach to the mixer using the same size O-ring joint.

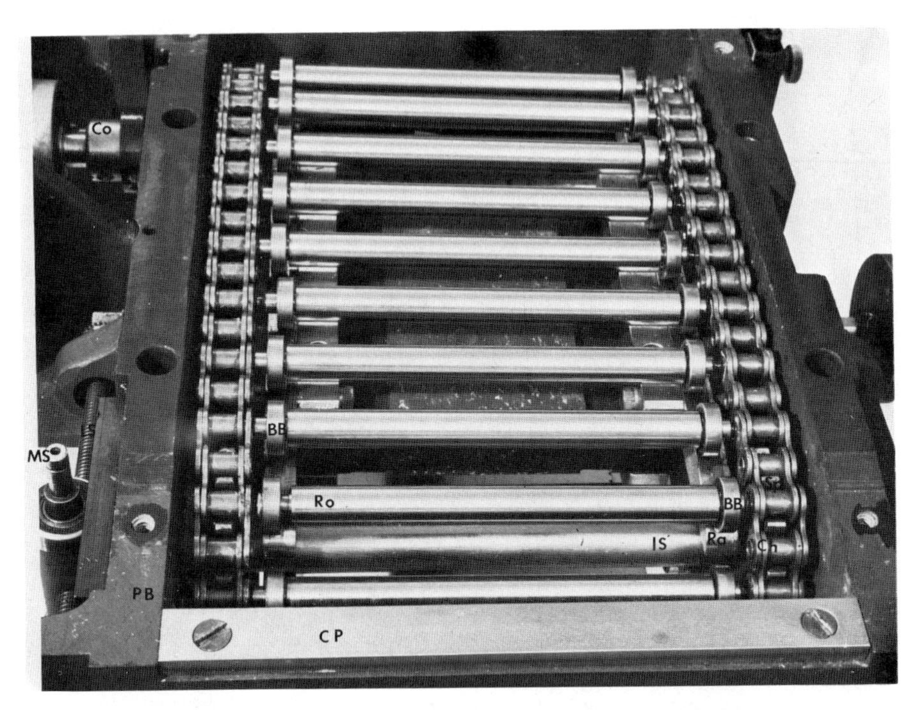

FIGURE 6. Top view of peristaltic pump with the pressure plate and pumping tubes removed. The clamping plate (CP) which secures the undulating diaphragm (not shown) is at the bottom of the figure. A second clamping plate (not shown) is located at the opposite end to the one shown. The two chains (Ch) are located next to the two sides of the pump body (PB) and are driven by a pair of sprockets (Sp) attached to the driveshaft (not shown) which extends from the coupling (CO) at the top left across to the top right. A second identical pair of sprockets are attached to the idler shaft (IS) which runs across the bottom of the pump. These shafts are supported by large ball bearings mounted in the sides of the pump body. The horizontal stainless steel rollers (Ro) are supported at both ends by miniature ball bearings (BB) which ride on the specially machined precision stainless steel ramps (Ra), as shown in Fig. 7, and are pulled by the hollow pin chains located on both sides next to the pump body (PB). The teeth from the idler sprockets (Sp) which drive the chains are shown at the bottom sides of the photograph. A movable tube stretcher (MS) with its lead screw is shown at the bottom left. The motor coupling is visible at the top left.

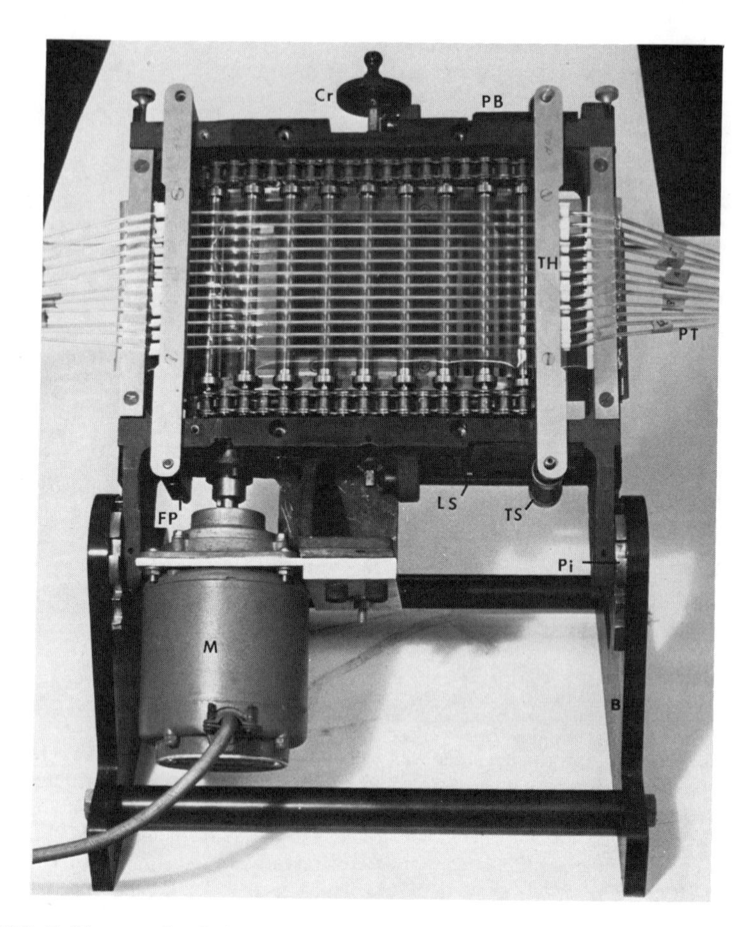

FIGURE 7. Photograph of the back of the peristaltic pump with the top pressure plate removed. This view is from the top back of the pump, which is tilted up. The Slo-syn stepping motor (M) is shown at lower left; the tube stretchers (TS) are at the extreme ends with the peristaltic pumping tubes (PT) between. The pumping tubes (PT) actually rest on a transparent plastic diaphragm which extends from left to right. The diaphragm rests upon stainless steel rollers which are in turn supported by miniature ball bearings at both ends. The rollers are driven by the hollow-toothed sprocketed chains adjacent to the walls of the casting. Since this is a back view the lead screw (LS) and tube stretcher (TS) are shown on the right and the crank (Cr) at the top. The pivot mechanism (Pi) is attached to the stand shown at the bottom.

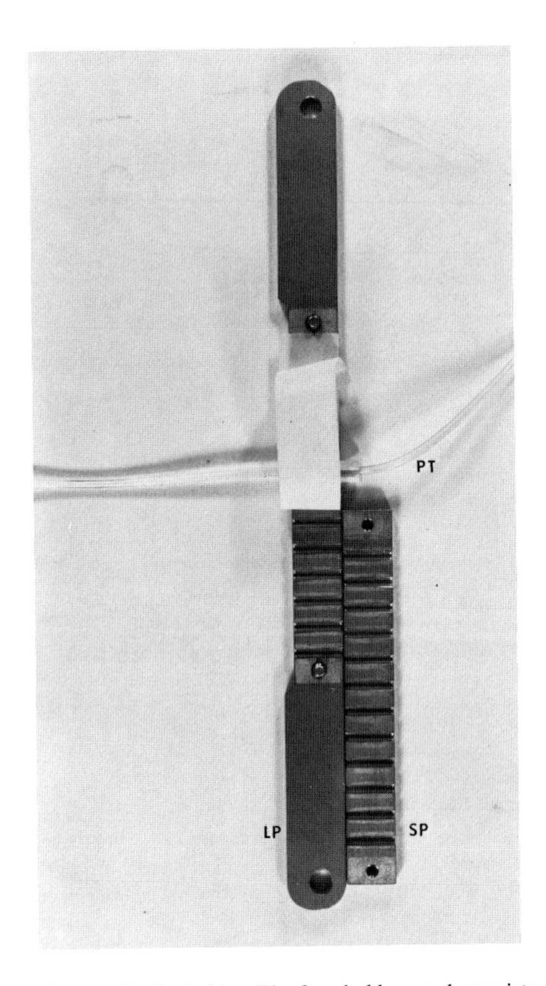

FIGURE 8. Stainless steel tube holder. The four holders each consists of a short piece (SP) and long piece (LP) with mounting holes. Both the underside of the long piece and the top of the short piece are grooved to hold the pumping tubes with the grooves of the long and short pieces facing and offset from each other. After the pumping tubes are inserted, they are held in each long and short piece by a piece of single-sided cellophane tape (top middle of the long piece). The long pieces are tapped to allow the two pieces to be screwed together.

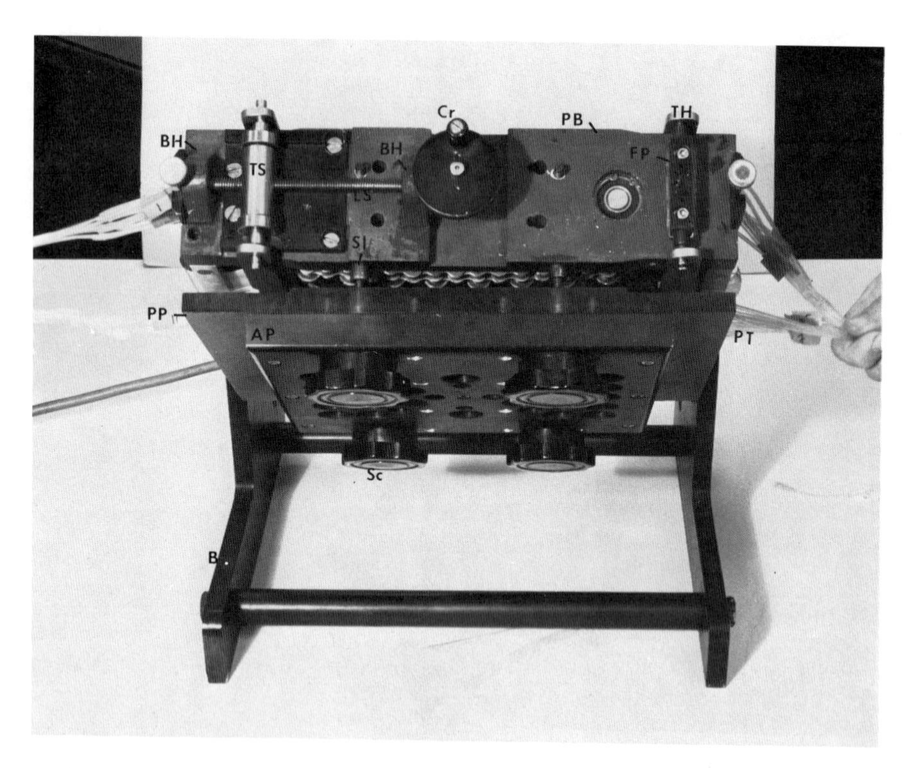

FIGURE 9. Front view of peristaltic pump (raised at 45° to show underside). The top pressure plate has been removed and the screws holding the bottom loosened to their maximum extent so that only two or three turns are in the slides (Sl) which protrude from the bottom of the pump body. The aluminum plate (AP), which has been lightened by drilling out several holes in it, is screwed onto the polycarbonate pressure plate (PP). The tube stretcher assembly is mounted on the left side of the pump. The crank (Cr) is attached to the crankshaft (not shown) which extends to the back of the pump body and connects to a second tube stretcher assembly. In both the front and back, a bevel gear (not shown) attached to the driveshaft couples to an identical gear attached to the lead screw (LS). Both lead screws are supported at each end in ball bearings mounted in bearing holders (BH) which were integrally cast with the pump body. The actual tube stretcher (TS) is supported by two ball bearings and advanced or retracted by the lead screw. The four tube holders (TH) are mounted on the pins of the two tube stretchers and the two tube holders. The pumping tubes are shown on both the top and bottom.

The digital controller (Fig. 10) controls the fraction collector (Fig. 11) and produces a pulse train determining the velocity of the stepping motor, which in turn propels the peristaltic pump. The number of steps per second (pulses) is determined by a digital potentiometer which controls the rate of the oscillator. The stepping motor is bidirectional; the pump proceeds forward to form the gradients and reverses to fractionate them.

The volume of each sample is determined by presetting one of the two scalers (Fig. 10), A or B. When the preset counter reaches the prescribed number of pulses, the output from the oscillator is disconnected from the stepping motor, which then stops; the sipper motor (SM) of the fraction collector (Fig. 12) is activated and elevates the sipper shaft (SS), which holds the sample tube (ST), to the top of its travel (Fig. 11) which closes the top-of-cycle microswitch (TCM). Then the tube advance motor (TAM) (Fig. 12) advances the fraction collector (Fig. 11) one step, producing a momentary opening of the tube new-position-reached microswitch (PRM).

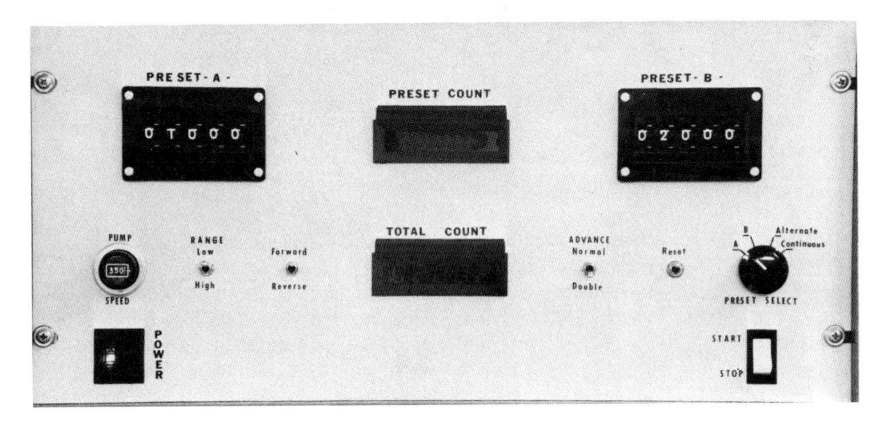

FIGURE 10. The digital controller consists of two presettable counters, A (upper left) and B (upper right). The PRESET SELECT switch (middle right) determines which of these presets will be active, whether they will alternate in producing two different size fractions, or whether the pump will be in continuous mode, which is employed for gradient formation. The PRESET COUNT continuously displays the number of pump counting units for each function. When the preset count is reached, this display is zeroed. The TOTAL COUNT is not zeroed and thus displays the summation of the counts. The switches and rheostat on the left at center height control the stepping motor. The "Forward/Reverse" switch determines the flow direction across the pump. This direction is switched for fractionation. The RANGE Low/High determines the pump speed range. It is presently used in the low speed mode. The PUMP SPEED control is a ten-turn digital-readout rheostat, which permits very accurate control of the pump motor oscillator.

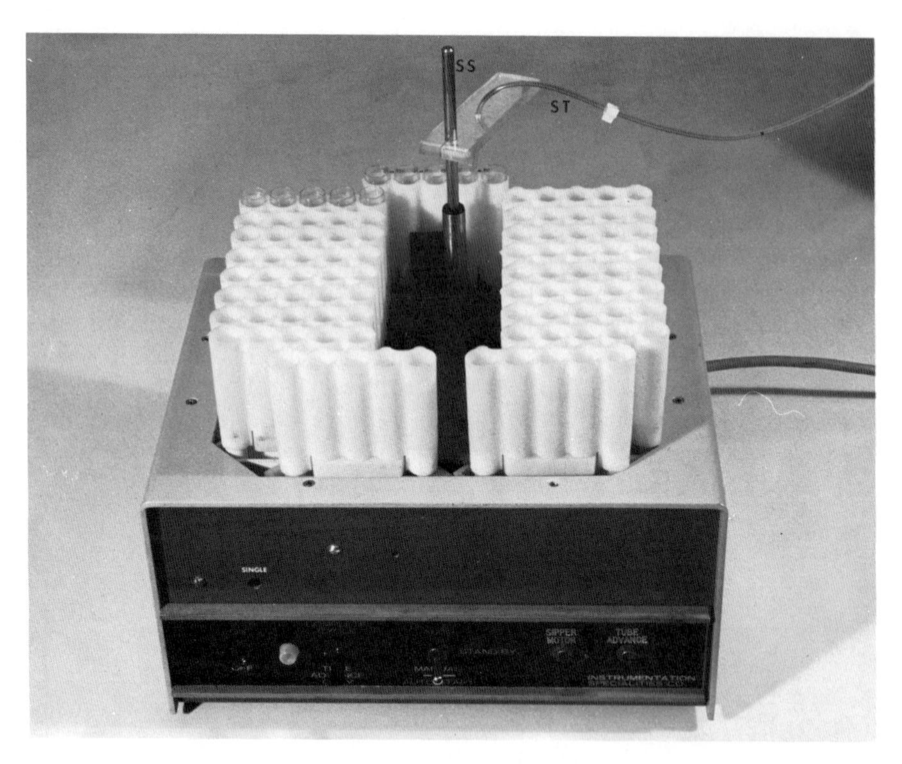

FIGURE 11. Top view, assembled modified ISCO OEM fraction collector. The stainless steel shaft (SS) (center back) is raised and lowered by the digital controller. The sample tube (ST) is mounted in the plastic plate which is friction-fitted to the shaft and thus is raised at the end of the preset count. The blocks which hold five clinical chemistry AutoAnalyzer-type cuvettes are then advanced one position and the stainless steel shaft is lowered, placing the sample tube into the next cuvette. The sample tube makes contact with the bottom of the cuvette and thus retains a negligible volume of gradient when it is subsequently transferred. All the manual controls have been left intact.

After this the sipper motor starts again and lowers the sample tube. When the sample tube is halfway down, the restart microswitch (RM) is closed, and the oscillator is reconnected to the stepping motor, thus restarting the pump. The sipper motor is stopped by the momentary closure of the bottom-of-cycle microswitch (BCM) when the sample tube has entered a new cuvette (Fig. 13). Overlapping the starting of the pump motor with the second half of the lowering of the sample tube results in a significant decrease in the amount of time it takes to fractionate a gradient.

A digital readout (Fig. 10) displays the amount of each gradient fraction pumped, and the total volume for the entire gradient is given by a second display.

The controller (Figs. 10, 14) has been designed to permit operating modes other than the collection of single constant-volume fractions. It will alternate the preset counts in the A and B scalers and will also advance the fraction collector two steps instead of one. The alternate mode will be useful if two aliquots of differing volume from each fraction are required for separate analysis, such as refractive index and flow microfluorometry and/or electronic cell volume analysis. The two-step mode permits two gradients to be fractionated simultaneously. The detailed electronics of the fraction collector controller are described in Appendix A.

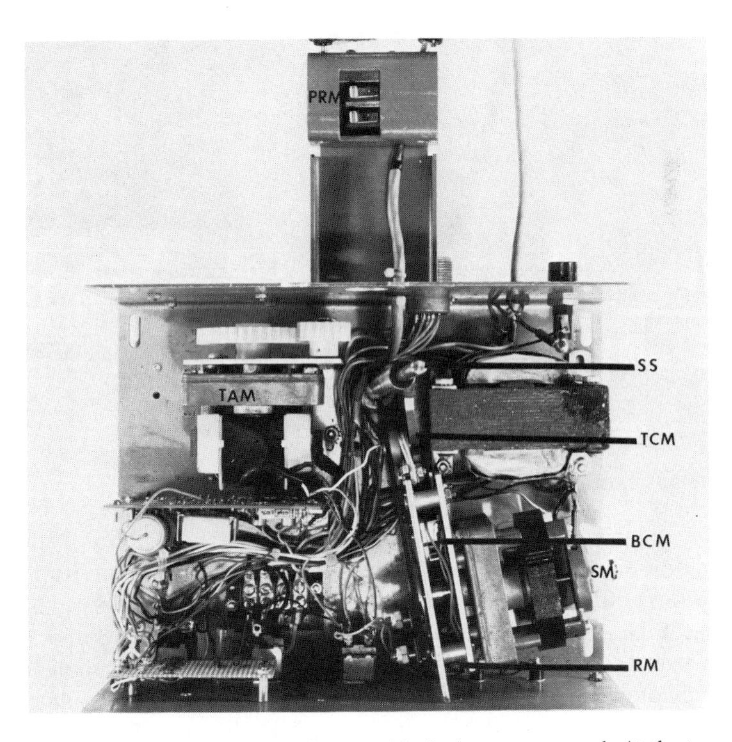

FIGURE 12. Underside of fraction collector with the bottom removed. At the top center is shown the new-position-reached microswitch (PRM). In the upper lefthand corner is shown a motor with a large white gear mounted on its shaft. This gear drives the adjacent small white gear which propels the blocks. The sipper motor (SM) on the lower right raises and lowers the stainless steel shaft (SS) and actuates the three microswitches: the bottom-of-cycle (BCM), top-of-cycle (TCM), and restart (RM) microswitches.

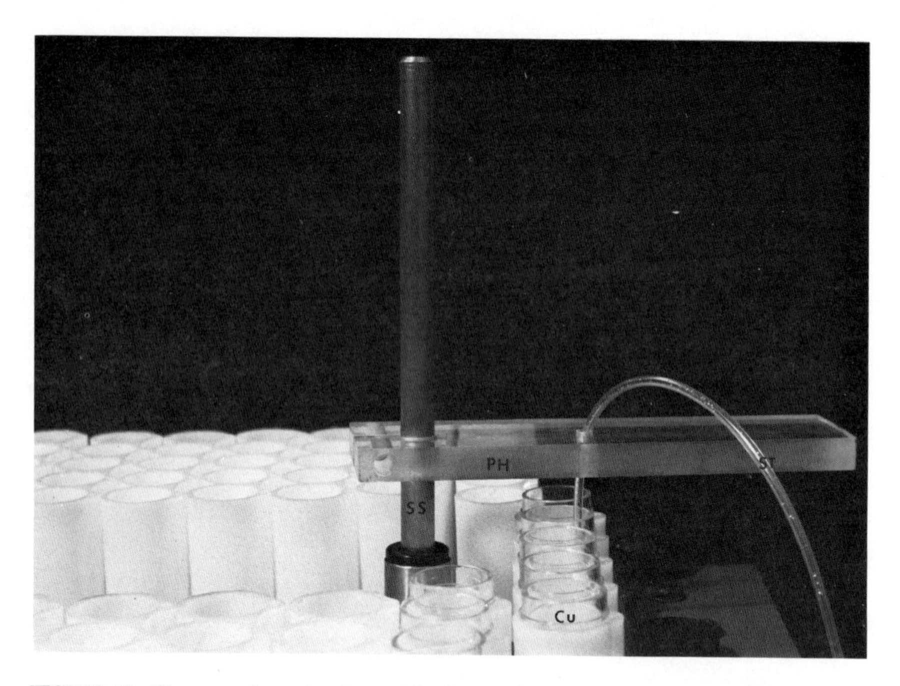

FIGURE 13. Close-up of sample tube positioning assembly (shown in Fig. 11). Plexiglass tube holder (PH) is attached to the stainless steel shaft (SS) and holds the sample tube (ST). The sample tube is raised to clear the rim and lowered to the bottom of the 2-ml disposable cuvettes (Cu). This eliminates random apportionment of the last drop which forms at the end of the sample tube in a conventional fraction collector.

E. Hydrodynamic and Wall Artifacts

After the gradient is formed the next step is the addition of the cells. Direct addition of the cells leads to droplet formation at the interface of the cells and the gradient and an excessive buildup of cells on the sides of the centrifuge tube. Similar hydrodynamic artifacts—streaming and turning over—associated with the layering of a suspension of macromolecules or cell particulates over a gradient of sucrose or other low-molecular-weight solute have been discussed in detail by both Brakke (1955) and Anderson (1955, 1956). The artifacts are due mainly to low-molecular-weight gradient material diffusing into the overlayered material at a greater rate than the high-molecular-weight overlayered material diffuses into the gradient. This results in density instability and the streaming of part of the overlayered solution downward through the gradient. Under the influence of a centrifugal force, the overlayered material can cause a density inversion, if it is

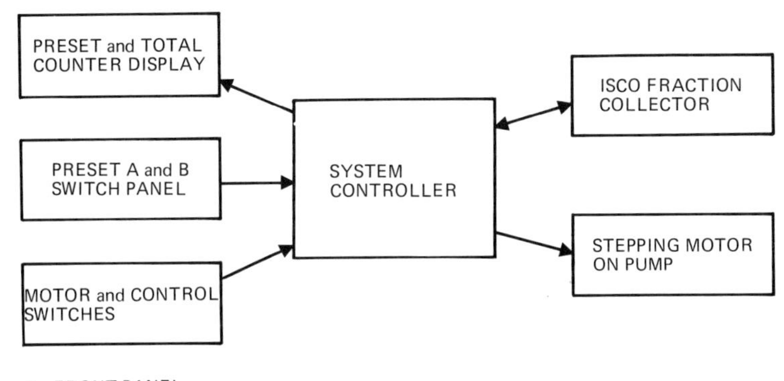

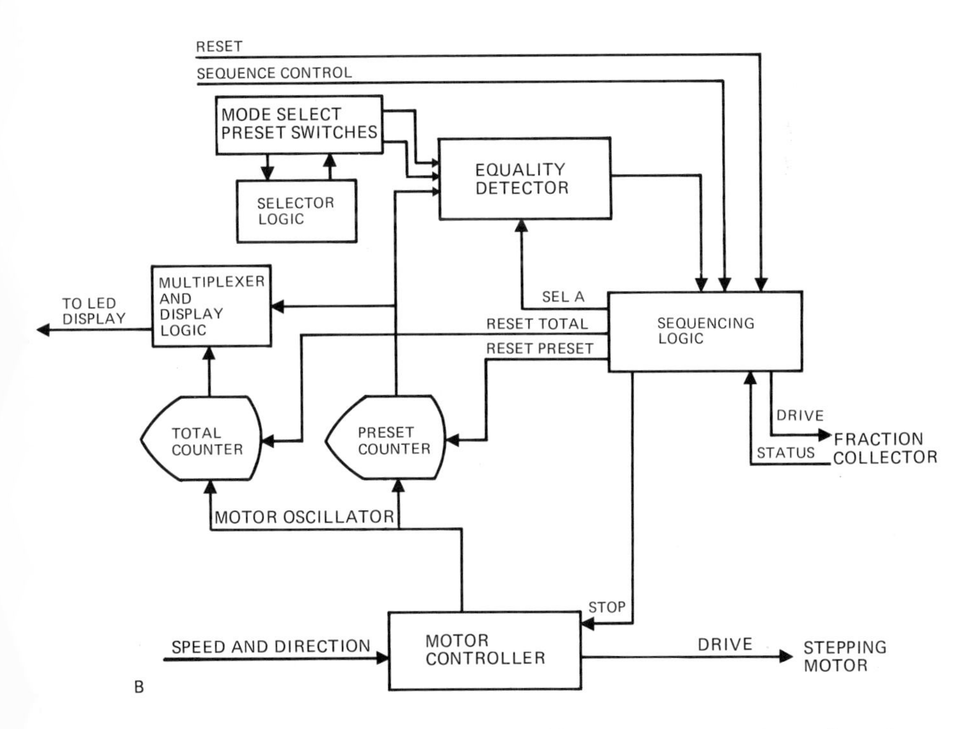

FIGURE 14. (A) Block diagram of digitally controlled fraction collector. The three units on the left and the system controller are all located in the digital controller unit. The modified ISCO fraction collector is described in Figs. 11 and 12. (B) Diagram of controller. When equality between preset counter output and preset switch input is detected, the controller halts the pump and cycles the fraction collector. At the end of the cycle the controller resets the preset counters and restarts the motor; it also modifies the cycle as dictated by switches on the front panel.

concentrated enough or becomes sufficiently concentrated as it enters the gradient. This inversion results in the bulk of the solution which contains the sample falling down through the gradient or along the walls of the centrifuge tubes. When cells are overlayered on gradients of BSA or other macromolecules, similar hydrodynamic artifacts have been observed. However, it is very unlikely that sufficient quantities of these macromolecules could diffuse into the overlayered cell-containing solution to generate density instabilities. In the case of cells, the streaming artifact can be explained by the retardation of the sedimentation of the cells at unit gravity as they enter the BSA gradient. This retardation causes the cells to pile up and to concentrate at or just below the interface between the layering medium and the BSA gradient. If a centrifugal force is then applied, the cells are concentrated in bulk at the interface, which then is of greater density than the lamella of the gradient beneath it, and the concentrated cell suspension at the interface turns over as a unit and sinks into the gradient. This situation is further complicated by the tendency of the cells to agglutinate in the layering medium, especially when they are in close proximity to one another. Rouleau formation of erythrocytes in plasma is a well-known phenomenon, causing erythrocytes to sediment faster than leukocytes, as seen in clinical sedimentation studies (Wintrobe, 1974).

In earlier work (Leif and Vinograd, 1964), the cells were first pelleted and then dispersed in the dense BSA solution, in order to eliminate the hydrodynamic artifacts and the wall effects and to maximize the number of cells that could be applied to the gradient. This solution was pumped into the gradient mixing chamber by the special peristaltic pump and mixed with the less dense BSA solution to form a gradient of cells that was linear and in the same direction as the BSA gradient. The concentration of cells even at the bottom of the gradient was very low in comparison with a conventional layered solution, and the majority of cells were focused inward and upward along a radial trajectory under a centrifugal field. This arrangement eliminated the hydrodynamic artifacts and minimized the wall effects . Although this technique has been successful with erythrocytes (Shortman, 1969a; Leif, 1970a; Leif and Vinograd, 1964), lymphocytes (Shortman, 1969a; Shortman *et al.,* 1967; Shortman, 1968), thymocytes (Shortman, 1968, 1969a), and erythroblasts (Shortman, 1969b), experiments with rat bone marrow cells revealed that about half the cells sank to the bottom of the centrifuge tube.

Since large "fragile" cells had to be applied to the top of the gradient, the methodology used to accomplish this consisted of two innovations (Leif *et al.,* 1972). First, the sample was placed in a floating polyethylene washer which confines the cells to the center of the tube, thus restricting the radial trajectory and minimizing collisions with the tube walls. Fox and Pardee (1970) have utilized a special aluminum cap with a hole in it to accomplish the same end. Second, the sedimentation velocity of the cells in the overlayering solution was greatly decreased by the addition of a viscous polymer. Since the BSA gradient is being used for isopycnic studies, the initial band width of the cells as they enter the gradient will have no effect on the end result except for the hydrodynamic artifacts. Inclusion of a high-molecular-weight polymer into the layering solution increases the viscosity without significantly increasing the density of the solution. This causes the sedimentation rate of the cells to increase as they enter the gradient, thus increasing the width of the cell zone and decreasing the concentration of cells.

The first high-molecular-weight polymer used to increase the viscosity of the layering solution was un-cross-linked polyacrylamide, but it agglutinated the erythrocytes. Since an uncharged macromolecule led to aggregation of the cells and the presence of negatively charged BSA molecules did not, DNA was then selected and used successfully to increase the viscosity.

Figure 15 shows a time study performed to demonstrate that the increase in viscosity due to the presence of the DNA was sufficient to prevent the streaming artifact. At 15 min, the maximum amount of time between layering and centrifugation, the movement of erythrocytes into the gradient is negligible. Figure 16 is an idealized picture of the effect of DNA and a less viscous layering media upon the movement of cells into a BSA gradient. A study to observe the combined effect of the streaming, turnover, and wall-effect artifacts is shown in Fig. 17. For this study, two identical 20-ml BSA-CMRL(CO_3) gradients were formed. The large-size polyethylene washer was placed onto one of the gradients. Then 1 ml of a cell suspension containing 0.25% DNA was layered into the center of this washer. This cell suspension was prepared by mixing a 0.50% wt/vol. DNA solution (Sigma Co., St. Louis, Mo., salmon sperm DNA) with an equal volume of the cell-containing suspending solution to give a final concentration of 0.25% DNA. A cell suspension prepared in the usual way, but without any DNA, was layered onto the other gradient. These gradients were centrifuged and fractionated. The wall effect on cells can be seen in Fig. 17, which was taken as the gradient was being pumped out. (It should be noted that using a higher-molecular-weight DNA aggregates the cells.)

Previously (Leif and Vinograd, 1964; de Duve *et al.*, 1959) it was reported that the swirling of BSA gradients could be eliminated by either very slow acceleration of a conventional swinging-bucket rotor or the utilization of the Sorvall HS rotor (Leif and Vinograd, 1964), which was

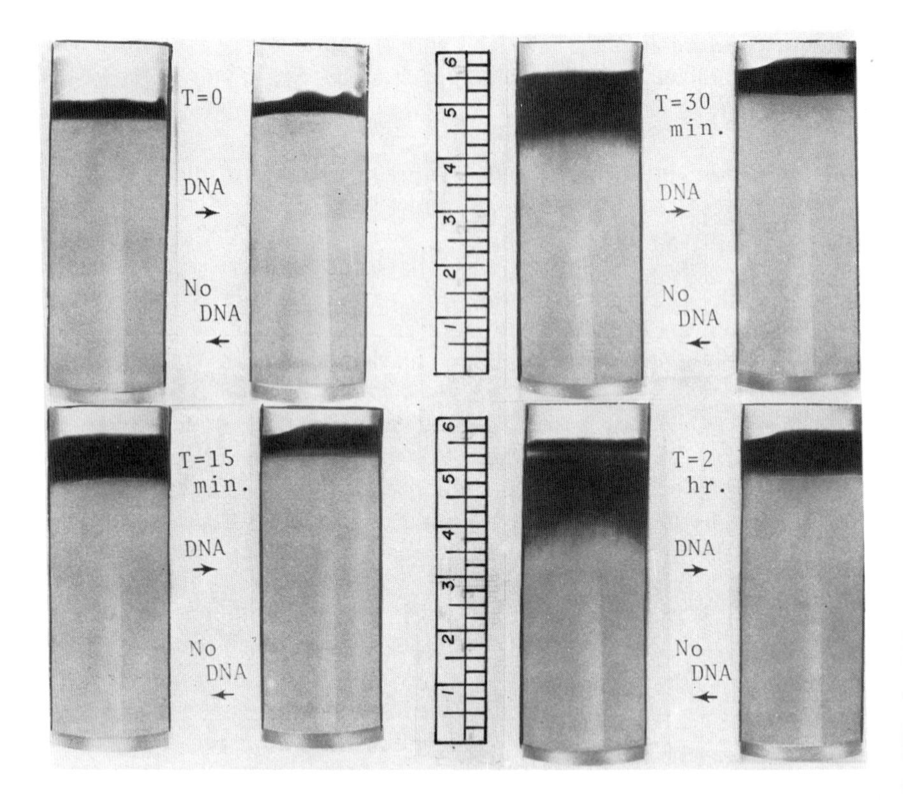

Figure 15. Effect after various time intervals of 0.25% DNA added to layering medium compared to behavior of cells in layering medium without DNA. Addition of DNA to layering medium retards movement of erythrocytes into gradient by increasing the medium's viscosity. Cells in layering media which do not contain DNA rapidly enter gradient.

free to move up and down as well as sideways. The HS rotor is no longer produced, and it was not designed for either high fields or large quantities of cells. A conventional International Equipment Corporation SB-110 swinging-bucket rotor was modified to permit sideways motion (Leif, 1970a) (Fig. 18) of the buckets in ball joints so that they were free to swing in the same way as the HS rotor (Fox *et al.*, 1968 patent). The buckets can thus align with the sum of the outward centrifugal force $\omega^2 r$ and the sideward forces due to acceleration or deceleration, $r d\omega/dt$, where r is the distance from the center and $d\omega/dt$ is the radial acceleration. This sum of forces is the effective force on the gradient. Because of the squared term in the centrifu-

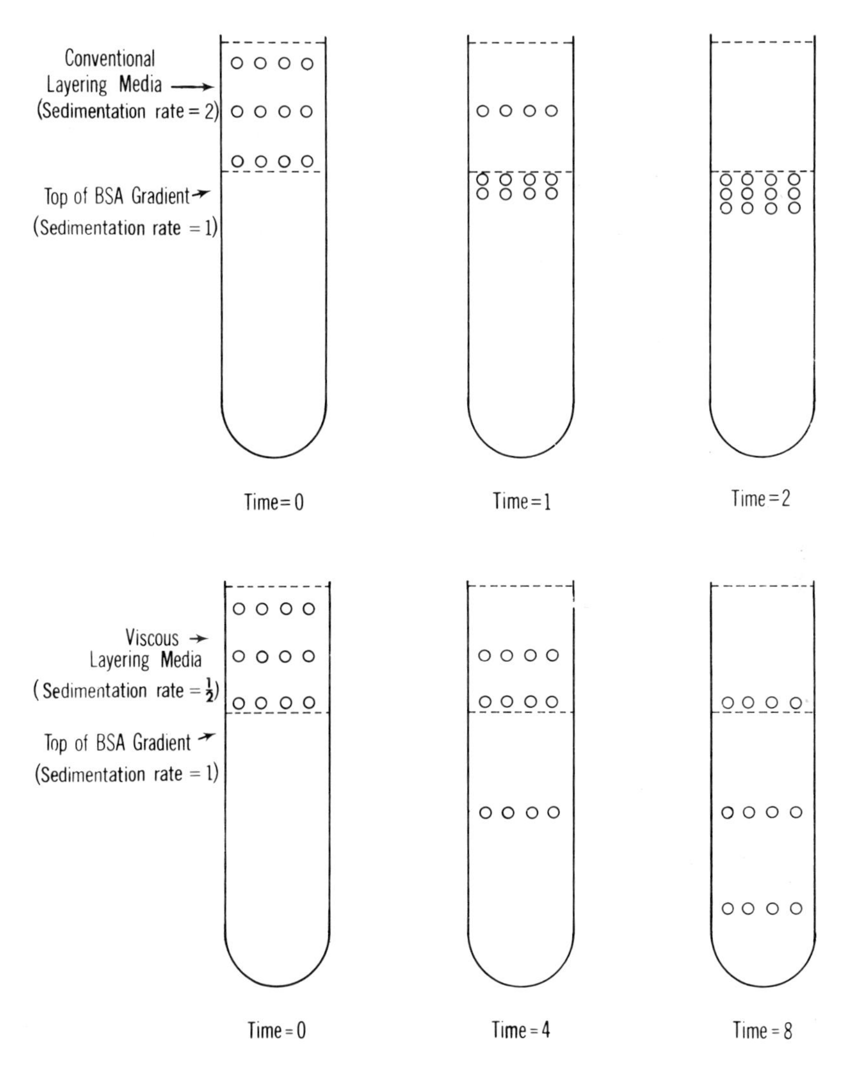

FIGURE 16. Idealized representation of movement of cells into BSA gradient from conventional (nonviscous) layering media and from viscous layering media. At the top is shown the concentration of cells at interface when they leave the less viscous layering media and enter the top of the more-viscous BSA gradient. The cells become crowded together and move as a packed mass into the gradient. At bottom is shown the dilution of cells as they leave the viscous layering media and enter the less-viscous top of BSA gradient.

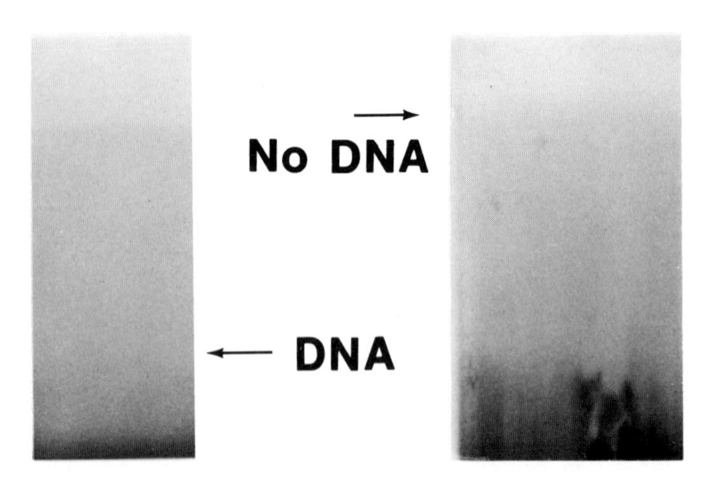

FIGURE 17. Photographs of two BSA gradients after major portion of band had been pumped out of each centrifuge tube. Only center of each centrifuge tube is shown. Left, BSA gradient with cells suspended in 0.25% DNA solution and overlayered in center of polyethylene washer. Right, deposition of erythrocytes on tube wall that occurs when DNA and polyethylene washer are omitted.

gal force expression, the contribution of the sideward forces is only significant at low speeds. This modified rotor is called the XYZ-40 rotor.

In order to look for the presence or absence of swirling in both the SB-110 and the XYZ-40 rotors, step gradients were employed. Step gradients were prepared from 1%, 2%, and 3% sucrose solutions. These were transported into the 25-ml special centrifuge tubes by the peristaltic pump to obtain sharp interfaces. The 2% sucrose solution contained 0.10% blue dextran. Two step gradients were prepared for each experiment.

One of the freshly prepared step gradients was then placed in the XYZ-40 rotor and very slowly accelerated from rest, with the door slightly ajar. The other identical gradient was allowed to stand at 4°C while the first was centrifuged, in order to serve as a control for the effect of diffusion on the broadening of the blue band. After being centrifuged at 10,000 rpm for 5 min, the first gradient was allowed to coast to a stop and then compared with the control gradient. The latter showed minimal band broadening. This control gradient was then placed in the XYZ-40 rotor, accelerated by setting the manufacturer's speed control at 10,000 rpm, centrifuged for 5 min at this speed, and allowed to coast to a stop. The slowly accelerated gradient was allowed to sit at 4° and was then compared with the rapidly accelerated gradient. The same procedure was then followed with new

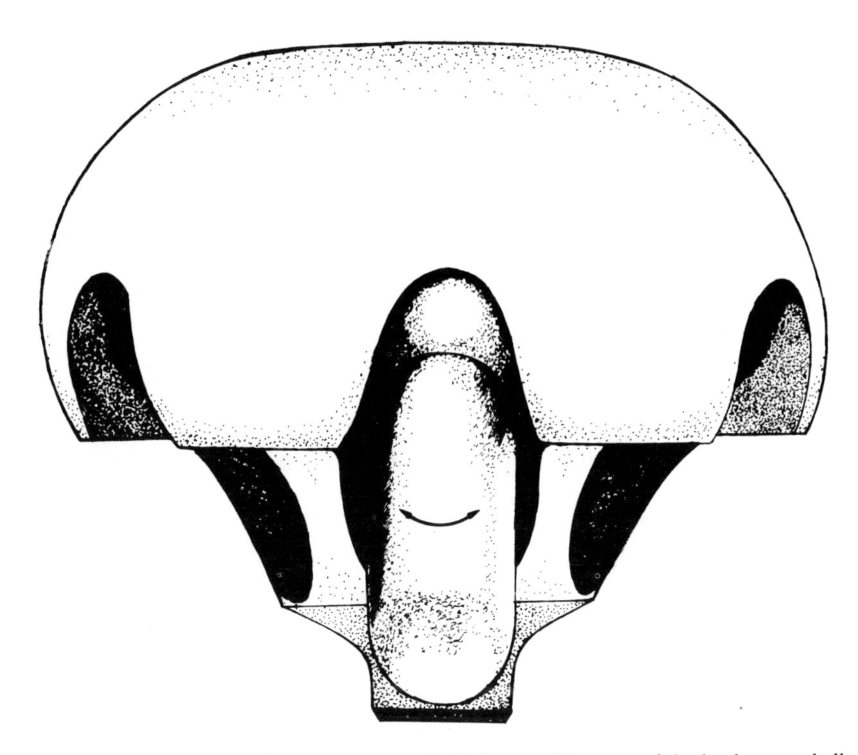

FIGURE 18. International Equipment Corp. XYZ-40 rotor. The tops of the buckets are ball-shaped and fit into the sockets in underside of the rotor. Only one bucket is shown in this drawing. The slots that extend from the sockets to the periphery of the rotor are shaped to permit both normal vertical motion of the bucket as it swings out and are relieved to permit horizontal motion shown by double-sided arrow. This second motion permits buckets to trail as rotor speed increases or decreases. Thus the bucket is aligned with the sum of the centrifugal and acceleration and deceleration forces. To function properly, rotor and buckets must be both anodized and permanently coated with molybdenum disulfide preparation as was done for these studies, or better yet, coated with Teflon.

gradients using the SB-110 rotor. The results before and after each centrifugation for each type of rotor are shown in Fig. 19.

It can readily be seen that neither rotor significantly broadens the band when accelerated very slowly, but that when they are accelerated rapidly the SB-110 rotor broadens the band considerably more than does the XYZ-40 rotor. Since slow acceleration and utilization of the XYZ-40 rotor both have been demonstrated to reduce or minimize swirling, the combination should virtually eliminate this artifact.

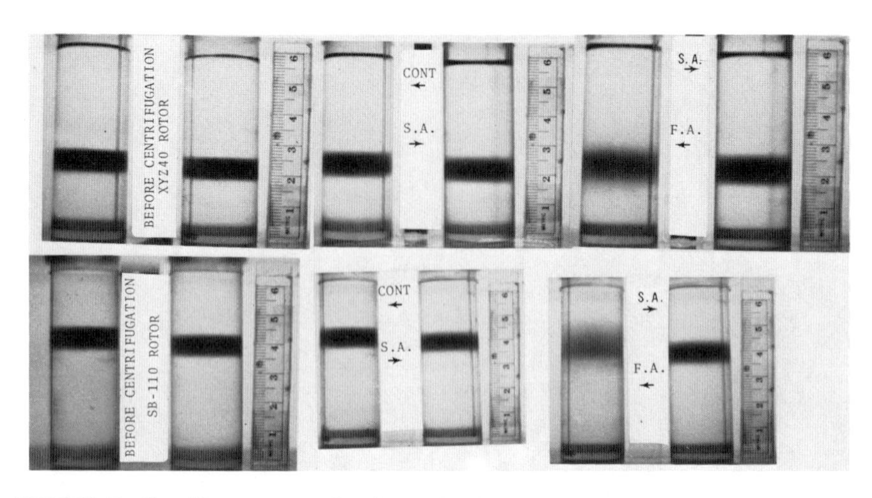

FIGURE 19. Centrifuge rotor acceleration study. Step gradients of 1%, 2%, and 3% sucrose solutions with 0.10% blue dextran in the 2% solution were utilized to test for swirling with International Equipment Corporation SB-110 and prototype XYZ-40 swinging-bucket rotors. CONT, control gradient; S.A. and F.A., slowly accelerated and rapidly accelerated gradients respectively.

In the case of a Spinco centrifuge which does not take these modified International rotors, swirling has been minimized by employing a simple acceleration control. The circuit is shown in Fig. 20.

The original density measurements were performed with a pycnometer and a microbalance (Leif, 1964; Leif and Vinograd, 1964). These measurements required more time than all of the rest of the experiment, and thus this technique is impractical for routine biological experiments. However, it was possible by these precise measurements to establish that the reproducibility of a buoyant density determination of the erythrocytes from one individual (R.C.L.) was 0.0005 g cm^{-3}.

Although Leif and Vinograd (1964) were the first to establish the relationship between refractive index and density, they favored the use of pycnometry. Later, more biologically oriented studies (Leif *et al.*, 1975c; Thornthwaite and Leif, 1974) required the use of refractive index measurements which do depend on the exact composition of the tissue culture medium which is added to the BSA. Shortman (1969a) employs bromobenzene–benzene density gradients. Theoretically, some of the tissue culture medium should partition into the organic phase, and the presence of the high concentration of BSA may increase the solubility of the bromobenzene and benzene in the aqueous phase, or the protein could bind to, and be partially denatured by, these organic materials.

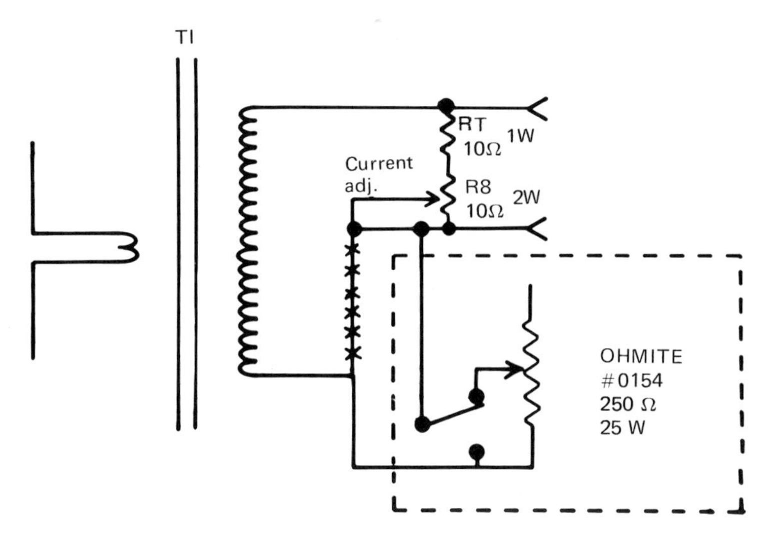

FIGURE 20. Centrifuge acceleration circuit schematic. The added rheostat is mounted in an external box and controls the acceleration between 0 and 1000 rpm.

Recently an obvious solution to this problem has been developed by Kratky *et al.* (1973). A flow-through digital densometer measures the period of a vibrating borosilicate glass "U" tube which is rigidly mounted at one end and acts as a pendulum. (These instruments are manufactured by Anton Paar, Austria and sold in the United States by Mettler, Hightown, N.J.)

F. Data Analysis

The data were analyzed and plotted by the CELL TYPE program. This program first calculates the density of the individual fractions, the number of cells present in each fraction, the total number of cells recovered from the gradient and the buoyant density distribution of the cells.

Table 2 defines the functions in the CELL TYPE program. The abbreviations used to describe them are given at the bottom of Table 2. The buoyant density ρ_4^4 of the individual fractions is calculated from the refractive index measurements of a less dense, a medium, and a dense fraction (Leif, 1970a). The average range of density of a fraction $\Delta\rho$ is also calculated. NUM CELLS IN FRACT is the total number of cells present in the fraction. The factor 2 in this calculation enters because the Coulter Counter counts a volume of 0.5 ml. The summation of NUM CELLS IN FRACT yields the total

TABLE 2
Functions Utilized in the CELL TYPE Program[a]

The number of cells in a fraction

$$\text{NUM CELLS IN FRACT} = 2(\text{DILUTION FACTOR})(\text{COULTER COUNTS} - \text{BACKGROUND})$$

The total number of cells recovered from a gradient

$$\text{NUM CELLS IN GRAD} = \sum_{i=1}^{n} \text{NUM CELLS IN FRACT}$$

The precentage of the total number of cells recovered from the gradient present in a given fraction

$$\%\ \text{CELLS IN FRACT} = 100\,\frac{(\text{NUM CELLS IN FRACT})}{(\text{NUM CELLS IN GRAD})}$$

The buoyant density distribution function

$$F(\rho) = \frac{(\text{NUM CELLS IN FRACT})}{(\Delta\rho)(\text{NUM CELLS IN GRAD})}$$

The percentage of the cells in a given fraction of one specific type

$$\%\ \text{COMP SP CELLS IN FRACT} = 100\,\frac{(\text{NUM SP CELLS COUNTED})}{(\text{TOTAL NUM CELLS COUNTED IN FRACT})}$$

The number of cells of a specific type in a fraction

$$\text{NUM SP CELLS IN FRACT} = \frac{(\%\ \text{COMP SP CELLS IN FRACT})(\text{NUM CELLS IN FRACT})}{100}$$

The total number of a specific cell type recovered from a gradient

$$\text{NUM SP CELLS IN GRAD} = \sum_{i=1}^{n} \text{NUM SP CELLS IN FRACT}$$

The percentage of cells of a specific type in a given fraction

$$\%\ \text{SP CELLS IN FRACT} = 100\,\frac{(\text{NUM SP CELLS IN FRACT})}{(\text{NUM SP CELLS IN GRAD})}$$

The buoyant density distribution function of a specific type of cell or a specific quantity such as radioactivity

$$F(\rho)_{\text{SP}} = \frac{(\text{NUM SP CELLS IN FRACT})}{(\Delta\rho)(\text{NUM SP CELLS IN GRAD})}$$

The percentage of the total cells recovered from the gradient which were of a specific type

$$\%\ \text{COMP SP CELLS IN GRAD} = 100\,\frac{(\text{NUM SP CELLS IN GRAD})}{(\text{NUM CELLS IN GRAD})}$$

The enrichment of a specific type of cell found in a given fraction

$$\text{ENRICHMENT FACTOR} = \frac{\%\ \text{COMP SP CELLS IN FRACT}}{\%\ \text{COMP SP CELLS IN GRAD}}$$

The buoyant density distribution function of a specific type of cells or quantity in terms of a specific group of cells such as all agglutinates

$$G_{(\rho)} = \frac{(\text{NUM SP CELLS IN FRACT})}{(\Delta\rho)\text{NUM SP CELLS IN GRAD}}$$

[a] COMP, composition: FRACT, fraction; $F(\rho)$, buoyant density distribution of total cells; $F(\rho)_{\text{SP}}$, buoyant density distribution of a specific type of cells; GRAD, gradient; i, fraction number; n, the number of the least dense fraction; NUM, number; SP, specific.

number of cells recovered from the gradient, NUM CELLS IN GRAD. Next the percentage of the total cells present in an individual fraction from the gradient, % CELLS IN FRACT, and the buoyant density distribution function $F(\rho)$ are calculated; $F(\rho)$ is the normalized distribution function, independent of both the total number of cells recovered from the gradient and of $\Delta\rho$, the range of the density fraction (Leif, 1970a; Leif and Vinograd, 1964). As Table 2 shows, $F(\rho)$ and % CELLS IN FRACT for any single experiment are directly related by the multiplicative constant, $\Delta\rho/100$.

Once the NUM SP CELLS IN FRACT is obtained from the product of % COMP SP CELLS IN FRACT and NUM CELLS IN FRACT, it is possible to analyze these data for each specific type of cell, which yields the total number of this cell type recovered, its percentage in an individual fraction, and its buoyant density distribution function. In the case of cells present in large concentrations, it is also possible to compare the % COMP SP CELLS IN GRAD with the composition percentages found in the "centrifugal cytogram" of the unfractionated cells. The enrichment factor is a measure of the purification accomplished with the gradient separation procedure. A useful fiducial point which describes the position of a band of cells in the gradient is the truncated median of the distributions of the cells in the gradient, ρt_{med}. This function is computed by disregarding the statistically unreliable tails on both sides of the distributions, $F(\rho) < 20$, and finding the median buoyant density where the number of cells on both sides of the truncated distribution are equal (Kneece and Leif, 1971).

A FORTRAN listing and detailed description of the CELL TYPE program including the plotting routines are given in Appendix B.

III. PAST PROCEDURES FOR THE PREPARATION OF FIXED STAINED CELLS FROM DILUTE SUSPENSIONS

Conventional smear techniques are unsuitable for the direct preparation of cells from dilute suspensions, e.g., those obtained by cell separation techniques, because the concentration of cells on the slide would be too low to be scanned successfully and many of the cells would be disrupted. The most common technique for concentrating and preparing cells is entrapment with microfilters like "Millipore" (Seal, 1956; Millipore Corp., 1966) or "Nucleopore" (Jansson *et al.*, 1967). Cells have also been sedimented onto glass slides with the Cyto-Centrifuge (Watson, 1966) or, with much less elaborate apparatus, onto cover glasses (Kolin and Luner, 1969; Van Dilla *et al.*, 1967). The technique of filtering cells onto microfilters, which is extremely popular and useful, is somewhat complex, however. Each cell suspension must be filtered separately, the filters must be attached to the slides, and the slow exchange of solvents from the filter requires that the slides must be processed by the techniques common for sections. Rendering the microfilters transparent and free of stains is often difficult and time-consuming. Because the cells are not flattened, detailed cytologic studies, especially of small cells, are not always possible. In the case of the Cyto-Centrifuge (Watson, 1966), which is a special instrument for preparing slides, the excess suspending solution is removed during centrifugation by absorption into a thick filter paper seal located between the slide and a special rotor. Unfortunately, many cells are lost by being forced into this seal. Zucker (1970) in a study of fetal mouse erythroid cells reported that "the Cyto-Centrifuge selectively plates nucleated cells on slides in preference to non-nucleated cells." It has also been reported that granulocytes are preferentially lost from leukocyte-enriched preparations of human blood cells (Oberjat *et al.*, 1970). All these previous centrifugation techniques have employed air-drying before fixation, which often causes distortion and loss of nuclear detail (Barrett and King, 1976).

Preston and Norgren (1971) have invented a centrifugal device for spreading blood on coverglasses. A coverglass is flooded with a layer of blood (either undiluted or diluted with 6% BSA) and then rotated in a plane parallel to the plane of rotation of the centrifuge about their common centers. The leukocyte differential counts are consistent in all regions of the coverglass. The number of broken or unknown cells is greatly reduced compared with smear preparations, and the leukocytes are well flattened by this procedure, which has made it possible to perform automated pattern recognition studies on blood (Ingram and Minter, 1969; Megla, 1973). Wolley *et al.*, (1976) have reported that this technique can be applied to cervicovaginal cells. However, the cells must be pelleted first and only one sample can be applied to each slide; thus this technique is not suitable for the preparation of fractions produced by cell separation procedures.

IV. CENTRIFUGAL CYTOLOGY

Centrifugal cytology (Leif *et al.*, 1971) is a new quantitative technique for producing glutaraldehyde-fixed dispersions of cells on conventional glass microscope slides or other substrates from dilute suspension. Although it was originally conceived for the sole purpose of analyzing buoyant density fractions, it has many applications for the preparation of fixed stained dispersions of cells on slides or other suitable surfaces, including cervical exfoliative cytology (Leif *et al.*, 1975a) and the dissociation of these cells for automated analysis (Leif *et al.*, 1977b), cell viability studies (Leif *et al.*, 1975b; Thornthwaite, 1974), high-resolution scanning electron microscopy (Goldman and Leif, 1973), and combined light and scanning electron microscopy (Thornthwaite *et al.*, 1976). It also has been possible with centrifugal cytology to produce fixed stained preparations,

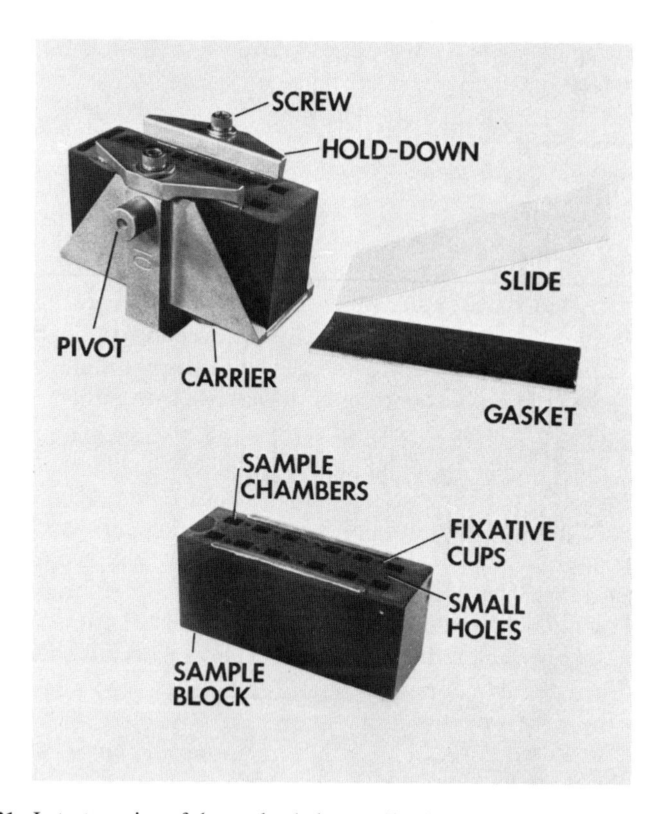

FIGURE 21. Latest version of the twelve-hole centrifugal cytology buckets. The completely assembled unit is shown upper left. The slide is placed on top of the intact gasket (upper right). The twelve-hole sample block is shown at the bottom. The glutaraldehyde fixative or D_2O–DMSO–saline are added to the fixative cups. The BSA-containing tissue culture medium or saline is withdrawn from the small holes. The use of this bucket should greatly facilitate the combined BSA-gradient/centrifugal-cytology studies where multiple underlayerings are necessary.

termed plaque cytogram assays, of specific types of cells involved in the immune response. A plaque cytogram assay has been developed for Jerne-plaque-forming cells (Thornthwaite and Leif, 1975; Leif *et al.*, 1975b) and allogeneic cytotoxic effector cells (Leif *et al.*, 1975b; Thornthwaite, 1977).

The latest version of the centrifugal cytology bucket (Leif *et al.*, 1977a) is described in Fig. 21. This design incorporates three major improvements over the previous model. (1) The distance from the pivots to the bottom has been lengthened by one inch; this increase in the moment arm improves the alignment with the centrifugal field and ensures that the buckets return to the vertical position when the centrifuge is stopped. (2) A new synthetic boundary valve overlayers the cells with fixative, producing very even dispersions of cells. This valve also eliminates the need for a special pipetting machine for the buckets; excess solution is removed via a small hole which accommodates a 20-gauge syringe needle and provides a fluid exit 1 mm above the slide. (3) The sample block hold-down mechanism has been redesigned to eliminate the removal of the tightening screws; pressure pads are now used instead to hold down the sample blocks. These pads rotate a full 180 degrees for removal of the sample block.

The bucket is assembled as follows (Fig. 21): a 3-in. gasket of 1-in. wide Scotch brand foam single-coated tape (1/16-in. thick, Cat. No. 4116; available from 3M Co., St. Paul, Minn. 55101) is placed backing-side-up on the flat surface of the aluminum carrier without peeling off the backing. On top of that is placed a plain, unfrosted glass microscope slide (prepared as described below). The gaskets (which do not stick to either surface) are replaced as needed, after every three uses approximately. The sample block is first pressed against an ink pad which has been lightly impregnated with Lubriseal stopcock grease (A. H. Thomas Co., Philadelphia, Pa.) and is then placed squarely upon the slide in order to avoid any smearing of the stopcock grease onto any areas of the slide which will subsequently be covered with cells. The hold-downs are now rotated 180° and the socket head screw tightened manually with the wrench (Fig. 21). It is advisable to retighten the screws after the initial centrifugation because it sometimes results in an irreversible compression of the gaskets. The bucket is disassembled in the reverse order. The screws are loosened, the hold-downs rotated 180°, and the sample block lifted straight up and out. Quite often the slide will remain attached by the grease seal to the sample block. This seal is easily broken by inserting the edge of a thin metal spatula between the slide and the sample block. Inversion of the sample block and slide prior to breaking the seal should be avoided. The sample blocks are cleaned by immersion in Zep detergent (Zep Mfg. Co., Hialeah, Fla.) in an ultrasonic cleaning bath (Heat Systems, Plainview, L.I., N.Y. 11803) and rinsed first in tap water for at least 5 min and then in distilled water for at least another 5 min.

Quantitative cell counts (Leif *et al.*, 1971) of known concentrations of blood cells have demonstrated that 89.2% of the cells are recovered in the mounted preparation. A reconstruction experiment utilizing various synthetic mixtures of human and tadpole blood cells established that there is no selection artifact in the ratio of these cells recovered on the entire slide nor any artifacts due to nondiscriminate cell placement. Cell size determinations of glutaraldehyde-fixed erythrocytes by both planimetry (Leif *et al.*, 1971) and electronic cell volume analysis (Thornthwaite *et al.*, 1978) indicate that 4% glutaraldehyde is approximately isosmotic.

The combined buoyant density-separation/centrifugal-cytology studies described below were performed with the predecessors of the present buckets and required the use of an elaborate and cumbersome multipipetting apparatus (Dunlap *et al.*, 1975) to underlayer the diluted BSA gradient medium with a 20% D_2O saline in order to avoid precipitation of the BSA by the glutaraldehyde fixative. The use of the new centrifugal cytology buckets which do not require the multipipetting apparatus will greatly facilitate this procedure.

The precise morphological assessment of the cells present in buoyant density fractions requires that the concentration of fixed stained cells present on the slide be controlled. This was accomplished by first counting the cells with a Coulter Counter and then diluting them according to a FORTRAN program (Dunlap *et al.*, 1975) which created a data table for looking up the appropriate dilutions. Today the use of a scientific hand calculator would be more reasonable. The cell concentration in the gradient (Cell conc) is calculated from the following equation:

$$\text{Cell conc} = 2(\text{Coulter counts} - \text{Bg}) \times \frac{\text{Vol. in vial}}{\text{Vol. of cell suspension}} \qquad (1)$$

where the factor of 2 is needed because the standard Coulter Counters employ a 0.5-ml manometer; Bg is the background obtained with the saline diluting solutions; "Vol. in vial" is the predetermined volume added to all the vials (usually 8–10 ml); and "Vol. of cell suspension" is the volume of each gradient fraction pipetted into the diluting vial. The last quantity can range from 0.010 to 0.150 ml and changes inversely with the concentration of cells in the gradient. It also is insignificant compared to the volume in the vial and thus has been omitted from the numerator of the preceding equation. If samples are counted sequentially, it is possible to anticipate these changes and to estimate the dilutions that will minimize coincidences and still permit a statistically valid count. The new AMAC sample valve described later in this chapter has been designed for this purpose. The volume of the cell suspension from the gradient which must be added to the diluting solution for each sample chamber (Vol. cent. cytol.) is

$$\text{Vol. cent. cytol.} = \frac{\text{Optimal counts per dispersion}}{\text{Cell conc.}} \qquad (2)$$

Combining the two equations:

$$\text{Vol. cent. cytol.} = \frac{\text{Optimal counts per dispersion}}{2(\text{Coulter counts} - \text{Bg})} \times \frac{\text{Vol. of cell suspension}}{\text{Vol. in vial}} \qquad (3)$$

For each dilution the two variables are the "Coulter counts" and the "Vol. of cell suspension."

Another constraint on the dilution is the requirement that the BSA concentration should never exceed 5% after dilution for centrifugal cytol-

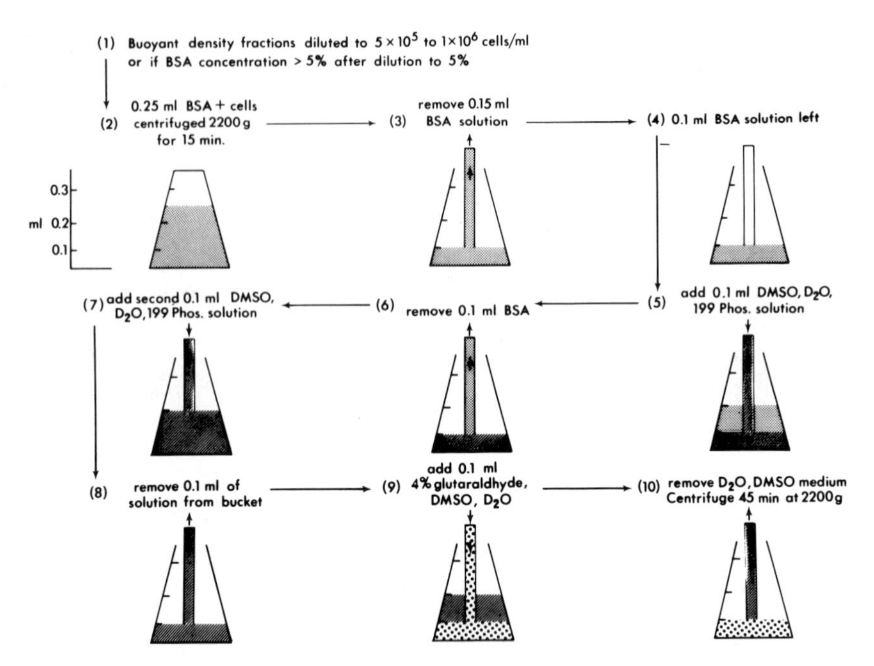

FIGURE 22. Diagram of the underlayering and fixation procedure. Bovine serum albumin fractions are first diluted to the desired concentration of cells (not to exceed a concentration of 5% BSA). After being loaded into the cytology buckets, the cell suspension is centrifuged for 15 min. Then 0.15 ml of the BSA solution is removed, as shown in step 3, leaving 0.1 ml BSA solution in the bucket (step 4), and 0.1 ml D_2O tissue culture medium is layered under this (step 5). In step 6, 0.1 ml of the BSA solution is removed at the interface; the cycle is repeated as shown in steps 7 and 8. After a 5-min centrifugation the glutaraldehyde solution is layered under the D_2O tissue culture medium (step 9), and the latter is removed at the interface (step 10).

ogy and preferably should be less than or equal to 4%. Even with the special manipulations described below, higher concentrations of BSA will result in a protein precipitate that obscures the cells.

As shown in Fig. 22, 0.25 to 1.00 ml of a cell suspension containing 12,500 to 250,000 cells as determined above are added to each of the twelve chambers of the centrifugal cytology rotor and then sedimented onto a slide at 2200*g* for 15 min. To remove the albumin which would normally be precipitated by the glutaraldehyde fixative, the cells are then overlayed with D_2O–dimethyl sulfoxide (DMSO) tissue culture medium (70% phosphate-buffered tissue culture medium, 20% D_2O and 10% DMSO by volume). This medium was underlayered twice beneath the BSA-containing tissue culture medium, which was removed each time. After a second such centrifugation, the cells are overlayed with a 4% glutaraldehyde solution containing 12% DMSO and 0.1% BSA. At present the 4% glutaraldehyde is buffered with 0.05 M Na cacodylate, brought up to pH 7.4 with 2 M HCl and containing 20% D_2O and 12% DMSO. The synthetic boundary valve and small liquid removal hole of the present centrifugal cytology bucket will greatly facilitate and expedite this procedure.

The final centrifugation with the fixative is 45 min. at 2200*g* at room temperature.

V. THE ISOLATION OF HETEROAGGLUTINATES

A. Introduction

If two cell types are allowed to interact with certain agglutinating agents (viruses, antibodies, or polymers), complex formation will be induced, as in the case of the ascites cells and erythrocytes. Because the two types of cells differ in buoyant density, only the complexes containing both kinds of cells would be expected to differ in buoyant density from the parental and self-agglutinated cells. In a gradient these heteroagglutinates would locate themselves at a unique position between the parental cells depending on the number and types of cells involved (Fig. 23). The self-agglutinated and nonagglutinated parental cells will be found at their original densities (Fig. 23). The density of the agglutinates will be determined

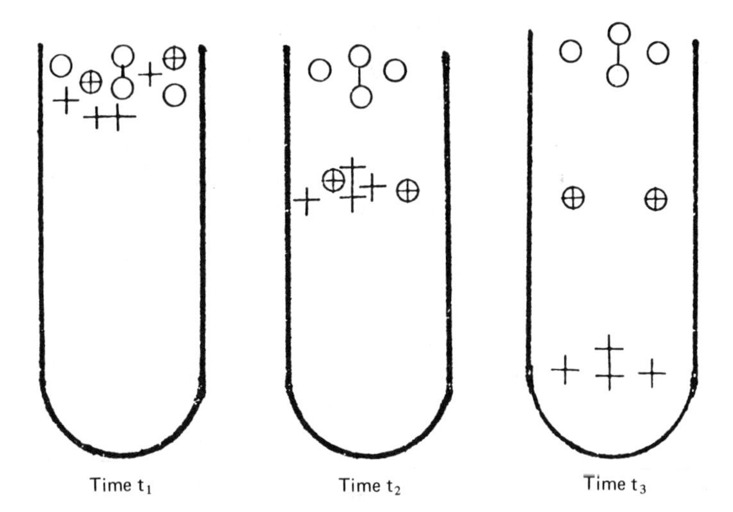

FIGURE 23. An idealized representation of the manner in which heteroagglutinated cells will distribute themselves in a BSA density gradient. The parental cell types (○ and +) and their respective homoagglutinates (○–○ and + +) sediment to their respective densities. Heteroagglutinates (⊕) composed of one cell from each parental type sediment to an intermediate density described by equation 7. It may be seen that cell complexes made up of different ratios of parental cells will sediment to a distinct and unique buoyant density due to the magnitudes of the specific volumes and buoyant densities of their various cellular components.

by the volume and mass fractions derived from each of the original cells. For instance, defining ρ_h as the buoyant density of the hybrid heteroagglutinates,

$$\rho_h = (M_1 + M_2)/(V_1 + V_2) \tag{4}$$

where M_1 and M_2 are respectively the total mass of the parental cells, and V_1 and V_2 are respectively the original volume of the parental cells combining to form the heteroagglutinates; and

$$M_1 = V_1\rho_1 \tag{5}$$

and

$$M_2 = V_2\rho_2 \tag{6}$$

where ρ_1 and ρ_2 are respectively the original densities of the parental cells. Combining Equations 1, 2, and 3,

$$\rho_h = (V_1\rho_1 + V_2\rho_2)/(V_1 + V_2) \tag{7}$$

Equation 7 shows, as stated above, that the effective buoyant density of a cell aggregate may be found from the density and specific volume of its cellular components. It should be distinct from that of the parental cell types and their homoagglutinates, which have densities identical to the parental cell types. Thus it should be possible to separate these aggregates on either step or continuous linear density gradients (Fig. 23).

B. Neutral Density Separations

In the initial experiments (Fig. 24), the two cell populations, the ascites cells and the erythrocytes, were found to have densities of approximately 1.070 to 1.075 g cm^{-3} and 1.045 to 1.055 g cm^{-3}, respectively; but while the erythrocyte distribution is very sharp, that of the ascites cells is usually broadened. The denser portion of the ascites population extends well into the regions between the two cell population peaks. As the heteroagglutinated cells were expected to fall between the two bands, it was necessary to reduce the ascites population by means of neutral density experiments to densities of less than 1.0495 g cm^{-3}, and thus to increase the volume of gradient separating the ascites cells from the erythrocytes.

The crude cell suspensions were washed twice with 199-P with Ca^{2+} and Mg^{2+} and pelleted at the bottom of 15-ml plastic graduated cylindrical test tubes. The supernate above this pellet was collected with a Pasteur pipette and discarded. Approximately one ml of BSA-B (density 1.0509 g cm^{-3}) was layered over the cell pellet and the cells resuspended by light vortexing. More BSA solution (enough to obtain a volume of liquid four to five times that of the original cell pellet) was then added and adequate mixing of cells was assured by passage of the cell suspension through a Pasteur pipet five to six times. The BSA solutions were then centrifuged for 15 min at approximately 3000 rpm × 1000*g* at 4°C. The light portion of ascites cells, which floated to the top of the BSA solution and formed an interface with the BSA, was collected, while the pellet and media were discarded. Typically the collected ascites cells were washed one or two times in 199-P with Ca^{2+} and Mg^{2+} and counted with the Coulter B Counter.

This "light" fraction of the ascites population has an increased tendency toward agglutination when exposed to hen erythrocytes with adsorbed virus (Warters and Leif, unpubl.; Warters, 1972). The amount of dense ascites contamination (cells with densities greater than 1.0495 g cm^{-3}) has been found to be very small after one such neutral density separation (see further on).

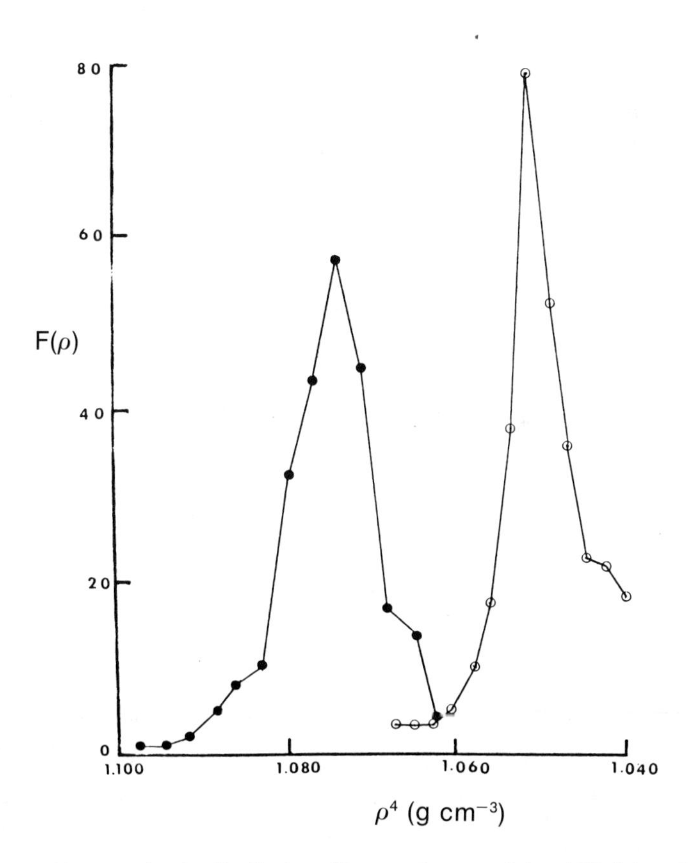

FIGURE 24. Buoyant density distribution of hen erythrocytes (•) and Ehrlich ascites tumor cells (○).

C. Control Experiment

The buoyant density fractions were prepared by centrifugal cytology and the hemoglobin stained by benzidine. The cells were counted and enumerated as described in the figure captions.

The control experiment, depicted in Figs. 25a,b,c, demonstrates a

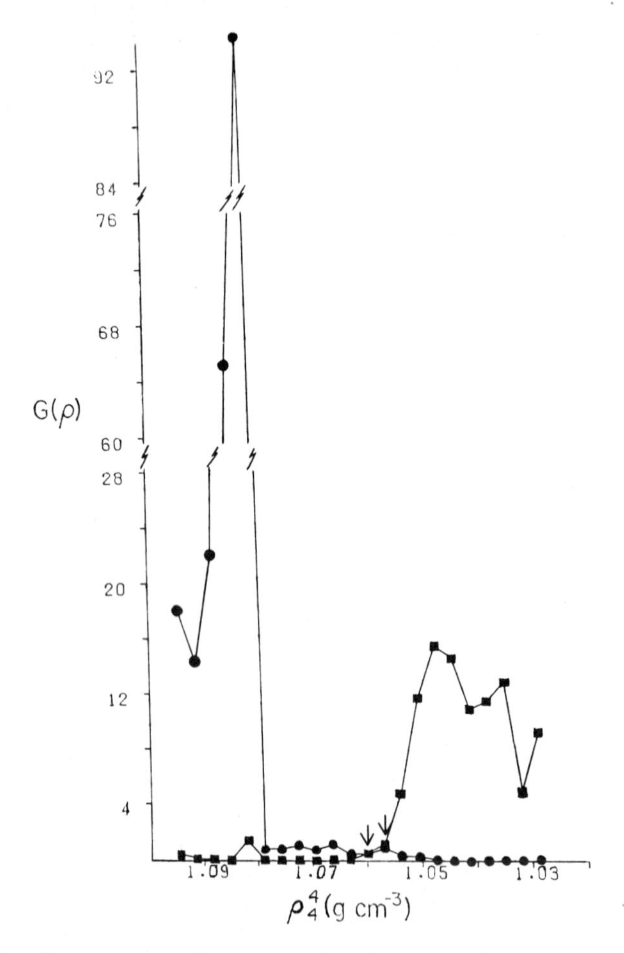

FIGURE 25a. Buoyant density distributions of single ascites cells (■) and single hen erythrocytes (•) in control experiment 111B. The cells were not virus treated. The gradient material was recovered as described under section VD. The function graphed as ordinate is the density distribution function $G(\rho)$, where $G(\rho)$ = (1/sum of ascites + erythrocytes) × (ascites or erythrocytes found in a fraction)/$\Delta\rho$. The denominator of the first term is the sum of the single ascites cells and hen erythrocytes recovered from the gradient and the numerator of the second term represents the number of single ascites cells or hen erythrocytes at a given buoyant density ρ. Arrows indicate the fractions referred to in Table 3.

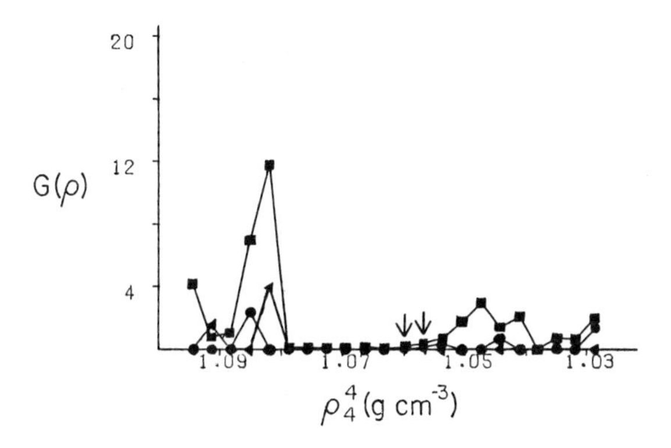

FIGURE 25b. Buoyant density distributions of heteroagglutinated ascites–hen-erythrocytes (AR, ■), ascites–ascites–erythrocytes (AAR, ●), and ascites–erythrocytes–erythrocytes (ARR, ▲) in control experiment 111B. The cells were not virus treated. The function graphed as ordinate is the density distribution function $G(\rho)$, where $G(\rho)$ = (1/sum of the agglutinates) × (AR, AAR, or ARR)/$\Delta\rho$. The denominator of the first term is the sum of all the agglutinated cell types recovered from the gradient and the numerator of the second term represents the number of agglutinates of a specific type at a given buoyant density ρ. Arrows indicate fractions referred to in Table 3.

generally sharp separation of both parental and non-virus-agglutinated cells. It is clear that these ascites cell populations made "light" by neutral density separations with BSA of density 1.0495 g cm^{-3} demonstrate band centers for both the single cells and the background agglutinated cells at densities from 1.040 to 1.045 g cm^{-3}, typically with few cells seen at

TABLE 3
Comparison of Fractions Containing the Largest Percent Yield of Heteroagglutinates

Exp. no.	Number of heteroag-glutinates in best 2 adjacent fractions (×10^3)	Density of fraction	% Heteroag-glutinates	% Heteroag-glutinates of total agglutinates	Total number of cells recovered from gradient (×10^6)
111	3.5	1.0599	1.6	80	36.7
Control	7.4	1.0568	1.3	100	
(linear gradient)					
108	571	1.0538	22.83	83	22.3
Virus	427	1.0491	29.34	89	
(linear gradient)					
109	398	1.0621	18.41	85	22.2
Virus	366	1.0555	7.63	85	
(linear gradient)					
Virus	140	1.0508–.0550	10.00	33	50.9
(step gradient)	270	1.0550–.0698	20.00	59	50.9

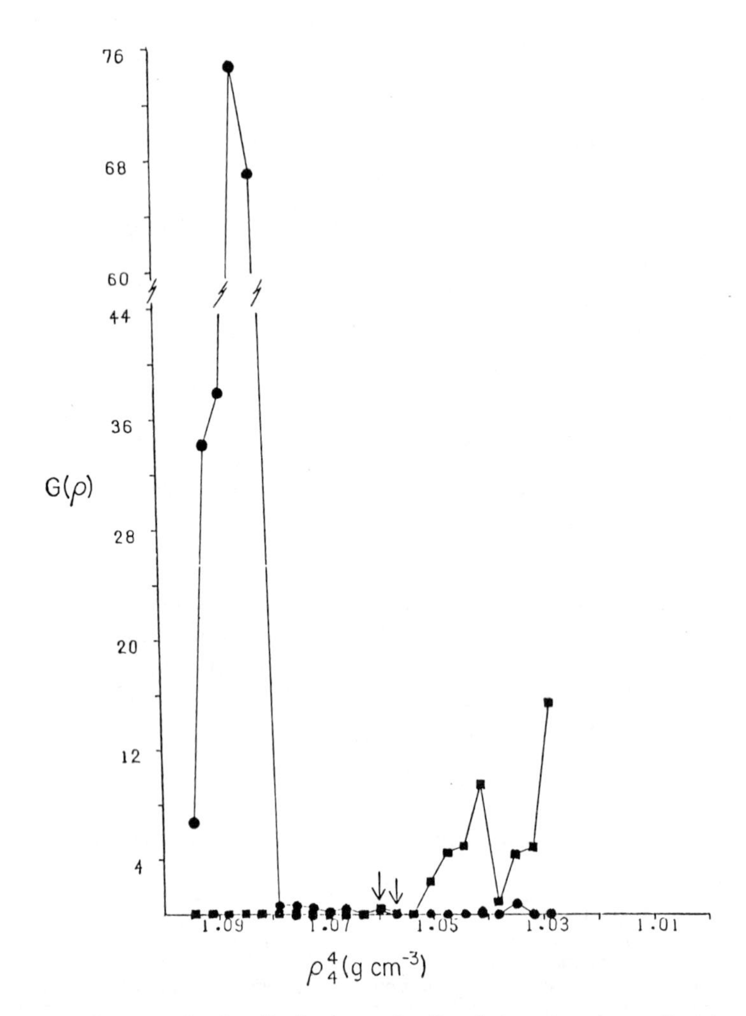

FIGURE 25c. Buoyant density distributions of self-agglutinated ascites cells (■) or hen erythrocytes (RBC, •) in control experiment 111B. The cells were not virus treated. The function graphed as ordinate is the density distribution function $G(\rho)$, where $G(\rho)$ = (1/sum of the agglutinates) × (AA or RR)/ρ. The denominator of the first term is the sum of all the agglutinated cell types recovered from the gradient and the second represents the number of agglutinates of a specific type (either ascites homoagglutinates or hen erythrocyte homoagglutinates in this case) at a given buoyant density ρ. Arrows indicate fractions referred to in Table 3.

densities greater than 1.050 g cm^{-3}. However, the distributions of these cell populations are not sharp; a neutral density procedure is not intended to produce a sharp cellular distribution but primarily to insure the removal of all cells with densities less than or, as in this case, greater than a given density. The background between the peaks is predominantly due to single hen erythrocytes which represent a very small fraction of the total number of erythrocytes. Very little background contamination from heteroagglutinated cells occurs in regions between the parental bands (Fig. 25b, Table 3); the majority fall under the peaks of the parental cells. This phenomenon is caused by an artifact inherent in the differential counting. It would be expected that there would be a very small background in those fractions containing principally either erythrocytes or ascites cells. However, if even a small percentage of background is found in such fractions, the total number of background cells computed will overshadow the number found in fractions containing considerably fewer cells. This is believed to be the case in these experiments. Due to the very large number of cells of either parental type in their respective bands and the much smaller number of cells found between these bands, any background within the parental bands will be greatly overestimated, overshadowing the lesser number of real heteroagglutinated cells found between the parental bands.

D. Method of Cell Agglutination

Hen erythrocytes were diluted to a concentration of approximately 3 to 5 $\times$ 10^7 cell per milliliter, and one milliliter was placed in a 15-ml plastic graduated test tube. The cells were pelleted and then added to a Sendai virus suspension. The volume of suspending medium varied slightly with the amount of virus used in a particular experiment; for instance, 3 $\times$ 10^7 cells were resuspended with 2000 HAU (hemagglutinating units) Sendai virus to give ½ ml of total suspending volume. The erythrocytes were incubated at 4°C with virus for 15 min, pelleted, and the supernatant discarded; they were then resuspended in ½ to 1 ml of a suspension of Ehrlich ascites cells containing 1.5 to 2.5 $\times$ 10^7 cells per milliliter. The mixture was incubated 15 to 30 min at 4°C with periodic shaking to allow agglutination prior to use.

E. Gradient Separation of the Heteroagglutinates

Since the volume between the ascites and the erythrocytes was expected to contain the heteroagglutinates, the conventional gradient separation was compared with a step gradient procedure. The conventional

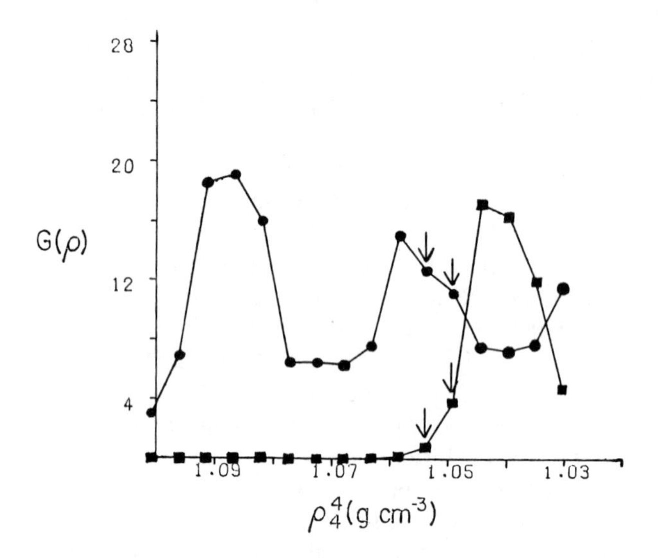

FIGURE 26a. Buoyant density distributions of single ascites cells (■) and single hen erythrocytes (●) in experiment 108B. These cells were exposed to virus as described in section VD. The function graphed as the ordinate is described in Fig. 25a. Arrows indicate fractions used in Table 3.

gradients (Fig. 26a,b,c,) demonstrate relatively sharp distributions, and thus relatively clean separations, of ascites cells and ascites homoagglutinates. The distribution of erythrocytes and erythrocyte agglutinates, however, shows a very pronounced broadening as compared to the control. A second peak of erythrocytes is found in the region of the heteroagglutinates

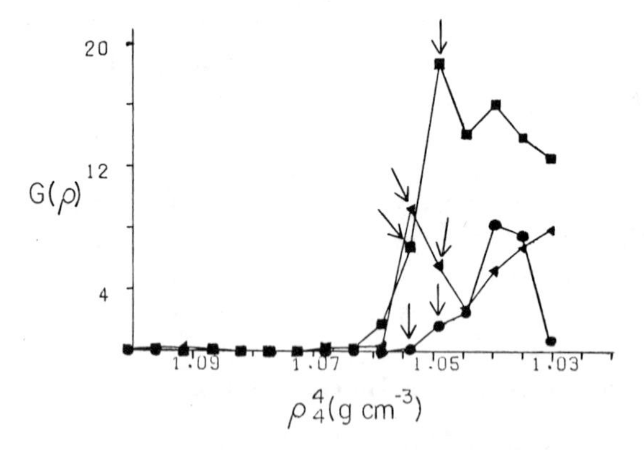

FIGURE 26b. Buoyant density distribution of heteroagglutinated ascites cells and erythrocytes (AR, ■; AAR, ●; ARR, ◀) in experiment 108B. These cells were exposed to virus as described in section VD. The function graphed as ordinate is described in Fig. 25b. Arrows indicate fractions used in Table 3.

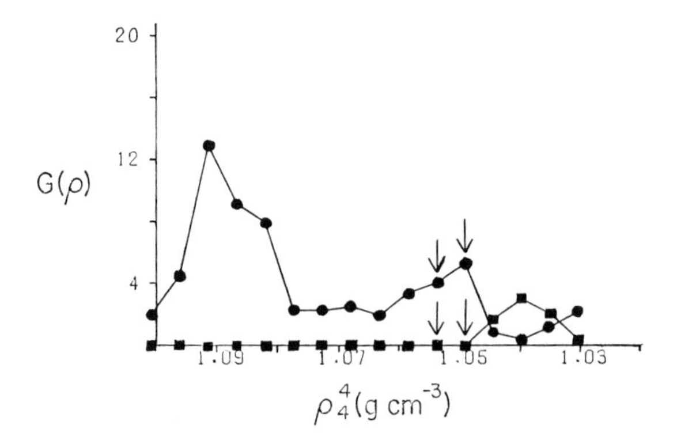

FIGURE 26c. Buoyant density distributions of self-agglutinated ascites cells (■) or hen erythrocytes (•) in experiment 108B. These cells were exposed to virus as described in section VD. The function graphed as ordinate is described in Fig. 25c. Arrows indicate fractions used in Table 3.

and the ascites cells. A small part of this background of erythrocytes, as noted above, can be explained by the wall effect, but not the peaks of erythrocytes found at densities less than typical for these cells, for instance at 1.055 to 1.060 g cm^{-3}. To determine the number of cells which deviate from what is expected, one may extrapolate the expected smooth curve from the one obtained experimentally and compare the two.

In the five fractions between densities of 1.040 and 1.055 g cm^{-3} of gradient 108B, there are approximately 2×10^6 more erythrocytes than would be encountered were the distribution smooth, or $1/7$ of the total number of erythrocytes applied to the gradient. These extra cells make up almost a third of the total cell types in these fractions. Gradient 109B contains 1.6×10^6 of these cells, or about 10% of the number of erythrocytes applied to the gradient and as much as $1/6$ of the total cells in these fractions. This contamination of the less dense regions of the gradient by erythrocytes may be explained by three non-mutually-exclusive possibilities: breakup of the heteroagglutinates during centrifugation, or when the cells were pumped out of the gradient, or during centrifugal cytology. Centrifugal cytology involves no shear forces; very large aggregates which are easily broken up by syringing, have been found still intact (Leif *et al.*, 1977b), We conclude, therefore, that the contribution of this last possibility to the breakup of the heteroagglutinates is minimal. It would also be improbable for the action of the peristaltic pump to be selective in breaking up only the heteroagglutinates in the less dense ascites band; the ascites homoagglutinates which are larger particles, should logically be more sensitive to the shear gradient than are the heteroagglutinates—and the peristaltic pump propels a bolus of liquid between the rollers which is subject to a minimal shear gradient. However, it is possible that some dissociation of the heteroagglutinates occurred during removal of the gradient. In addition, since preliminary experiments demonstrated that the yield of these virus-induced heteroagglutinates decreased with increasing centrifugal force, it must be presumed that centrifugation can break them up.

The three types of heteroagglutinates are the one-to-one heteroagglutinates of an Ehrlich ascites cell (A) and a hen erythrocyte (R), designated AR; the heteroagglutinates which contain two ascites cells and one erythrocyte designated AAR; and one ascites cell and two erythrocytes, ARR. The distribution of the one-to-one heteroagglutinates (AR) peaks just below the ascites distribution and continues into it. The ARR band peak is in the next denser fraction and the AAR band in the second less dense fraction. Approximately 10% and 14% of the total cells recovered on experiments 108 and 109B were heteroagglutinates. These values are somewhat greater than the values expected. In the two best fractions of these experiments (Table 3), yields of approximately 29% and 18% were obtained; this table also shows the total number of heteroagglutinates found in this fraction, the density of the fraction, the percent of heteroagglutinates found, and the percentage of the agglutinates which are heteroagglutinates. Expanded differential counts of these fractions of greater interest are included in Table 4.

One of the major reasons that the technique is successful is that the homoagglutinates, especially the ascites cells, are very thoroughly eliminated from the region between the parental cells (Fig. 26c). The percentage of the total agglutinates which were heteroagglutinates ranged between 83% and 89%. The heterokaryocytes which form at 37°C are larger than the parental cells, and since these are homogeneous density cuts, velocity separation which is based only on the combination of size and shape should then be sufficient to produce virtually pure fractions of heterokaryocytes. The heterokaryocytes can be readily identified in centrifugal cytology preparations since they are large cells which often stain for hemoglobin (Fig. 27) and contain two morphologically distinguishable nuclei.

A step gradient was attempted in order to compare the results with the linear gradient separation. A cell suspension composed of hen erythrocytes and the "less dense" ascites cells was exposed to 6000 HAU of virus and suspended in a BSA solution of density 1.0508 g cm^{-3}. This cell suspension was layered over a step gradient composed of three additional BSA shelves with densities of 1.0550, 1.0698, and 1.0800 g cm^{-3} respectively. Above the cell suspension layer was added a layer of phosphate-buffered saline (Dulbecco). The step gradient was centrifuged for 10 min at 3000 rpm at 4°C, and four fractions were taken. Fraction one was composed of the top PBS layer containing any cells which had floated upward from the original BSA cell suspension. The second, third, and fourth fractions were composed of the BSA layers having densities of 1.0508, 1.0555, and 1.0698 g cm^{-3}

TABLE 4
Expanded Differential Counts of Fractions Utilized in Table 3[a]

Exp. no.[b]	Density	A	AA	AR	AAR	ARR	RR	R	Total	Agglutinates[c] % Hetero	Agglutinates[c] % Homo
111	1.0599	461	2	7	2			312	789	1.1	0.3
Control	1.0568	620	9	5	2			40	676	1.0	1.3
108	1.0538	105	1	134	15	42	35	313	645	29.6	5.6
Virus	1.0491	464	14	105	19	21	6	201	830	18.0	2.4
109	1.0621	370	8	110	17	10	17	212	744	18.4	3.4
Virus	1.0555	460	5	46	8	1	2	199	721	7.6	1.0

[a]The counts were expanded for greater statistical accuracy. It was found that these counts were approximately identical to the nonexpanded counts.
[b]All gradients are linear.
[c]Out of total cells found.

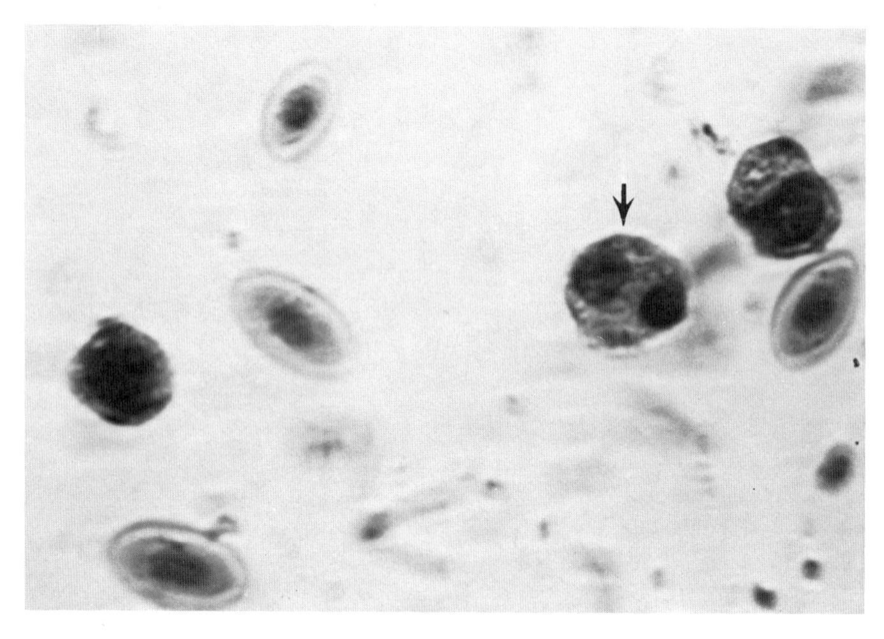

FIGURE 27. Centrifugal cytology preparation of virus-agglutinated cells which have fused on the microscope slides. The oval cells are hen erythrocytes; the round mononucleate cells are Ehrlich ascites cells, and the binucleate cell (arrow) is a hemoglobin-containing heterokaryon.

respectively. Complete recovery of each layer necessarily resulted in a small amount of contamination by the underlying layer.

This step gradient separation of a cell suspension did result in some purification of the heteroagglutinated cells. Table 5 shows that cells generally distributed themselves as equation 7 predicts. The single ascites cells and ascites self-agglutinates (having densities effectively identical to the parental ascites cells) were found in the top two fractions at densities less than 1.0508 g cm^{-3}. The single erythrocytes and erythrocyte self-agglutinates were found predominately in the bottom two fractions at densities greater than 1.0698 g cm^{-3}. The heteroagglutinates composed of two ascites cells and one erythrocyte (AAR) or of two hen erythrocytes and one ascites cell (ARR) were found in the middle two fractions and the bottom two fractions respectively. The heteroagglutinates composed of one ascites cell and one erythrocyte (AR) were found throughout the entire gradient.

Although no single type of heteroagglutinates showed a clear separation, there was a pronounced tendency for similar types to cluster and to separate from parental types. There was a maximum 2.5 $\times$ increase in purity of heteroagglutinated cells by this technique. However, the two intermediate density steps yielded only 33% and 59% compared to the 83–

TABLE 5
Results of Exposure of Agglutinated Cells to a BSA Step Gradient[a]

	Fraction no.			
	1	2	3	4
Density	1.0508	1.0508–1.0550	1.0550–1.0698	1.0698
Total number of cells	13×10^6	1.5×10^6	1.4×10^6	35×10^6
Percent of total cells	25.00	3.00	3.00	69.00
Percent of cells in each fraction found as heteroagglutinates	3.30	9.33	19.2	0.30
Total number of heteroagglutinates	4×10^5	1.4×10^5	2.7×10^5	1×10^5
Total number of homoagglutinates	4×10^6	3×10^5	2×10^5	6×10^6
Percent of agglutinates in each fraction found as:				
AA	90	66	22	0
AR	4	14	33	2
AAR	6	19	15	0
ARR	0	0	10	0
RR	0	1	19	98
Percent of heteroagglutinates in each fraction found as:				
AR	41	42	56	52
AAR	59	58	26	5
ARR	0	0	18	43

[a]The step gradient was centrifuged for 10 min at 3000 rpm at 4°C.

89% for the linear gradient of the agglutinates as heteroagglutinates, indicating that the linear gradients have a much higher degree of resolution. However in retrospect in this case, since the density of the cells is known, the optimum gradient procedure would be first to employ a rapid step gradient to eliminate the vast majority of the parental cells and homoagglutinates and then to use a linear gradient to separate out the heteroagglutinates from the other cells.

VI. COMBINED BSA GRADIENT CENTRIFUGAL CYTOLOGY STUDIES

In addition to the isolation of the heterokaryon precursors described above, studies have been performed on guinea pig bone marrow, chicken erythrocytes, bovine pituitary, and Jerne-plaque-forming cells.

Approximately 40 cell types were observed in guinea pig bone marrow (Leif *et al.*, 1975c). Cells with definitive morphologies such as erythrocytes, the neutrophilic series (Fig. 28), the binucleate blast megakaryocyte precursors, and cells in mitosis banded as virtually single peaks. Cells

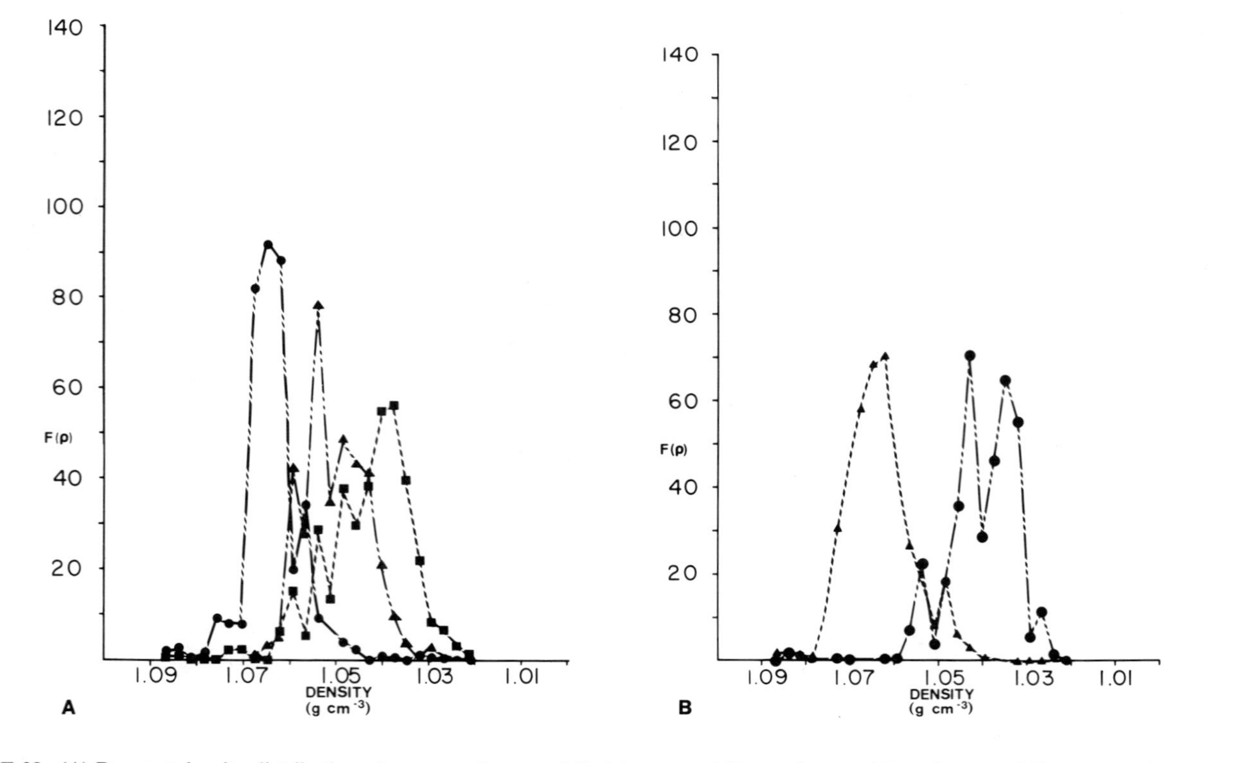

FIGURE 28. (A) Buoyant density distribution of segmented neutrophils (●), neutrophilic myelocytes (■), and neutrophilic metamyelocytes (▲). (B) Buoyant density distribution of progranulocytes (●) and neutrophilic band cells (▲).

TABLE 6
[^{3}H]Thymidine Incorporation into DNA during Erythroid Cell Development (Bone Marrow)

Gradient area pooled	Cell stages found	Density range	Number of cells (× 10^8)	cpm in DNA	cpm/10^8 cells
Top layer	Immature erythroblasts	1.03–1.05	2.6	4890	1880
Medium layer	Late erythroblasts and polychromatic erythrocytes	1.05–1.07	4.1	7123	1737
Bottom layer	Reticulocytes and mature erythrocytes	1.07–1.09	3.8	1097	289

which were parts of continua or could easily be misclassified were found in multiple peaks. The small lymphocytes which are known to be polydisperse were found as five peaks. This distribution of erythroblasts was complex due either to the very strong benzidine staining by the glutaraldehyde-fixed hemoglobin, which resulted in some of the erythroblasts being wrongly staged, or to the presence of a separate population of macrocytes. In any event two separate bands of hemoglobin-containing cells were very often observed on the gradients. In general, the rule that the younger cells are always less dense than the mature cells was followed. These results were our first indication that morphology is a good first approximation of reality.

Buoyant density studies of chicken blood and bone marrow cells, in collaboration with Drs. Cieplinski and Huang of the Johns Hopkins University, resulted in the separation of these cells according to age. The individual fractions were pooled into three major fractions containing respectively from top to bottom, the very immature cells, the intermediate cells including the polychromatic erythrocyte stage, and the reticulocytes and mature erythrocytes. Viability of the cells was conserved and useful studies of isotope incorporation to study histone biosynthesis were performed at all stages; histone V did not appear until the intermediate cell stage and was then present in all later stages (Cieplinski, 1972; Cieplinski *et al.* unpubl.). DNA synthesis was measured by [^{3}H]thymidine incorporation (Table 6). These studies make it possible to study the function of histone V and the possibility of correlation with the control of hemoglobin gene transcription and with the process of heterochromatinization.

The distribution of pituitary cells in the gradient was monitored by centrifugal cytology for morphology and by radioimmune assay for specific hormone content. These studies (Hirsch *et al.*, 1979) demonstrated that when cells can be identified both in terms of morphology and specific hormone content by radioimmune assay and fluorescent antibody staining, the two distributions always agree on the major morphology peak (Fig. 29). However, the buoyant density distributions of the hormones were truly unimodal and were usually narrower than the distribution obtained by morphology, which often contained shoulders at either end of the distribution. The main morphological peaks always overlapped the radioimmune distribution.

These studies were made possible by the development of a special procedure for dissociating the bovine pituitary into single cells. The procedure was as follows: The pituitary glands were sectioned at 225 μm with a Smith Farquhar Tissue Slicer. This greatly increased the surface area of the tissues available to enzyme action while damaging only approximately 10% of the cells. The washed slices were then suspended in a 6-ml cold enzyme mixture which contained trypsin and pancreatin and placed in a special

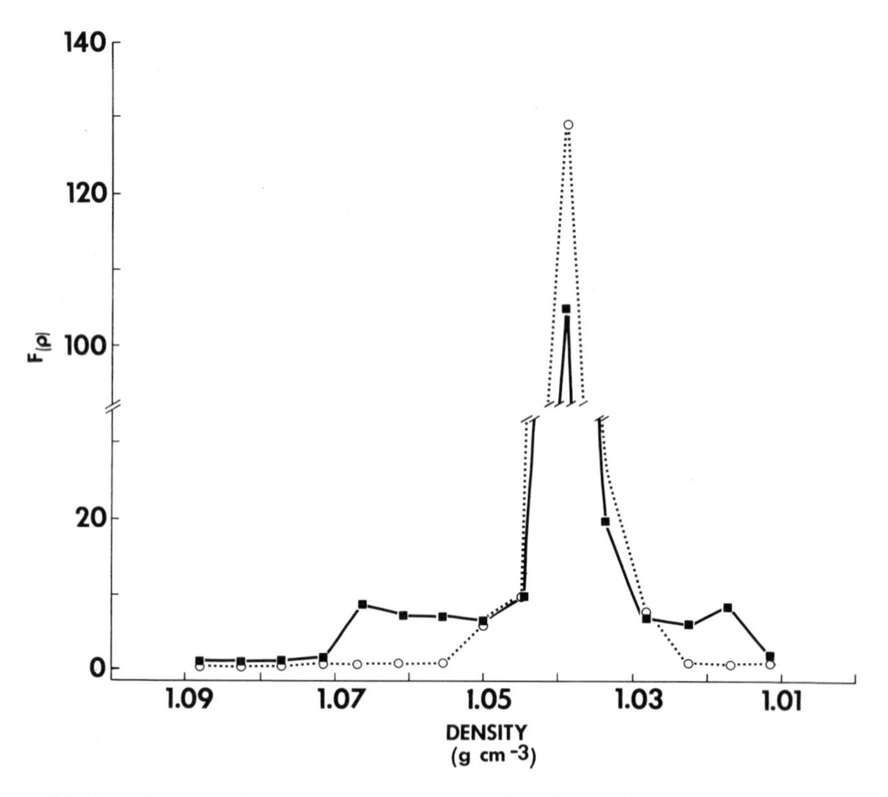

FIGURE 29. Buoyant density of bovine pituitary gland. Follicle-stimulating-hormone-producing cells as determined by morphology (■) and radioimmune assay (○). Notice that the outlying shoulders in the morphology distribution are not found in the radioimmune assay distribution.

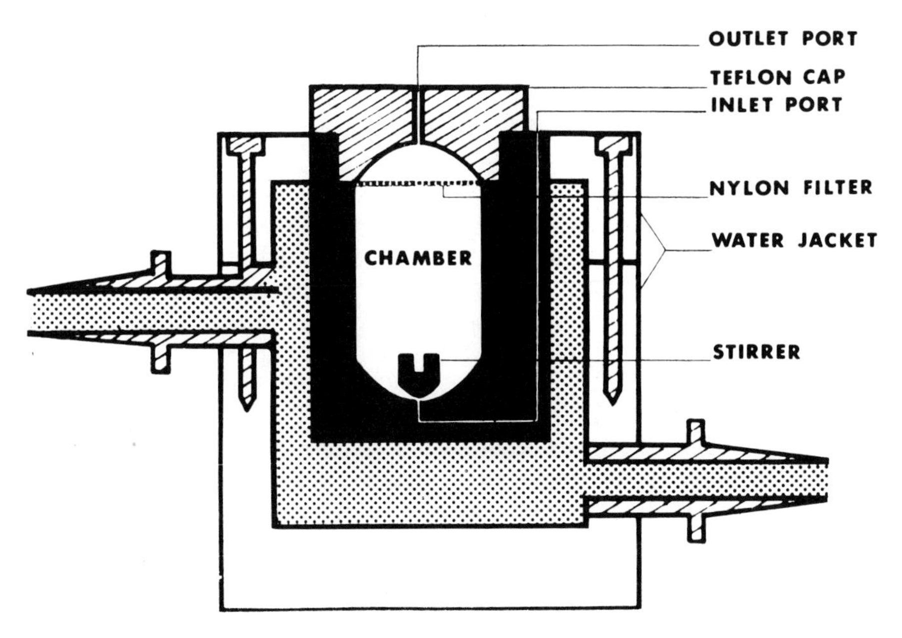

FIGURE 30. Continuous-flow tissue dissociation chamber. The conical Lexan chamber (9 ml volume) has an inlet port on the bottom and an overflow port located on the parabolic-shaped Teflon cap. Incoming enzyme solutions flow around a Teflon magnetic centrifugal spectrophotometer cell stirrer which provides vertical and horizontal mixing with a minimum of vortexing; centrifugal pumping action generated by the cross channels (in the upper face of the stirrer) mixes without aeration. The continuous upward fluid flow causes dispersed cells and small clumps of cells to float up and out of the chamber. A 149-μm nylon monofilament screen placed across the top of the chamber prevents large cell clumps and tissue fragments from escaping and clogging the outlet port. The cells may be pumped from one chamber directly into another chamber or into tissue culture media which can contain enzyme inhibitors. Kel-F tubing (0.040 in. o.d.) can be used to interconnect several chambers or directly connect a chamber to a pump. Constant temperature of the incubation vessel is maintained by a water jacket surrounding the vessel. The rate of fluid flow through the chamber can be controlled either by a peristaltic or an infusion pump.

continuous-flow dispersal chamber preheated to 37°C (Fig. 30). A mixture of DNase and RNase was added to the suspension. A Teflon magnetic stirrer was placed in the chamber and a 149-μm nylon monofilament "Nytex" screen was placed across the top of the chamber before the system was sealed with the parabolic Teflon cap. Kel-F tubing was connected to the inlet and outlet parts of the chamber. The trypsin-pancreatin enzyme mixture was placed in a syringe and pumped through a 0.22-μm Millipore filter at 0.5 ml/min into the inlet part of the dissociation chamber

Every 8 min, the nuclease medium which was presumably digested by the proteolytic enzymes was replenished. The effluent of the chamber, which consisted of cell aggregates less than 150 μm was collected in cold saline. The entire procedure usually took less than 40 min. Since the small aggregates were collected and chilled virtually immediately after they crossed the Nytex cloth, the period of actual contact of the cells with the proteolytic enzymes was minimized. The dispersed cell clumps were washed by centrifugation to remove the proteolytic enzymes and finally dissociated with a mixture of collagenase and hyaluronidase in the continuous-flow dissociation chamber. Incubation was performed at 20°C for 20 min; the monodisperse cells were again collected in the cold (4°C) and washed to remove any residual enzymes. The cells were now ready for subsequent experimentation.

This sequential enzymatic dissociation utilized the "hard" enzymes such as trypsin to break up the slices and the "soft" enzymes collagenase and hyaluronidase to produce the monodisperse cell suspension. The separation of the steps eliminated the problem of the trypsin digesting the soft enzymes.

Thornthwaite and Leif (1974) described a method for preparing fixed stained dispersions of plaque-forming and rosette-forming cells using centrifugal cytology (plaque cytogram assays). Both light and scanning electron microscopy studies demonstrate that both of these types of cells are pleomorphic. Also, three different types of plaques and rosettes were described. One very interesting finding of this study is that plaque-forming cells which produce hemolytic antibody have smooth surfaces and rosette-forming cells are rough-surfaced or have microvilli. Since antibody-forming cells are B cells and the other cells are presumably T cells, this result is a counterexample to the results of Polliack *et al.* (1973). However, our source of cells was spleen rather than blood, and the animal was mouse rather than human. Human T lymphocytes which form rosettes with sheep erythrocytes also have numerous microvilli.

In a subsequent study (Thornthwaite and Leif, 1975), the plaque cytogram assay for Jerne-plaque-forming cells (PFCs) was combined with linear BSA gradients to show the correlation between the morphology and buoyant density of immunocompetent cells. Ten types of PFCs (Fig. 31) and four types of plaques have been identified and enriched in the density gradients. This combined buoyant-density/morphology study verified that both the observed pleomorphism of the plaque-forming cells and the density heterogeneity previously reported by Williams and Shortman (1972) were real. Reproducible density profiles of mouse erythrocytes, lymphoid cells, and PFCs were also obtained in these BSA gradient studies.

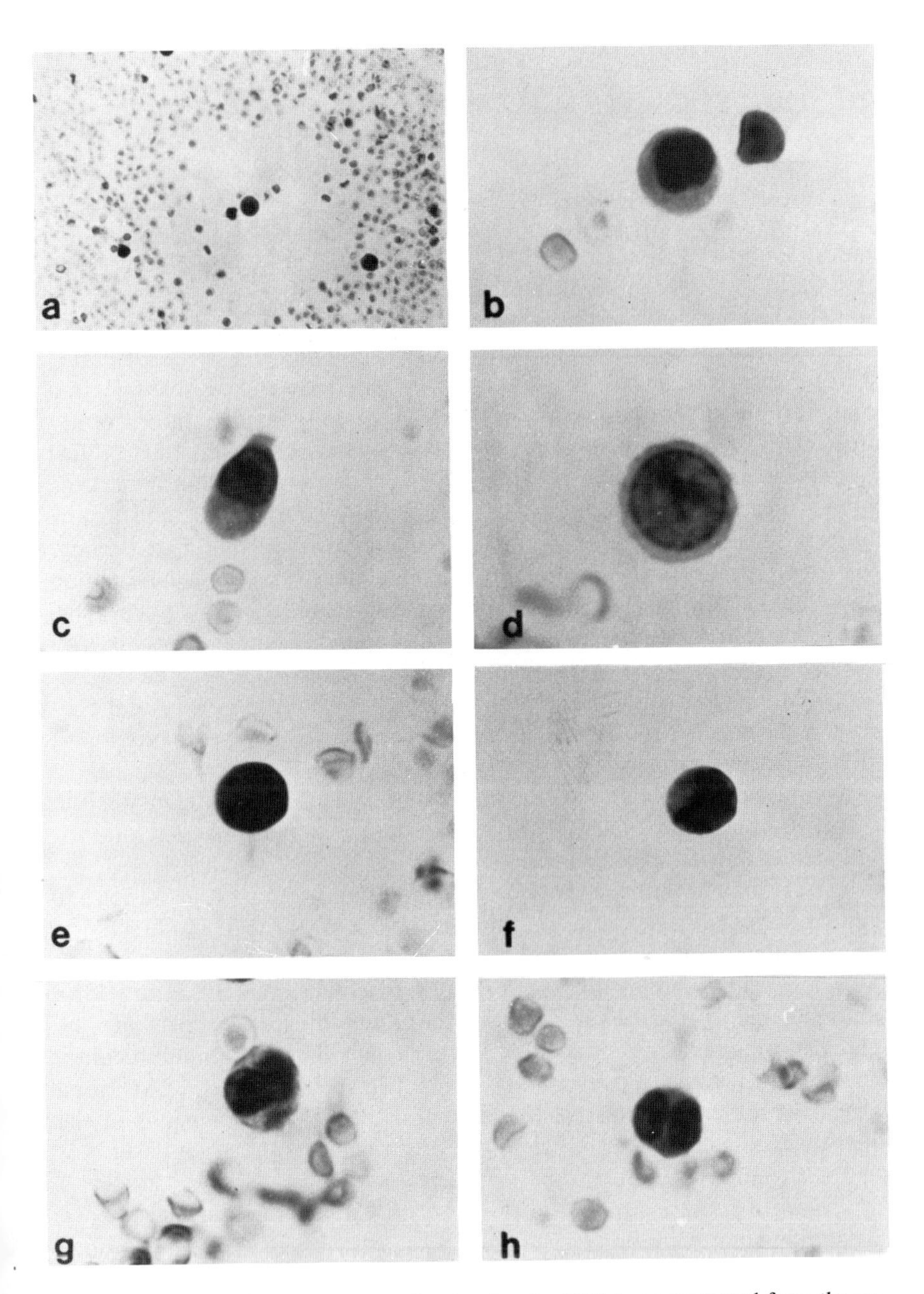

FIGURE 31. Light microscopy composite showing the PFC types recovered from the gradient. (a) typical lysed SRBC plaque, 300x; (b) plasma cell, 1000x; (c) plasmablast 1000x; (d) lymphoblast, 1300x; (e) lymphocyte, 1000x; (f) eccentric, indented nucleus, 900x; (g) segmented nucleus, 900x; (h) binucleated, 750x.

VII. THE DESIGN AND IMPLEMENTATION OF A FLOW ANALYZER FOR CELL SEPARATION STUDIES

The automated multiparameter analyzer for cells (AMAC) (Leif, 1970b) was conceived as a multipurpose electrooptical flow analyzer for clinical analysis of blood leukocytes and exfoliated cells and for characterizing the results of cell separation studies.

The latest version of this instrument, the AMAC III, consists of a 100-μ square orifice with sensing electrodes at each end (Fig. 32) (Leif *et al.*, 1977c; Thomas *et al.*, 1977). It is similar in electrode and sample injection configuration to the previous nonoptical AMAC II laminar flow Coulter effect transducer (Thomas *et al.*, 1974) but permits simultaneous optical measurements. The AMAC III (Fig. 33) is presently capable of measuring fluorescence, light scattering, electronic cell volume (ECV), and a new physical parameter developed by Coulter and Hogg (Coulter and Hogg, 1970) which reflects the change in AC impedance amplitude modulation generated by the presence of a cell or other particle in an orifice. This change is transformed into an intrinsic property termed "opacity" by dividing it by the standard DC Coulter electronic cell volume. The AMAC III is unique in that all of these measurements can be performed simultaneously with a single multipurpose transducer. Since there is a possibility with sequential measurements of scrambling the data from two nearly coincident cells, simultaneous acquisition of all parameters eliminates the complexity and uncertainty of correlating data obtained from such nonsimultaneous downstream measurements.

The orifice of the AMAC III is presently illuminated with a Series 550 Control Laser Corp. neon laser which emits 0.5 W at the 333- and 338-nm doublet; it was previously filled with argon for the preliminary studies described below. A long-working-distance 50-power objective lens with a numerical aperture of 0.60 is used to gather the fluorescence emission. The light scattering pattern produced by the undeflected beam is predominantly a single spot with an approximately symmetric speckle pattern. No strong vertical or horizontal spots or lines attributable to the dimensions of the square orifice were observed when the beam waist of the argon laser was kept below about 30 μm.

Figure 34 demonstrates the results with Coulter fluorescent spheres. The coefficient of variation (CV) for ECV measured with the AMAC bridge circuit was 2.87, and was 5.71 for the fluorescence detected with a photodiode. The same batch of spheres produced a CV of 5.29 with the Coulter TPS-1. Fluorescence distributions (Fig. 35) were obtained from propidium-iodide-stained EL4 ascites cells (Krishan, 1975) but since this staining protocol destroys the resistivity of the membrane and consequently the

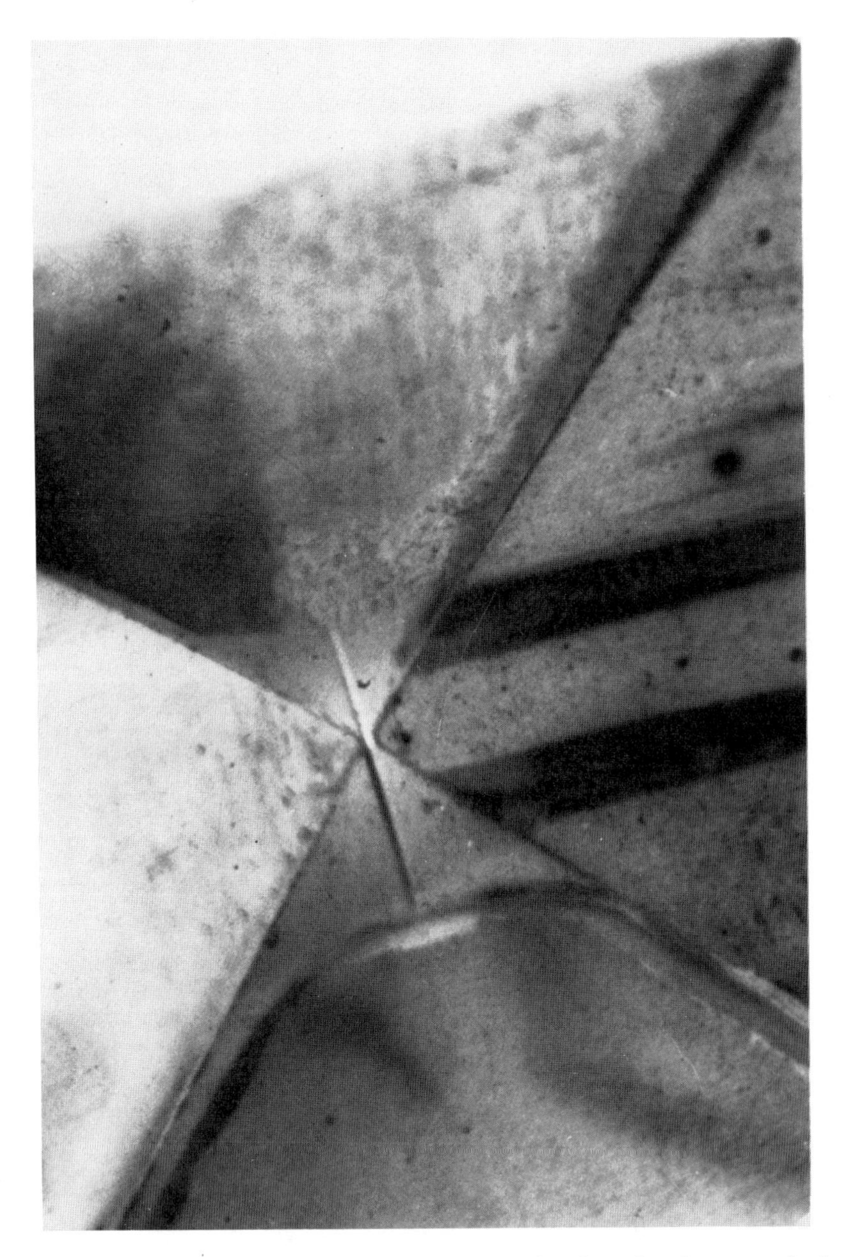

FIGURE 32. AMAC III square orifice showing two sensing electrodes. A narrow wire has been inserted into the water-filled orifice to demonstrate the optical quality of the transducer.

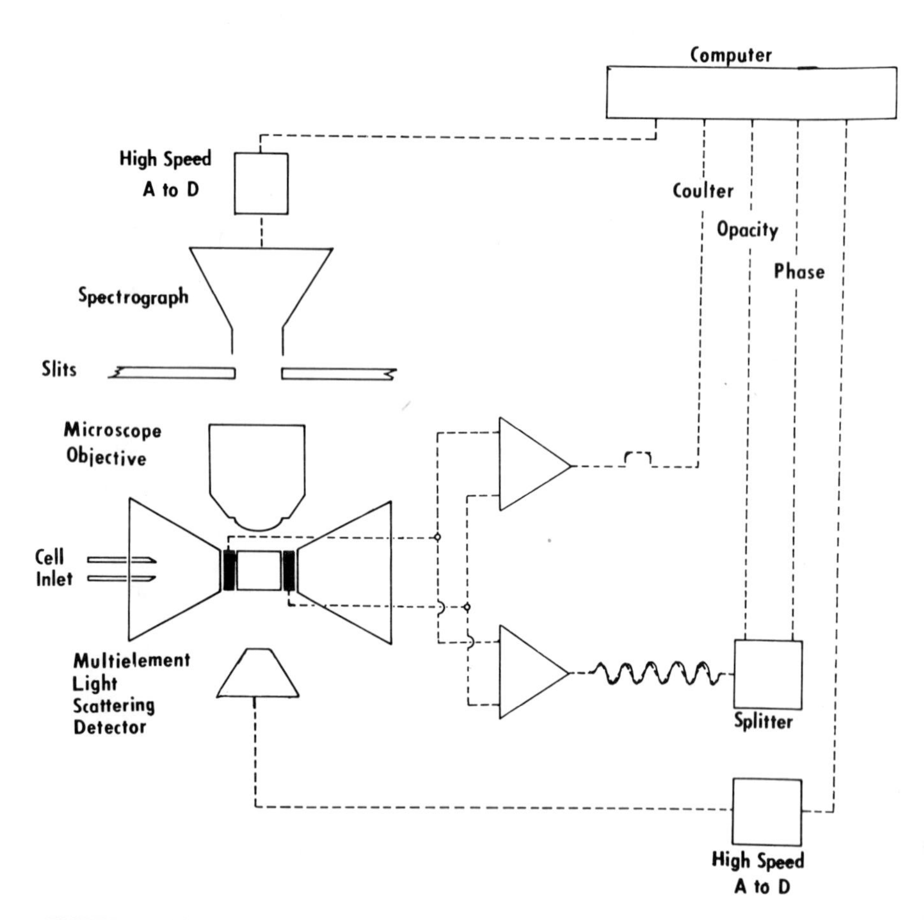

FIGURE 33. The cell inlet to the square orifice is shown at the lower left. The laser beam is pointed up through and vertical to the figure. The fluorescence emission from the cell is focused on the movable slit (wavelength selector) located in front of the spectrograph. The output is limited to one emission at present. In the future a multielement detector will be interfaced to a high-speed analog-to-digital converter (A to C). The forward-scattered light will eventually be sensed by a multielement light scattering detector, which will be interfaced to a high-speed ADC. Simultaneously with the optical measurements the electronic cell volume, opacity, and perhaps phase measurements will be performed. The solid lines shown at the edges of the orifice are the sensing electrodes employed for these studies.

electronic cell volume distribution, it is unsuitable for combined electrooptical analysis of cells.

Electronic cell volume studies with the AMAC III on human erythrocytes obtained a CV of 13.3 (Fig. 36); while this is considerably greater than the 9 to 10% obtained with the AMAC II (Thomas *et al.*, 1974), it must be emphasized that a 100-μm square orifice is much larger than the 70-μm

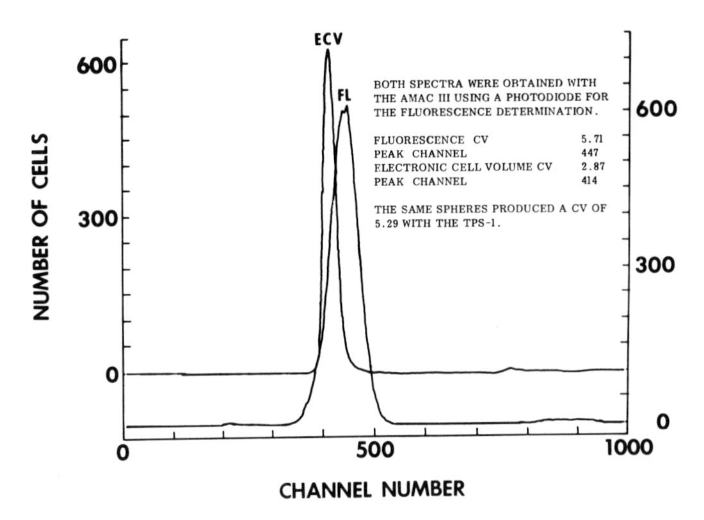

FIGURE 34. Comparison of the electronic cell volume (ECV) and fluorescence spectra (FL) of Coulter spheres. The gain settings were adjusted to place the maxima of the two distributions near each other.

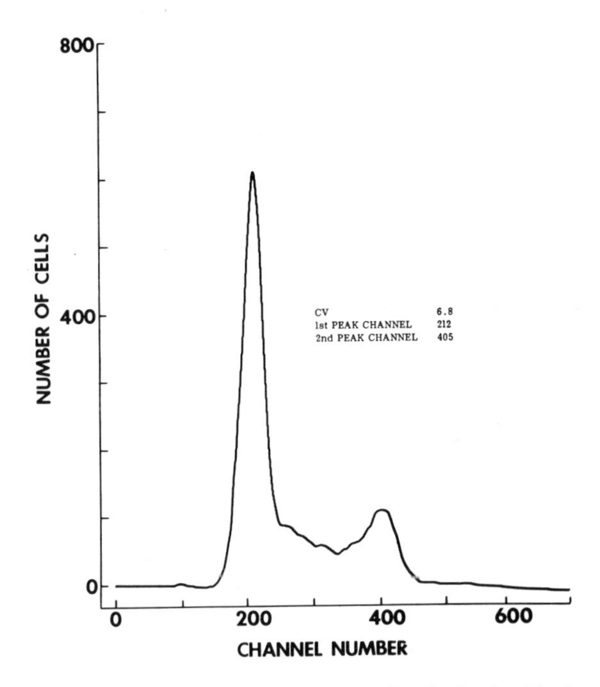

FIGURE 35. Fluorescence distribution of EL4 cells obtained with the AMAC III. The propidium iodide staining procedure renders the cells conductive and thus destroys the electronic cell volume spectrum. The fluorescence emission was detected with a photodiode.

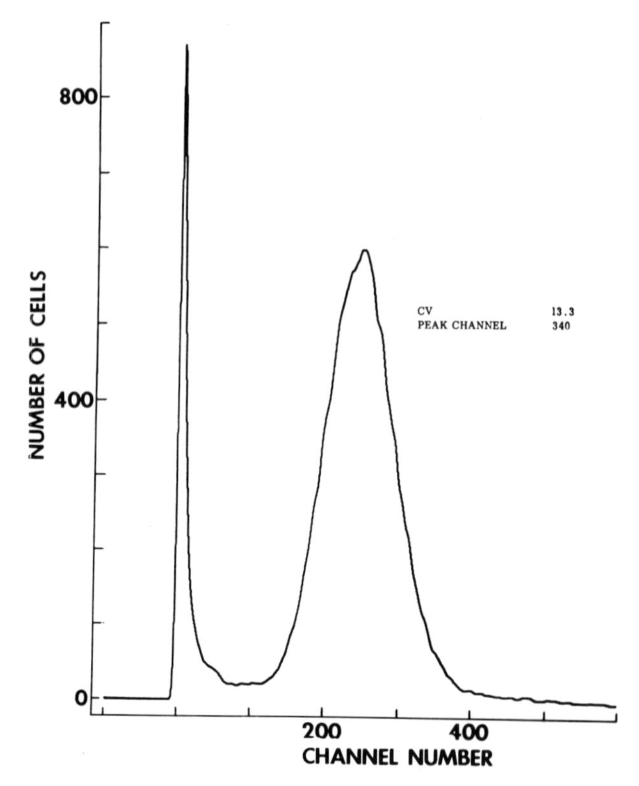

FIGURE 36. A human erythrocyte ECV distribution obtained with the AMAC III.

round orifice, and the expected relative decrease in signal due to the size differential would be 7:1. The laser did not introduce significant noise into the system; the CV with the laser on was 13.9. Recent studies with a new power supply have narrowed the CV to 11.5%.

Finally, with electronic circuitry developed by Coulter Electronics it was possible to obtain combined opacity and ECV measurements of human erythrocytes with the AMAC III transducer (Fig. 37). Because of the use of the 100-μm square orifice, the opacity distribution is artificially broadened from that observed with the standard Coulter instrument.

Since it has been possible to perform fluorescence, ECV, and opacity measurements separately with the AMAC III and since the design is suitable for multiple-angle light scattering studies, it should be feasible in the near future to perform all four studies simultaneously on each cell. These several classes of variables should provide sufficient dimensionality to characterize cells uniquely.

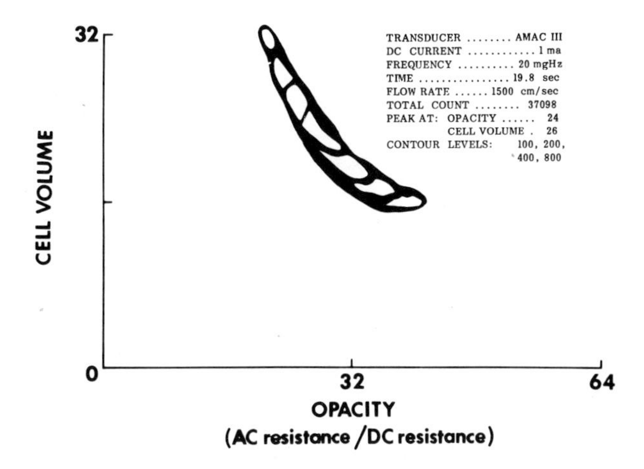

FIGURE 37. Two-dimensional analysis (ECV versus opacity) of erythrocytes, produced with the use of both Coulter electronics and computer systems. The opacity distribution is artificially broadened by the use of the 100-μm square orifice.

In the latest version of the optical system (Fig. 38), the emission from the objective is passed through a pair of slits to reduce scattered and stray laser light. The light is collected by a holographic grating, which focuses a dispersed spectrum onto an end-on photomultiplier tube. A second pair of slits can be positioned laterally in front of the phototube to obtain all or only a portion of the signal from the dispersed emission.

A. Fluid System

The fluid system (Leif *et al.*, 1977c; Leif and Thomas, 1973; Thomas *et al.*, 1974) was designed to deliver a selected sample volume of cells over the range from 10 to 250 μl at a controllable rate with the volume delivered remaining constant and reproducible from experiment to experiment. For this purpose a special multivolume manual sample valve had to be constructed and mounted (Fig. 39). The samples are stored in any one of several drill holes of different sizes located in the rotor. (Outside loops cannot be used in this system, because the cells tend to settle out, and the range of required sample volumes made construction extremely difficult.) Since the sample holes are vertical, settling of the particles on the walls is not a problem.

Both hemoglobin dilution (Table 7) and reproducible cell-count studies (Table 8) have been performed with the new sample valve. In the cell-count experiments we used both fixed and unfixed erythrocytes in phosphate

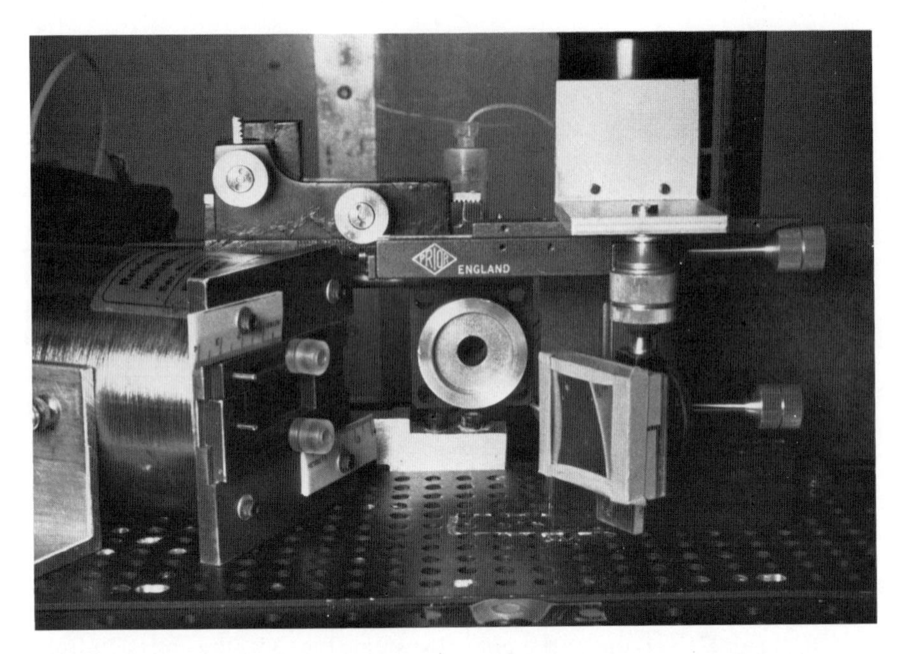

FIGURE 38. The AMAC III optical system. This consists of a photomultiplier (left), transducer (center rear), long-working-distance microscope objective with its housing (center), and a concave holographic grating (right). The grating is normally centered 13 cm behind the microscope objective and 9.30 cm from the photomultiplier at a 30.8° angle to both. Fluorescence emission from the transducer is gathered by the microscope objective and simultaneously focused vertically and spectrally dispersed horizontally by the grating. The slit assembly mounted on the front of the photomultiplier is adjustable to permit selection of the emission wavelength to be studied. Another pair of slits located behind the objective is at an image plane and thus serves to remove most of the light scattered and internally reflected in the quartz of the AMAC III transducer. The system is focused through a 6-power microscope eyepiece (not shown) located at center front. The grating is retracted to permit focusing and viewing of the orifice and flowstream, and is centered when spectra are gathered.

TABLE 7
Results of Hemoglobin Dilution Studies (Seven Samples Per Sample Chamber)

Sample chamber	Chamber vol., μl	Mean absorbance	SD	SD/mean, %
1	9.5 ± 0.5	0.120	0.004	3.1
2	22 ± 0.5	0.260	0.002	.8
3	53 ± 2	0.608	0.016	2.6
4	78 ± 2	1.002	0.027	2.7
5	222 ± 1	2.47	0.016	.6

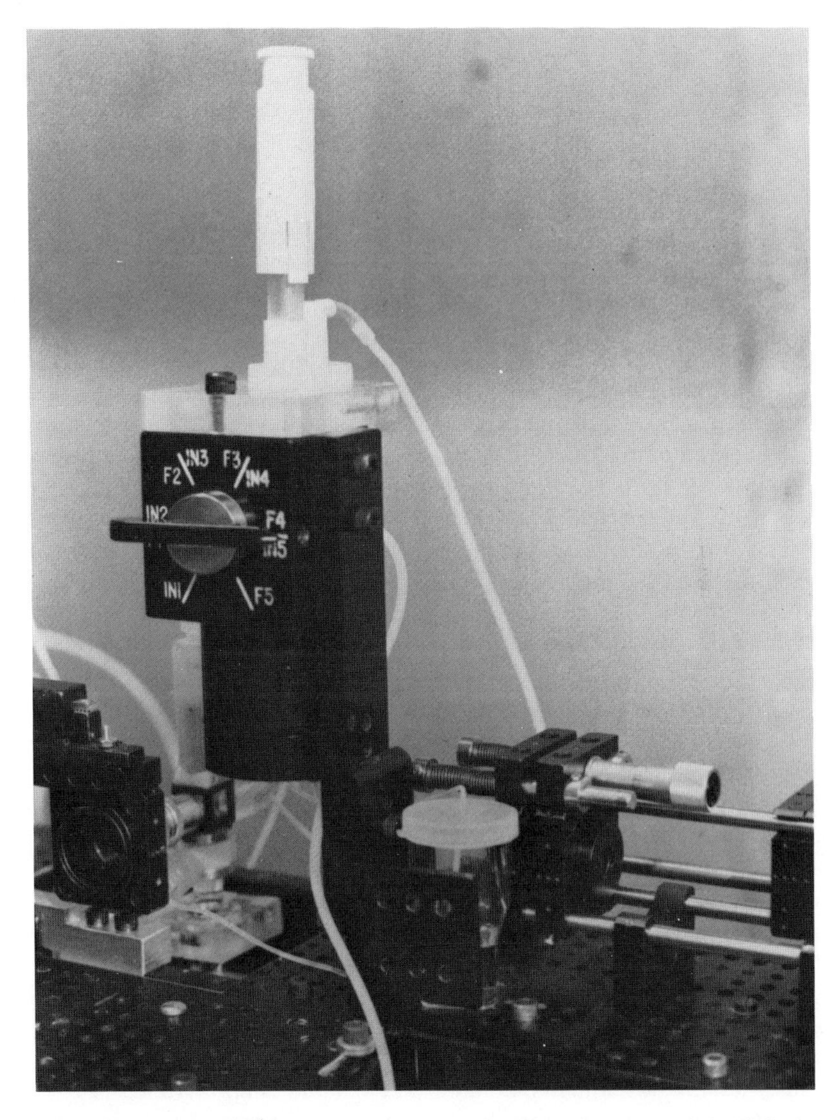

FIGURE 39. The AMAC III is shown to the lower left of the valve. A sample bottle is shown on the right. The valve has five different positions which correspond to the five holes in the Teflon rotor, each of which holds a different volume of sample. In the input mode the sample is pumped from the sample bottle through a connecting tube and up through the valve rotor, and the excess is discharged out of the outlet part of the constant-volume pipettor. This pipettor serves as the pump. The valve is then rotated from the inlet position to the flow position and the contents of the drill-hole in the rotor are delivered to the inlet of the AMAC III. The drill-hole in the inlet position is continuously washed by saline which passes through the needle valve. This flow of saline first pushes the bolus of sample out of the drill-hole, then washes the drill-hole clean.

TABLE 8
Results of Cell-Count Studies (Eight Samples Per Sample Chamber)

Sample chamber	Chamber vol., μl	Erythrocytes	Mean cells	SD (cells)	SD/mean, %
2	22 ± 0.5	Fixed	42,718	699	1.6
4	78 ± 2	Fixed	242,841	7349	3.0
5	222 ± 1	Unfixed	302,997	7455	2.5

buffer, pH 7.4. For the hemoglobin dilution studies, the hemoglobin solution was aspirated into the valve and the sample chamber delivered into a 1-ml volumetric flask with Drabkin's solution. The absorbance at 540 nm was then measured with a Zeiss (PMQII) spectrophotometer. As can be seen in the results for both calibration techniques, the worst standard deviation was 3.1% (Table 7), which is still acceptable for cell counts.

The use of this new sample valve finally permits the simultaneous enumeration of the number of cells present in a gradient fraction and production of multiparameter electrooptical spectra.

VIII. CONCLUSION

The capacity to separate cells is but one step in the development of a complete system for establishing the taxonomic relationship of differentiating normal and neoplastic cells. In addition to developing the cell separation instrumentation to a very high state of precision and reliability, it has been essential to implement the rest of the system: centrifugal cytology for morphological assessment of the cells present in the fractions and flow analysis with the AMAC for objective cell classification and rapid counting. Fast, accurate enumeration of the cells also expedites dilution of the fractions for centrifugal cytology.

Conventional morphologic assessment and flow analysis are complementary techniques which should both be used in characterizing cell separation study results. The relationship between morphological assessment and flow analysis is analogous to that of Newtonian and quantum physics under the "principle of correspondence." Each must give correct results in the region for which it alone is a valid measurement; and in regions of overlap both must give similar or identical results.

Because of the greater statistical accuracy of flow analysis, results obtained by this technique will be more precise than those obtained by morphological enumeration. However, the populations described by flow analysis should each be readily correlated with a given morphologic class or be a definable subpopulation of a morphologic class, such as T lymphocytes. It should be cautioned that characterizing cell populations by flow analysis alone, without adequate morphological assessment, for instance, by a single parameter such as low-resolution electronic cell volume analysis, is a procedure which maximizes the data and minimizes the information.

APPENDIX A. FRACTION COLLECTOR CONTROLLER CIRCUIT

By S. N. Lefkove, T. A. Yopp, K. Leeburn, R. A. Thomas, D. H. K. Hindman, and R. C. Leif

The circuitry used to control the fraction collector is divided into four subsystems: selector, detector, sequencing, and display. All logic is TTL; zero voltage is low and 2.2 V or more is high. Four modes of fraction collection are possible: (1) a predetermined number of steps selected by setting the PRESET counter A on the front panel, (2) similar operation with PRESET counter B, (3) alternate collection of separately determined counts in both A and B, and (4) continuous operation.

The selector logic determines which of the two front panel banks of thumbwheel switches (PRESET A or PRESET B) is activated. If the system starts up in the ALTERNATE mode (having been cleared), it will match the present counts in counter A first and the preset counts in B on the second cycle. It will then go back to A, and continue alternating between the two. In this case and case (4) as well, flip-flop U22B, whose Q-output is the $\overline{\text{B PRESET}}$ COMMON line (Fig. 40), will change state at every PRESET REACHED: if it was high, it will go low and vice versa. This input is from U16A, pin 6, which is reset each time PRESET REACHED occurs. This logic uses a 7474D flip-flop (U22B), a 7421 AND gate (U24A) and the output of 7474 flip-flop U16A mentioned before. For cases (1) and (2), the PRESET and CLEAR inputs to U22B will determine the output.

Enabling the A bank of thumbwheel switches is done by applying a low input to its common and a high to the B bank's common, by means of two pairs of inverters (Fig. 40) in parallel; (59C and 59D on the A side, 59E and 59F on the B side). Initially, the Q-output from flip-flop 22B will be low and $\bar{Q}$ will be high, regardless of the A or B bank settings. Since negative logic is being used, A is low and B is high when the selector switch is in the A position (Fig. 41). This puts a low on the clear input of flip-flop U22B and a high on the PRESET input. As shown in the accompanying truth table for the two relevant states of a D flip-flop (Table 9) this produces a low on the Q-

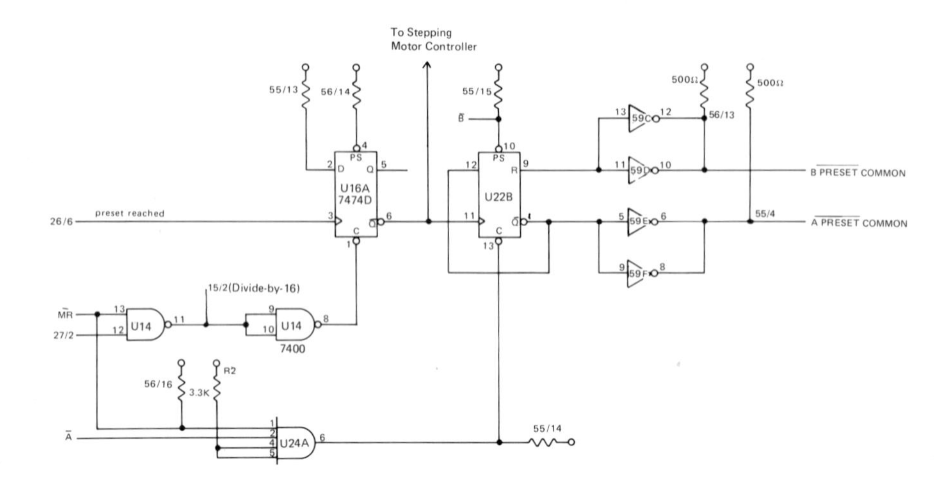

FIGURE 40. The PRESET switch logic enables the thumbwheel switches by putting a logical low on their common lines. Only one of the two groups of switches is operative at a time. Flip-flops U16A and U22B, located at the center of the figure, perform this function.

output and a high on the $\bar{Q}$; the result is a high on the $\overline{\text{B PRESET COMMON}}$ output and a low on the $\overline{\text{A PRESET COMMON}}$, enabling the A thumbwheel switches. Similarly, when the selector switch is in the B position, then signal B is low and signal A is high. According to the truth table, the Q output will then be high and the Q output low, making the $\overline{\text{B PRESET}}$ $\overline{\text{COMMON}}$ low and the $\overline{\text{A PRESET COMMON}}$ high and enabling the B thumbwheel switches. Activating one bank causes its common lines to be terminated to ground; terminating it high inactivates the bank and presents a logical one to the input AND gates of the next stage, the detector circuit.

The detector logic is a coincidence circuit which presents each of the five binary-coded decimal (BCD) digits of the thumbwheel switch to a bank

TABLE 9
Truth Table of 7474D Functions Used to Control Flip-Flop U22B

Counter enabled	Signal on common		Inputs				Outputs	
	A	B	PR	CLR	CLK	D	Q	$\bar{Q}$
A	L	H	H	L	X	X	L	H
B	H	L	L	H	X	X	H	L

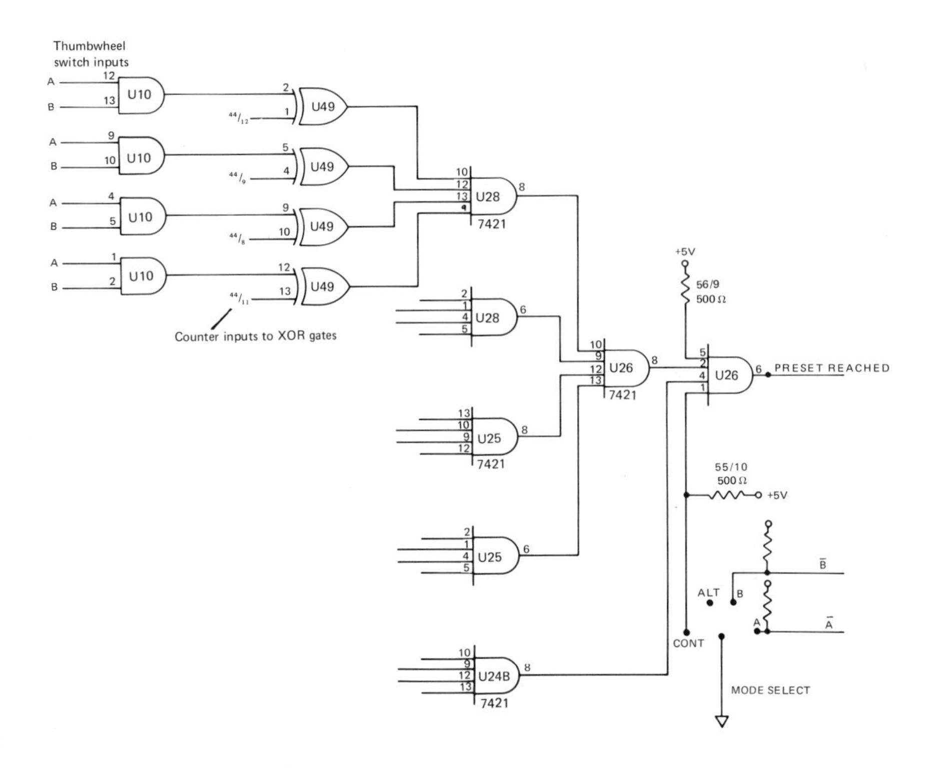

FIGURE 41. Coincidence detector logic of the preset and total counters. At the top left is shown one of the five banks of AND gates and corresponding exclusive OR gates; since the circuitry of the other four banks is identical, they have been omitted. Their inputs come from the front panel thumbwheel switches and from the preset counters (Fig. 42), U40–U44, respectively. Since the thumbwheel switches use negative-true logic and the counters use positive-true logic, we have used exclusive OR gates for the match condition. When the twenty XOR gates show matches (logic 1 output), the output of each AND gate will go high, indicating coincidence. Pin 6 of U26 will then give a logic 1 output. This four-input terminal AND gate is controlled by the MODE SELECT switch (pin 1) as well as by inputs 2 and 4, which go high when coincidence occurs; pin 5 is tied permanently high.

of four AND gates (Fig. 41). Each AND gate inputs to an exclusive OR (XOR) gate whose other input comes from the preset counter (Fig. 42). This bank of twenty XOR gates forms the comparator which detects coincidence between the switch and preset counter outputs. The resulting outputs go to a second bank of five AND gates; the first four, representing the four least significant digits of the count, are summed by another AND gate (U26, pin 8), while the fifth, representing the most significant digit, appears at the output of the fifth AND gate (U24B, pin 8). Both these signals go to the terminal AND gate (U26, pin 6) which is also controlled by the permanently high input from pin 5 and by the MODE SELECT switch; if all inputs are high

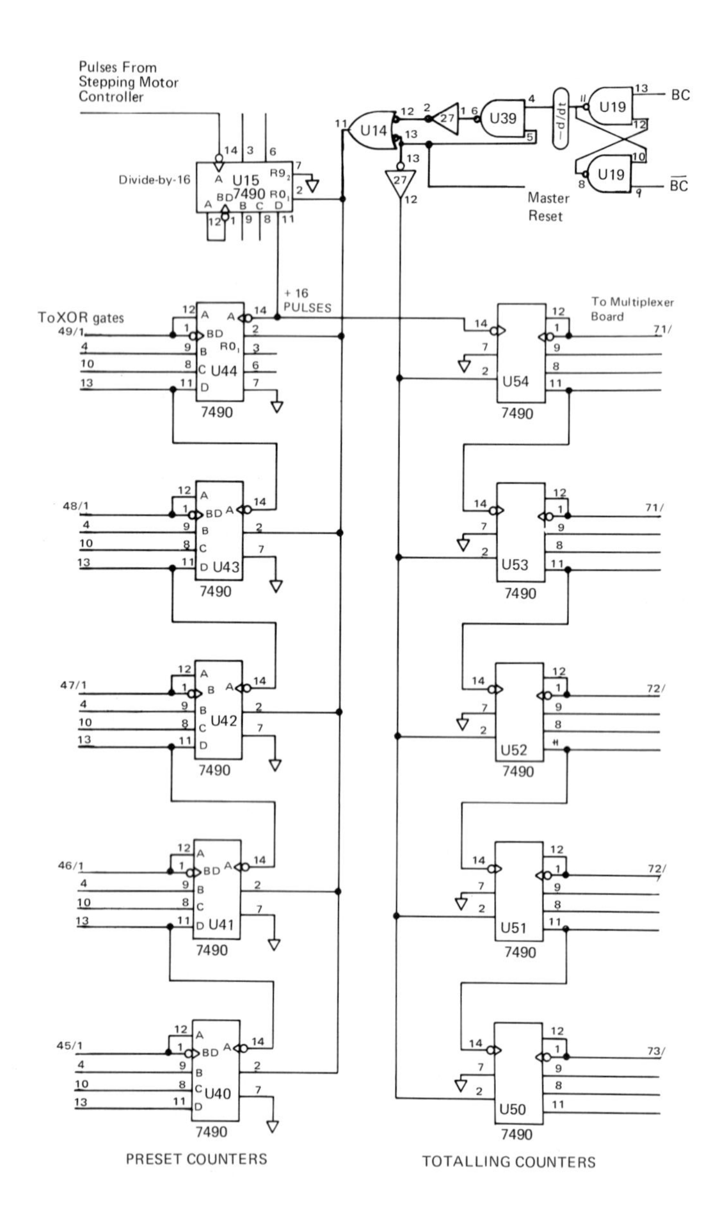

FIGURE 42. Preset and total counter logic. The five counters which make up the bank of preset counters (left side) are labeled U40–U44 with U44 holding the least significant decade. The totaling counters are labeled U50–U54 with U54 holding the least significant decade. Both counters are advanced one count simultaneously by a pulse from U15 after every sixteenth pulse it receives from the stepping motor. Outputs from the preset counters go to the exclusive OR gates (Fig. 41) and display board (Fig. 45) which handles multiplexing and display on the LEDs as well as character decoding. Outputs from the totaling counters go only to the display board (Fig. 46). All ICs are 7490s except inverter U27, which is a 7404.

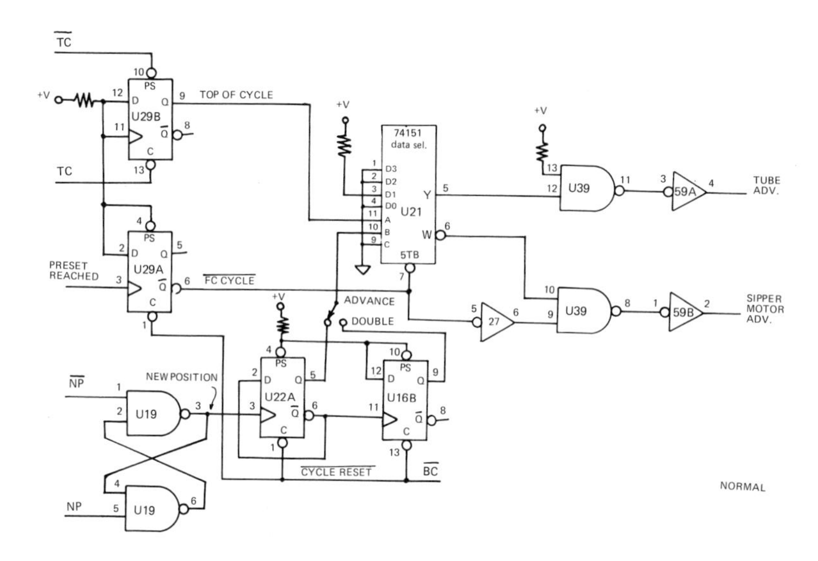

FIGURE 43. Sequencing logic. The main logic elements are 7474D flip-flops U29A and B, U22A, and U16B which are strobed by the fraction collector microswitches and in turn input to the 74151 data selector (U21), which controls the sipper motor and tube advance.

(logical one), the output will be high, indicating PRESET REACHED, which starts the sequencing logic (Fig. 43). In CONTINUOUS mode, however, MODE SELECT will be low, so that PRESET REACHED cannot occur and the sequencing logic is inactivated. In this case the stepping motor will run continuously.

The preset counters (Fig. 42) are U40 and U44, with the most significant decade in the former and the least significant in the latter. The totaling counters are U50 to U54; U54 has the least significant decade and U50 the most significant. The counters are driven by a +5-V pulse train (Fig. 44) at the same frequency as the motor oscillator. The output from the preset counters goes to the exclusive OR gates of Fig. 41 and to a set of multiplexing and LED display circuits on a separate board (Figs. 45 and 46), as does the ouptut from the totaling counter; this board also does character decoding. The PRESET REACHED signal is applied to the U16A flip-flop clock, taking the Q-output high and $\bar{Q}$ low. Low $\bar{Q}$ stops the stepping motor clock (Fig. 44) which in turn halts the preset and totaling counters (see multiplexer and display logic, Figs. 45 and 46). This also begins the sequencing logic (see below and Fig. 43).

The preset and totaling counters (Fig. 42) differ only in the way they are cleared. Inverting the MASTER RESET signal through inverter U27 (pin

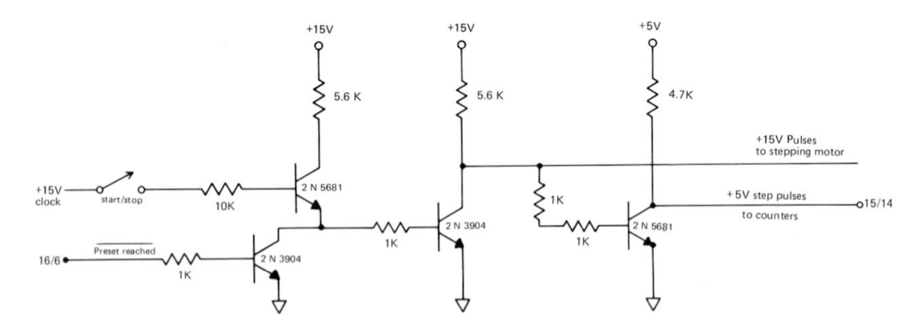

FIGURE 44. The stepping motor interface. This circuit gates the output of the variable oscillator Slo-syn stepper motor controller and provides a parallel pulse stream at TTL logic levels (5 V) to drive the counters (Fig. 42).

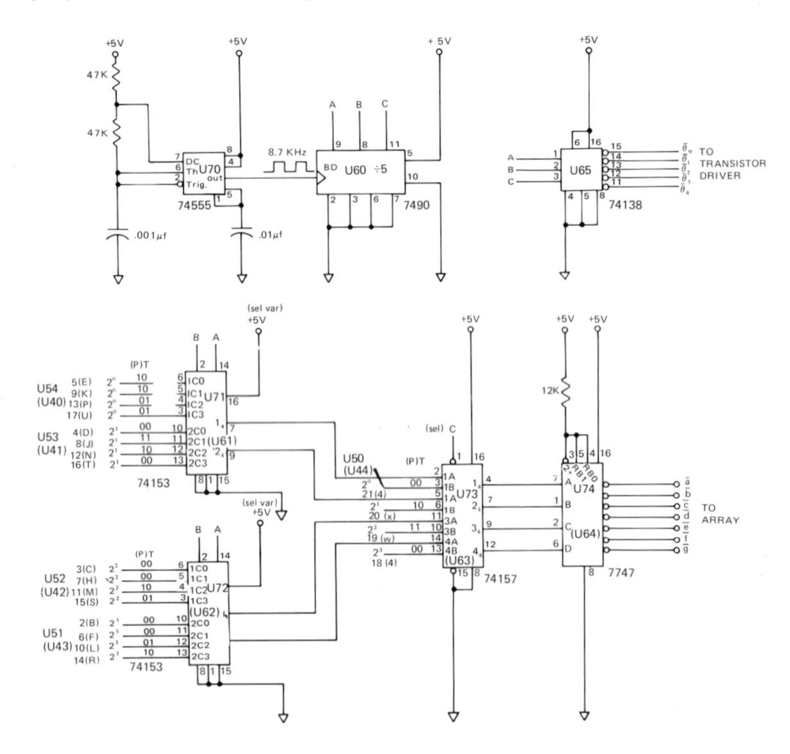

FIGURE 45. The display outputs are acquired by multiplexing the outputs from the preset and totaling counters. Since the two devices are identical, only one is shown. The circuit logic consists of a clock (U70), a ÷5 counter (U60), a 74138 transistor driver (U65) controlled by the divide-by-5 counter, and two identical multiplexer sections. The one shown here takes the output from the preset count. It consists of two IC 74153s (U71 and U72), an IC 74157 (U73), and an IC 7447 (U74); only one section is shown here. The second, which accepts the output from the totaling counters, consists of U61, U62, U63, and U64. Figures in parenthesis on the drawings refer to inputs to the multiplexer sections not shown and the ICs themselves.

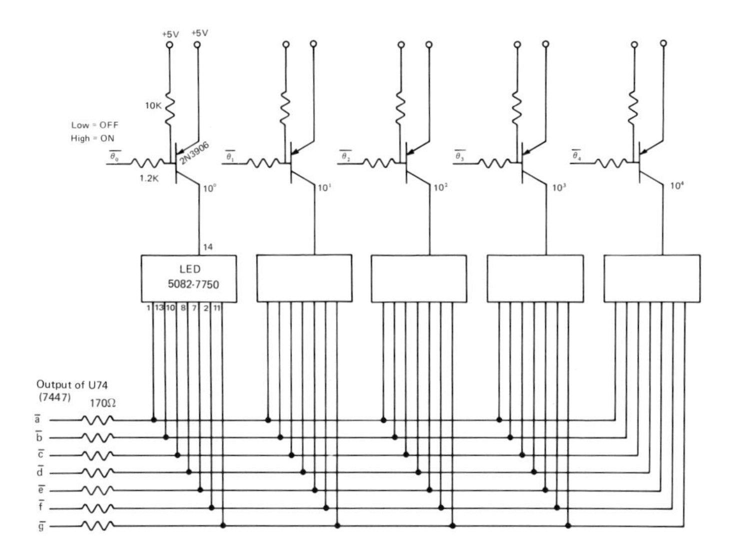

FIGURE 46. A seven-segment decoder produces the proper display pattern for each of the five sequencing decades from the two 74157s, U63 and U73 of Fig. 45, which control the LED array (5082–7750). The sequencing is handled by advancing the ÷5 counter (U60, Fig. 45). Simultaneously, a driver transistor (U65) is switched on which activates the desired LED. The bit pattern to be displayed is governed by the output from the 7447s, U64 (not shown) and U74 (Fig. 45).

12) clears the totaling counters, and the preset counters are cleared (from U14, pin 11, Fig. 42) by one of two signals, either by $\overline{\text{MASTER RESET}}$ from the front panel switch or by a counter clear from the bottom-of-cycle (BC) microswitch on the fraction collector. The cross-coupled NAND gate pair U19 debounces the BC switch output (top right).* U14's operation can be seen in Fig. 42 as a negative-input OR gate. The number of pulses that go to the stepping motor is divided by 16 (U15) before entry to both counters, which are advanced simultaneously.

The PRESET REACHED signal starts the sequencing logic (Fig. 43), which immediately turns on the sipper motor. The sipper motor rises until it activates a microswitch near the top of its travel, which signals the sequencing logic to stop it when it reaches the top and to start the tube advance motor instead, which will advance either one or two positions depending upon the advance switch position. The normal position means an advance of one tube position; the double position, an advance of two. When this is finished, the logic will stop the tube advance motor and begin the sipper motor again. The sipper motor cam will eventually engage

*The differentiator (−d/dt) produces a positive-going pulse in response to a negative-going input but does not respond to a rising edge.

another switch called the bottom-of-cycle switch and the cycle will start again by clearing the 7474 flip-flop which was clocked by PRESET REACHED (U16A of Fig. 40). The count accumulated in the preset counters will also be set back to zero, so that the coincidence condition no longer exists and the cycle begins again.

The sequencing logic is described in Fig. 43 The A and B inputs and strobe (STB) of the 74151 data selector (U21) control its Y and W outputs, which turn the tube advance and sipper motors respectively to the ON state. Initially, a test tube is in place and the fraction collector is between the bottom-of-cycle and top-of-cycle positions (if necessary it is advanced manually); it will go to the top-of-cycle position when turned on. Flip-flop 29B and the two cross-coupled NAND gates are used to debounce the outputs of the NEW POSITION microswitch located inside the fraction collector. The initial state of the fraction collector causes TOP OF CYCLE (TC) to be low, the complement of BOTTOM OF CYCLE ($\overline{\text{BC}}$) to be high, and NEW POSITION (NP) to be high. While the stepping motor is driving the peristaltic pump, both the sipper motor and the tube advance motor are inhibited. This state is the complement of FRACTION COLLECTOR CYCLE ($\overline{\text{FC CYCLE}}$), which will be high until the preset count is reached and the stepping motor is stopped, whereupon it goes low to begin the cycle. At this point the A and B inputs to the data selector are both low, causing the data at input DO (which is tied low) to appear in its true form (low) at the Y output and in its complemented form (high) at the W output. The effect of this is to turn on the sipper motor, which continues to run until the top-of-cycle microswitch is closed. TOP OF CYCLE now goes high, causing the data at input D1 (which is tied high) to appear at the Y and W outputs. This will stop the sipper motor and start the tube advance motor. NEW POSITION, initially high, will go low as the tube that has just been filled moves out of position. This has no effect on flip-flop 22A which responds only to low-to-high transitions of its clock input. When the next tube moves into position, NP goes high, causing the output of U22A, pin 5 to go high. If the advance switch is in the NORMAL position the B input to the data selector will now go high. This causes the data at input D3 (which is tied low) to appear at the Y and W outputs, stopping the tube advance motor and restarting the sipper motor. If the advance switch is in the DOUBLE position, the B input to the data selector will not go high until two tubes have been advanced. The output of U22, pin 6, which is the complement of pin 5, will initially be high. The first low-to-high transition of NP (which causes pin 5 of U22 to go high) will cause pin 6 of U22 to go low, which has no effect on flip-flop U16. However the next low-to-high transition of NP will cause a low-to-high transition of pin 6 of U22. At this point output pin 9 of U16 (which is now the B input of the data selector) will go high, stopping the tube advance motor while restarting the sipper motor. Next, TC will go low, causing input

D2 to appear at the Y and W outputs, but this will have no effect since D2 is the same as D3. When the sipper reaches the bottom-of-cycle position $\overline{\mathrm{BC}}$ will go low. This causes a positive-going spike to appear at the pin 4 input of NAND gate U39, but since this gate is biased so that this signal does not affect the gate output, $\overline{\mathrm{MR}}$, the complement of Master Reset, stays high during the entire cycle. Once the sipper motor has passed the bottom-of-cycle position $\overline{\mathrm{BC}}$ will go high. This causes a negative-going spike to appear at the input of NAND gate U39 (pin 4), which propagates through the gate and the inverter following it, causing $\overline{\mathrm{CYCLE\ RESET}}$ to go low momentarily. This reset signal causes $\overline{\mathrm{FC\ CYCLE}}$ to go high and causes both pin 5 of U22 and pin 9 of U16 (inputs to the advance switch) to go low. The cycle stops immediately as both the sipper motor and the tube advance motor are inhibited. The preset counters are cleared and the stepping motor on the peristaltic pump is restarted. Notice that the fraction collector is stopped in exactly the initial configuration described above.

The outputs of the totaling and preset counters are multiplexed on the board which handles the display logic (Fig. 45). This board consists of an 8.7-KHz clock, a divide-by-5 counter, a 74138 (used as a transistor driver) whose outputs are controlled by the state of the divide-by-5 counter, and two identical sections which multiplex the preset and total inputs. The A, B, and C outputs from the divide-by-5 counter go to the 74138 transistor driver and to the multiplexers. Both sections consist of a pair of 74153 4-to-1 multiplexers, a 74157 two-line-to-one-line multiplexer, and a 7447 seven-segment decoder, which takes a four-digit binary-coded decimal input and produces signals to control the segments of a LED display. The 74153s process the less-significant decades of the counts and are fed by 16 of the 20 signal lines from each bank of counters. Their output is controlled by the state of the A and B outputs of the divide-by-5 counter. When both A and B are low, for example, it transfers the signal on the zero input line to its output; when A and B are 01, it transfers the signal from the 2 input, and so on, so that each of the four combinations of A and B therefore transfers one of the four possible inputs to the output.

The remaining four signals, representing the most significant decade, go to the B side of the 74157 multiplexer, which is controlled by the C output of the counter. For the first four counts of its divide-by-5 sequence this C output is low and the 74153 outputs are transferred to the output of the 74157. On the last count, C is high, transferring the input on the B side of the 74157 to the output. In this way the seven-segment decoder produces the proper display pattern for each of the five decades in the sequence while a drive transistor is simultaneously switched on (Fig. 46) which then turns on the particular LED which is to be illuminated. At the same time the 7447 output has the bit pattern for decade 0, the decade 0 transistor driver is turned on. When decade 1 is to be displayed, only the decade 1 transistor is turned on and so on; these are scanned in sequence by advancing the 7490 which is the divide-by-5 counter (U60). Since the fundamental frequency of the clock (U70), which is a 555 timer used in the astable mode, is 8.7 kH, this means that the entire scanning sequence takes place in roughly 70 ms.

APPENDIX B. BUOYANT DENSITY DISTRIBUTION PROGRAM

By Suzanne B. Leif and Robert C. Leif

Three FORTRAN programs were written to analyze the data from the BSA gradient separation experiments. The first is the DENSITY DISTRIBUTION program which calculates the buoyant density distribution, both in terms of total cells and specific cell types. The second determines the ENRICHMENT of each specific type of cell and the third outputs the distribution for PLOTTING on a standard plotter such as a Cal Comp. The first step in the DENSITY DISTRIBUTION program is to determine the Coulter Counter background. A calibration reading without any cells is taken before and after the experiment, and these two values are averaged for Coulter count background. During the experiments the Coulter count was obtained for each sample (CCAD), and the average background on the Coulter Counter for that day (Z), the pump setting (volume counting unit or VOLCNT) and the milliliters per pump counts (F) were noted. (A glossary of terms following this Appendix describes the short abbreviations such as CCAD which were used in the program.) For each fraction a record was kept of the initial diluent added, the volume of diluent and the Coulter counts. After the first several experiments the initial diluent was never used. For three fractions in each experiment the refractive index was found. All of these data were entered on punch cards.

The next step was to enter the data obtained from the centrifugal cytology distributions prepared from each fraction. The individual distributions on the slides were then counted manually under the microscope to determine the cellular composition (the "cytogram") of the individual density fraction, and these data were punched on cards for the second half of the main program.

The first half of the DENSITY DISTRIBUTION program calculates the buoyant density in terms of total cells, and prints out the original data and the percentage of individual cell types in each cytogram. The second half prints out the distribution of individual cell types for the whole array of fractions.

In most of the experiments an automatic pump count was used and the computer calculated the increments from fraction to fraction. The program is flexible, however, and allows the entry of individual pump counts for each fraction.

It then scans the data and finds the three manually determined refractive indices. From these it calculates the average $\Delta\rho$ for the experiment and the individual ρ values for each fraction.

The dilution factor, *DF*, is given by the following equation:

$$DF = \frac{\text{(Vol. fract. aliquot)} + \text{(Vol. diluent)}}{\text{(Vol. aliquot)}} \tag{1}$$

In terms of the program names (cf. Glossary) this is as follows (note: all equations with A suffixes give the actual program coding):

$$DF = \frac{[\text{PUMPCN(I)*F}] + [\text{IDA(I)}]}{\text{PUMPCN(I)*F}} \tag{1A}$$

The number of cells in each fraction is found using the following formula:

$$\text{Num. cells in fract.} = 2\text{(Dilution factor)(Coulter counts} - \text{Coulter count background)} \tag{2}$$

$$\text{TCELL(I)} = \text{TDIL(I)*CCNOBK(I)*PUMPCN(I)*F} \tag{2A}$$

(The factor of 2 enters because the Coulter Counter's sample volume is 0.5 ml.)

The total number of cells in the entire experiment is then the sum of the number of cells from each fraction.

From these numbers the density distribution $F(\rho)$ can then be calculated:

$$F(\rho) = \frac{\text{(Num. cells in fract.)}}{(\Delta\rho)\text{(Num. cells in grad.)}} \tag{3}$$

$$\text{FRHO(I)} = \frac{-\text{TCELL(I)}}{\text{SUMCEL*AVRNO } [\text{PUMPCN(I)} - \text{PUMPCN(I} - 1)]} \tag{3A}$$

At this time the first charts are printed. The leader page contains experiment identification and date, comments, and the refractive indices. The main chart lists the buoyant densities in terms of the total cells. If only half the program is run, it will terminate with this chart printing. This half of the program can be run alone by inserting an END card after the calculation of the dilution factors and $F(\rho)$ (card 151).

The second half of the program analyzes the individual cell type counts and finds the buoyant density distribution of each morphological class of cell.

It also reprints the original data (the differential count) as an aid in checking for typographical errors on the punch cards.

The percent composition of specific cells in each fraction is calculated from the following formula:

$$\% \text{ Comp. sp. cells in fract.} = 100 \frac{(\text{Num. sp. cells counted in fract.})}{(\text{Tot. num. cells})} \tag{4}$$

$$\text{PTCELL} = 100 \frac{[\text{SPCELS(J,I)}]}{(\text{SUMCEL})} \tag{4A}$$

This array is then printed.

The number of specific cells in the fraction is found by taking the result from equation 4, multiplying by the number of cells in the fraction, and dividing by 100. Then the number of specific cells in the entire gradient is found by adding the array for that cell for all of the fractions.

Equation 5 gives the buoyant density distribution for each morphological class of cell:

$$F(\rho) \text{ Sp. for each cell type} = \frac{(\text{Num. sp. cells in fract.})}{(\Delta\rho)(\text{Num. sp. cells in grad})} \tag{5}$$

$$\text{FRHO(I)} = \frac{-\text{SPCELS(J,I)}}{\text{SUMCEL*AVRHO*PUMPCN(I)}} \tag{5A}$$

The percent of specific cells in each fraction is found by dividing the number of specific cells in each fraction by the number of specific cells in the gradient and multiplying the result by 100. A running subtotal of the percent of specific cells in each fraction is kept and a chart is printed for each cell type found in the experiment.

The calculation of an enrichment factor is performed in a separate FORTRAN "ENRICHMENT" program. "PUNCH" commands for the needed arrays for this enrichment program were inserted in the original DENSITY DISTRIBUTION program to permit it to run without an operator at the keyboard.

To find the enrichment factor, data from the fractions are compared to the total number of those cells recovered from the gradient.

The percent composition of specific cells which were recovered from the gradient is then calculated to determine cell recovery:

$$\% \text{ Comp. sp. cells recov. from grad.} = \frac{100\,(\text{Num. sp. cells in grad})}{(\text{Num. cells in grad})} \tag{6}$$

$$\text{Y(I)} = \frac{\text{TSUB(I)}}{\text{SUMCEL}} \tag{6A}$$

This array is then printed, and the enrichment factor found by:

$$EF = \frac{\%\ \text{Comp. sp. cells in fract.}}{\%\ \text{Comp. sp. cells recovered from grad}} \tag{7}$$

$$\text{ENRICH(J,I)} = \frac{\text{A(J,I)}}{\text{Y(J)}} \tag{7A}$$

Also calculated is the percent of specific cells in each fraction:

$$\%\ \text{Sp. cells in fract.} = \frac{\text{Num sp. cells in fract.}}{\text{Num sp. cells in grad.}} \tag{8}$$

$$\text{PTCELL} = \frac{\text{SPCELS(J,I)}}{\text{TSUB(J)}} \tag{8A}$$

It is also possible to calculate the recovery of each specific cell type from the percent composition of specific cells which were recovered from the gradient, as calculated in equation 6. This quantity can be divided by the percent composition of each specific cell in the unfractionated aliquot, which is calculated as shown in equation 9, to yield the specific cell type recovery.

$$\%\ \text{Com. sp. cells in unfract. aliquot} = 100\ \frac{\text{(Num sp. cells counted)}}{\text{(Tot. num. cells counted)}} \tag{9}$$

$$\text{UNFRAC(II)} = \frac{\text{UNFRAC(II)}}{\text{X}} \text{ where X} = 0 \text{ to start}$$
$$\text{X} = \text{UNFRAC(II) X for each II} \tag{9A}$$

The third program was a standard Cal Comp program which plotted out the buoyant density distributions. Since it is just a series of standard Cal Comp calls, it has been omitted from the listings.

These programs are essentially portable, except for slight differences in the FORTRAN compilers between various computers. For instance, the CDC 6400 allowed a seven-character name and the others allowed only six characters. They also used different delimiters for literals in the format statements. DO loops were allowed to start with 0 on the CDC but not on the IBM 370. Changing from EBCDIC to ASCI represented no real problem since the machines were equipped with translation programs. This program uses a great deal of core with all of its arrays. No effort was made to optimize its use of space or running time as additions and revisions were frequently being made at the time of writing and the emphasis was on rapid completion of a functional program. These programs are to be revised to be implemented on a minicomputer.

```
                              MAIN PROGRAM                                000100
                                                                          000200
C  THIS PROGRAM IS TO ANALYZE DATA FROM GRADIENT RUN                       000300
C  THE VERY FIRST CARD OF THE DATA SHOULD TELL NUMBER OF RUNS             000400
C  THE DATA CARDS FOR THIS PROGRAM SHOULD BE AS FOLLOWS...                000500
C  CARD 1 REFA10Z1,Z2,VOLCNT 3F5.0,F 10.7,NO I5,DATE NAME TIME SPEED 4A10 000600
C  CARD 2 START OF DATA . . X,TWOND,CCAD,N, AND PUMPCOUNT                 000700
C  CARD 3 NCYTOS AND   NTYP  2I2                                          000800
C  CARD 4 CELTYP DATA  16 TO A CARD IN F4.0 FORMAT                        000900
      DIMENSION CNA(50),NTITL(50),NTI(50),NT(50)                          001000
      DIMENSION  PUMPCN(50),N(50),SPCELS(50,50)                           001100
      DIMENSION CELTYP(50,50),AA (50,50),NTITLE(50),NTIT(50)              001200
      DIMENSION CCAD(50),X(50),TWOND(50),DRHO(6,6)                        001300
      DIMENSION  REF(3),DAT(3),NAME(3),CTIME(3),CSPEED(3)                 001400
      DIMENSION RHO(50),TDIL(50),FRHO(50),CCNOBK(50),TCELL(50)            001500
      DIMENSION NAMCEL(50),TSUB(50)                                       001600
       REAL N                                                             001700
      READ (5,1,END=777) NORUNS                                           001800
 1     FORMAT (I2)                                                        001900
 2     DO 82  MN=1,NORUNS                                                 002000
C TO CLEAR THE ARRAYS                                                     002100
      DO  3  I=1,50                                                       002200
      CCAD(I) = 0.0                                                       002300
      X(I) = 0.0                                                          002400
      TWOND(I) = 0.0                                                      002500
      RHO(I) =0.0                                                         002600
      TDIL (I) =0.0                                                       002700
      FRHO(I) = 0.0                                                       002800
      TCELL(I) =0.0                                                       002900
      PUMPCN(I) =0.0                                                      003000
      CCNOBK (I) =0.0                                                     003100
      NAMCEL(I) =0.0                                                      003200
 3    N(I) =0.0                                                           003300
      NC = 0                                                              003400
C THE NEXT STATEMENT IS TO READ THE SINGLE DATA CARD WITH THE             003500
C  REFERENCE NUMBER.                                                      003600
C THE COULTER COUNTS  BACKGROUND BEFORE AND AFTER ARE CALLED              003700
C  Z1 AND Z2.  THE VOLUME PER COUNTING UNIT IS CALLED VOLCNT.             003800
C  F WHICH IS ML PER PUMPCOUNT IS FOUND BY USING                          003900
C  THE TUBE SIZE, NUMBER OF TUBES ETC.  NO IS THE                         004000
C  NUMBER OF FRACTIONS USED IN THE EXPERIMENT.                            004100
      READ(5,4,END=777)REF,Z1,Z2,VOLCNT,F,NO,DAT,NAME,CTIME,CSPEED        004200
 4    FORMAT(2A4,A2,3F5.0,1F10.7,1I5,4(2A4,A2))                           004300
 5    DO 6 I=1,NO                                                         004400
 6     READ(5,7,END=777)X(I),TWOND(I),CCAD(I),N(I),PUMPCN(I)              004500
 7    FORMAT(14X,2F10.3,1F10.0,2F10.3)                                    004600
 8    WRITE (6,9)                                                         004700
 9     FORMAT(1H1,'DATE      NAME      NOTEBOOK        CENTRIFUGATION     004800
     C   COULTER BACKGROUND    VOLUME PER      GRADIENT MATERIAL AND REMA 004900
     CRKS')                                                               005000
      WRITE (6,10)                                                        005100
 10    FORMAT(1H ,21X,'REFERENCE         TIME    SPEED         BEFORE     005200
     CAFTER    COUNTING UNIT',/)                                          005300
       WRITE(6,11)DAT,NAME,REF,CTIME,CSPEED,Z1,Z2,VOLCNT                  005400
```

```
 11   FORMAT(1H0,3(2A4,A2),6X,2(2A4,A2),F5.0,6X,1F5.0,7X,1F6.0,/////)     005500
C THIS IS TO CHECK IF THE PUMPCOUNTS HAVE BEEN ENTERED WITH THE DATA      005600
C IF NOT IT WILL FORM PUMPCOUNTS USING THE VOLUME COUNT AND THE          005700
C  FRACTION NUMBER.                                                      005800
       I = 1                                                             005900
      IF(PUMPCN (I).NE.0.)  GO TO  13                                    006000
       DO 12  I=1,NO                                                     006100
 12    PUMPCN (I)= I* VOLCNT                                             006200
C THIS WILL WRITE OUT THE HEADINGS FOR  THE N AND RHO                    006300
 13   WRITE (6,14)                                                       006400
 14   FORMAT(1H ,'    FRACTION NUMBER   X     N      X     RHO')         006500
C THIS SECTION  WILL FORM THE DRHO S  FROM THE THREE GIVEN N VALUES      006600
C  AND PRODUCE THE RESULTS.                                              006700
      M = 1                                                              006800
      DO  15  I=1,NO                                                     006900
      IF(N(I).EQ.0.)  GO TO 15                                           007000
      J = 1                                                              007100
      TEMP = (N(I) - .7022)/.633                                         007200
      DRHO(M,J)=I                                                        007300
      J = J+1                                                            007400
      DRHO(M,J) = TEMP                                                   007500
      M = M+1                                                            007600
      WRITE (6,16) I,N(I),TEMP                                           007700
 15    CONTINUE                                                          007800
 16   FORMAT(1H0,8X,1I3, 10X,  1F7.2,5X,1F10.5)                          007900
C THIS SECTION WILL FIND THE AVERAGE RHO AND PRINT THE RESULT            008000
      I = 1                                                              008100
      K = 1                                                              008200
       DO 18  L= 1,3                                                     008300
      J = DRHO(I,K)                                                      008400
      IF(J-1.EQ.0)  GO TO  17                                            008500
      CNA(L) = PUMPCN (J-1)+(PUMPCN (J)-PUMPCN (J-1))/2.                 008600
       GO TO 18                                                          008700
 17   CNA(L) = PUMPCN(J) /2.                                             008800
 18    I=I+1                                                             008900
      L = 2                                                              009000
      CNA(L)=(DRHO(K,2)-DRHO(K+1,2))/(CNA(L-1)-CNA(L))                   009100
C   STORES DRHO/DV IN THE SECOND SLOT                                    009200
      CNA(L+1) =(DRHO(K,2) -DRHO(K+2,2))/(CNA(L-1) - CNA(L+1))           009300
      AVRHO =  (CNA(L)+CNA(L+1))/2.                                      009400
C THIS SECTION WILL FIND THE DRHOS FOR EACH FRACTION                     009500
      WOW = CNA(1)                                                       009600
       DO  20 J=1,NO                                                     009700
      IF(J-1.EQ.0)  GO TO  19                                            009800
      CNA(J)=PUMPCN(J-1)+(PUMPCN(J)-PUMPCN(J-1))/2.                      009900
       GO TO  20                                                         010000
 19   CNA(J)  = PUMPCN(J)                                                010100
 20    RHO(J)=AVRHO*(CNA(J)-WOW)  +DRHO(1,2)                             010200
      Z = (Z1 +Z2)/2.                                                    010300
C TO FIND THE TOTAL DILUTION                                             010400
       DO 23  I=1,NO                                                     010500
      IF (I-1.EQ.0) GO TO 21                                             010600
      CNA(I) = PUMPCN (I) - PUMPCN (I-1)                                 010700
       GO TO 22                                                          010800
```

```
 21   CNA(I)  =  PUMPCN(I)                                                    010900
 22   FIRST = (CNA(I)*F) /(CNA(I)*F)                                          011000
      SECOND = (X(I)+TWOND(I))/X(I)                                           011100
 23    TDIL(I) = FIRST * SECOND * 2.                                          011200
C COULTER COUNTS AFTER DILUTION                                               011300
       DO 24  I=1,NO                                                          011400
 24    CCNOBK (I) = CCAD(I) - Z                                               011500
C TO FIND THE TOTAL NUMBER OF CELLS                                           011600
       DO 25  I=1,NO                                                          011700
 25    TCELL(I) = TDIL(I) * CCNOBK (I) * CNA(I) * F                           011800
C THIS IS TO FIND THE F(RHO)  FOR EACH FRACTION                               011900
      SUMCEL  = 0.0                                                           012000
       DO 26   I=1,NO                                                         012100
 26    SUMCEL  = SUMCEL  + TCELL(I)                                           012200
      WRITE(6,27)   AVRHO, SUMCEL                                             012300
 27   FORMAT(1H0,20X,'AVERAGE RHO =  ',1F15.10,'    SUMCELL =   ',1F10.0)    012400
      DO 29 I=1,NO                                                            012500
      IF (I-1.EQ.0)  GO TO 29                                                 012600
      FRHO(I) =-TCELL(I)/(SUMCEL *AVRHO*(PUMPCN (I)-PUMPCN (I-1)))            012700
      GO TO 29                                                                012800
 28    FRHO(I) = -TCELL(I) / (SUMCEL*AVRHO*PUMPCN(I))                         012900
 29   CONTINUE                                                                013000
C THE NEXT GROUP OF STATEMENTS WILL FORM THE CHART HEADINGS                   013100
      WRITE (6,30)                                                            013200
 30   FORMAT(1H1,'  CUMULATIVE    FRACTION                    SECOND DILUT   013300
     CION         TOTAL        COULTER         MINUS     TOTAL CELLS          013400
     CF(RHO)')                                                                013500
      WRITE(6,31)                                                             013600
 31   FORMAT(1H ,' PUMP COUNTS AT X NUMBER X   RHO           1ST DIL          013700
     C 2ND DIL   DILUTION  COUNTS AFTER  BACKGROUND  IN FRACTION')            013800
      WRITE (6,32)                                                            013900
 32   FORMAT(1H ,'  FRACTION END                                              014000
     C                         DILUTION ')                                    014100
C THIS IS TO PRINT OUT THE RESULTS                                            014200
      DO 33  I=1,NO                                                           014300
 33   WRITE(6,34) PUMPCN(I),I,RHO(I),X(I),TWOND(I),TDIL(I),                   014400
     CCCAD(I),CCNOBK (I),TCELL(I),FRHO(I)                                     014500
 34   FORMAT(1H0,5X,F6.0,8X,1I3,6X,1F7.4,12X,1F5.4,3X,1F5.2,7X,               014600
     C1F6.0,5X, 1F6.0,5X,1F6.0,7X,1F10.0, 5X,1F10.5)                          014700
      PUNCH 35, (RHO(I), I=1,NO)                                              014800
 35     FORMAT (2X, 13F6.4)                                                   014900
      PUNCH 36, (TCELL(I),I=1,6)                                              015000
 36    FORMAT ('UNFRACTIONATED CELLS', 6F10.0)                                015100
      PUNCH 37, (TCELL(I),I=7,NO)                                             015200
 37    FORMAT (8F10.0)                                                        015300
C  NCYTOS IS THE NUMBER OF CYTOGRAMS.  NTYP IS THE NUMBER OF THE CELLTYPE     015400
C  NC    IS THE NUMBER OF CARDS OF DATA  FOR EACH CYTOGRAM                    015500
C   THIS WILL READ IN THE MATRIX OF NUMBERS  FROM ALL OF THE CYTOGRAMS        015600
      READ (5,38,END=777) NCYTOS,NTYP                                         015700
 38   FORMAT (2I2)                                                            015800
       DO 39  MOO=1,NCYTOS                                                    015900
 39   READ(5,40)(CELTYP(I,MOO),I=1,NTYP)                                      016000
 40   FORMAT(16F5.1)                                                          016100
      DO 41 I=1,NTYP                                                          016200
```

```
 41    READ(5,42) NTITLE(I),NTITL(I),NTIT(I),NTI(I),NT(I)                  016300
 42    FORMAT(5A4)                                                         016400
       WRITE(6,43)                                                         016500
 43    FORMAT(1H1,15X,' ARRAY OF ORIGINAL DATA ')                          016600
       DO 44  I=1,NO                                                       016700
 44    CCAD (I) = RHO(I) - 1                                               016800
       WRITE (6,45) (CCAD(I), I=1,18)                                      016900
 45    FORMAT (21X,18F6.4)                                                 017000
       IF (NCYTOS.LT.19) GO TO 47                                          017100
       NUM = 18                                                            017200
       NC = 1                                                              017300
       GO TO 48                                                            017400
 47    NUM = NCYTOS                                                        017500
 48    DO 49  MAN = 1,NTYP                                                 017600
 49    WRITE(6,50)NTITLE(MAN),NTITL(MAN),NTIT(MAN),NTI(MAN),NT(MAN),       017700
      C(CELTYP(MAN,MOO),MOO=1,NUM)                                         017800
 50     FORMAT(1H0,5A4,1X,18F6.0)                                          017900
       IF(NC.EQ.0) GO TO 54                                                018000
       WRITE (6,51)(CCAD(I),I=19,NO)                                       018100
 51     FORMAT (//,21X,18F6.4)                                             018200
       DO 52 MAN=1,NTYP                                                    018300
 52    WRITE(6,53)NTITLE(MAN),NTITL(MAN),NTIT(MAN),NTI(MAN),NT(MAN),       018400
      C(CELTYP(MAN,MOO),MOO=19,NCYTOS)                                     018500
 53    FORMAT(1H0,5A4,1X,18F6.0)                                           018600
C  THE X ARRAY WILL CONTAIN THE TOTAL NUMBER OF CELLS FOR EACH CYTOGRAM    018700
 54    DO 55  II=1,NCYTOS                                                  018800
       X(II) = 0.0                                                         018900
       DO 55  JJ=1,NTYP                                                    019000
 55    X(II)=CELTYP(JJ,II)  + X(II)                                        019100
C  AA WILL BE THE ARRAY OF NUMBERS CELTYP(I,J) / TOTAL NUMBER OF CELLS     019200
C   FOR CYTOGRAM                                                           019300
       DO 57  II=1,NTYP                                                    019400
       DO 57  JJ=1,NCYTOS                                                  019500
       IF (X(JJ).NE.0.0) GO TO 56                                          019600
       AA(II,JJ) =0.0                                                      019700
       GO TO 57                                                            019800
 56    AA(II,JJ) = CELTYP(II,JJ) / X(JJ)                                   019900
 57    CONTINUE                                                            020000
C  PRINT THE ARRAY  AA                                                     020100
       WRITE (6,58)                                                        020200
 58    FORMAT(1H1,15X,' PERCENT OF INDIVIDUAL CELL TYPES IN EACH CYTOGRAM  020300
      C')                                                                  020400
       WRITE (6,59)(CCAD(I),I=1,18)                                        020500
 59    FORMAT (21X,18F6.4)                                                 020600
       DO 60 I-1,NTYP                                                      020700
 60    WRITE(6,61)NTITLE(I),NTITL(I),NTIT(I),NTI(I),NT(I),(AA(I,J),J-1,NU  020800
      CM)                                                                  020900
 61    FORMAT(1H0,5A4,1X,18F6.0)                                           021000
       IF (NC.EQ.0) GO TO 65                                               021100
       WRITE (6,62)(CCAD(I),I=19,NO)                                       021200
 62    FORMAT (//,21X,18F6.4)                                              021300
       DO 63 I=1,NTYP                                                      021400
 63    WRITE(6,64)NTITLE(I),NTITL(I),NTIT(I),NTI(I),NT(I),(AA(I,J),J=19,   021500
      CNCYTOS)                                                             021600
```

```
 64   FORMAT(1H0,5A4,1X,18F6.3)                                          021700
C THIS SECTION WILL FIND THE FRHO FOR THE EACH CELL TYPE                 021800
 65       DO 66 I=1,NCYTOS                                               021900
       DO 66 J=1,NTYP                                                    022000
 66   SPCELS (J,I) = TCELL(I) * AA(J,I)                                  022100
      DO 82  J=1,NTYP                                                    022200
      SUMCEL = 0.0                                                       022300
      DO 67  I= 1,NCYTOS                                                 022400
 67   SUMCEL = SUMCEL + SPCELS(J,I)                                      022500
      DO 70  I= 1,NCYTOS                                                 022600
      IF (CELTYP(J,I).NE.0.0) GO TO 68                                   022700
      FRHO(I) =0.0                                                       022800
      GO TO 70                                                           022900
 68   IF (I.EQ.1)  GO TO 69                                              023000
      FRHO(I)=-SPCELS(J,I)/(SUMCEL*AVRHO*(PUMPCN(I)-PUMPCN(I-1)))        023100
      GO TO 70                                                           023200
 69   FRHO(I)=-SPCELS(J,I)/(SUMCEL*AVRHO*PUMPCN(I))                      023300
 70   CONTINUE                                                           023400
 71   WRITE(6,72) NTITLE(J),NTITL(J),NTIT(J),NTI(J),NT(J)                023500
 72   FORMAT(1H1,20X,'DISTRIBUTION OF ',5A4,//)                          023600
      WRITE (6,73)                                                       023700
 73   FORMAT(1H0,'FRACTION     ORIGINAL      RHO       PERCENT     NO SP 023800
     C CELL     SUBTOTAL     PERCENT        SUB TOTAL    FRHO:'/': NUMBER 023900
     C        NUMBER                    CELL TYPE  IN FRACTION     OF TCELL 024000
     C       TCELL        OF PERCENT')                                   024100
      DO  74 M = 1,50                                                    024200
 74   IDA(M) = 0.0                                                       024300
C   THIS SECTION WILL FIND THE DISTRIBUTION OF SPECIFIC CELL TYPES       024400
      SUBPER = 0.0                                                       024500
      SUBTOT = 0.0                                                       024600
      DO 79  I=1,NCYTOS                                                  024700
      SUBTOT = SUBTOT + SPCELS (J,I)                                     024800
      IF (SUMCEL.NE.0.0)   GO TO  75                                     024900
      PTCELL = 0.0                                                       025000
      GO TO 76                                                           025100
 75   PTCELL = SPCELS  (J,I)  / SUMCEL                                   025200
 76   SUBPER = SUBPER +PTCELL                                            025300
      WRITE(6,78)I,CELTYP(J,I),RHO(I),AA(J,I),SPCELS(J,I),SUBTOT,PTCELL, 025400
     CSUBPER,FRHO(I)                                                     025500
 78    FORMAT(1H0,1I3,10X,1F6.0,6X,1F6.4,6X,1F6.4,7X,1F10.0,5X,1F10.0,   025600
     C3X,1F10.6,2X,1F9.5,6X,1F9.5)                                       025700
 79   CONTINUE                                                           025800
      TSUB (J) = SUBTOT                                                  025900
 80   FORMAT (5A4,6F10.0)                                                026000
      PUNCH 80, NTITLE(J),NTIT(J),NTI(J),NT(J),(SPCELS(J,I),I=1,6)       026100
      PUNCH 81, (SPCELS(J,I),I=6,NCYTOS)                                 026200
 81   FORMAT (8F10.0)                                                    026300
 82   CONTINUE                                                           026400
 777  CALL EXIT                                                          026500
       END                                                               026600
```

```
                      ENRICHMENT PROGRAM                                 000100
                                                                         000200
       DIMENSION  AA(50,50), SPCELS(50,50), ENRICH(50,50),RHO(50)        000300
       DIMENSION Y(50), UNFRA(50), NTIT(5,50), TSUB(50)                  000400
```

```
       SUMCEL = 297982344.                                              000500
       READ(5,1) NO,NTYP,NCYTOS                                         000600
 1     FORMAT (3I2)                                                     000700
       READ (5,5) (RHO(I), I=1,NO)                                      000800
 5     FORMAT (2X,13F6.4)                                               000900
       DO 10  J=1,NTYP                                                  001000
       READ (5,10)  TSUB(J)                                             001100
 10    FORMAT (1F10.0)                                                  001200
       DO  25  J=1,NTYP                                                 001300
       READ(5,15)(NTIT(K,J),K=1,5),(SPCELS(J,I),I=1,6)                  001400
 15    FORMAT (5A4,6F10.0)                                              001500
       READ(5,20) (SPCELS(J,I),I=6,NCYTOS)                              001600
 20    FORMAT (8F10.0)                                                  001700
       READ (5,25) (AA(J,I),I=1,NCYTOS)                                 001800
 25    FORMAT (16F5.4)                                                  001900
       DO 30  I=1,NTYP                                                  002000
       READ (5,30) UNFRA(I)                                             002100
 30    FORMAT (1F5.1)                                                   002200
C FIND THE PERCENT FOR THE UNFRACTIONATED CELLS                          002300
        X = 0.0                                                         002400
       DO 35  II=1,NTYP                                                 002500
 35     X =  UNFRA(II)  +  X                                            002600
       DO 45   II=1,NTYP                                                002700
       IF  (UNFRA(II).NE.0.0) GO TO 40                                  002800
       GO TO  45                                                        002900
 40     UNFRA (II)  =  UNFRA (II)  / X                                  003000
 45    CONTINUE                                                         003100
C  FIND THE PERCENT OF SPECIFIC  CELLS RECOVERED                         003200
       DO 50  I=1,NTYP                                                  003300
 50     Y(I) = TSUB(I) / SUMCEL                                         003400
C   PRINT THE PERCENT  ARRAY                                            003500
       WRITE (6,55)                                                     003600
 55    FORMAT(1H1,20X,'PERCENT OF INDIVIDUAL CELL TYPES IN EACH CYTOGRAM 003700
      C',///)                                                           003800
       WRITE(6,60)(RHO(I), I=1,15)                                      003900
 60    FORMAT (22X,15F7.4)                                              004000
        DO 70  I=1,NTYP                                                 004100
      WRITE (6,70)(NTIT(J,I),J=1,5),(AA(I,J),J=1,15)                    004200
 70    FORMAT (1H0,5A4,1X,15F7.3)                                       004300
       WRITE (6,75) (RHO(I),I=16,NCYTOS)                                004400
 75    FORMAT(1H1,20X,10F7.4,'  UNFRACT  NUM SPCEL  PERCENT SPCEL',/,93 004500
      CX,'CELLS   IN GRADIENT  RECOVERED')                              004600
       DO 80  I=1,NTYP                                                  004700
       WRITE (6,80)(NTIT(J,I),J=1,5),(AA(I,J),J=16,NCYTOS),UNFRA(I),    004800
      CTSUB(I),Y(I)                                                     004900
 80    FORMAT(1H0,5A4,11F7.4,2X,1F10.1,3X,1F10.7)                       005000
       DO 105  J=1,NTYP                                                 005100
       WRITE (6,85)(NTIT(K,J),K=1,5)                                    005200
 85    FORMAT(1H1,30X,'DISTRIBUTION OF ',5A4,//)                        005300
       WRITE (6,86)                                                     005400
 86    FORMAT(1H0,'FRACTION      RHO       PERCENT SPECIFIC          NO  005500
      CSP CELL           PERCENT SPECIFIC          ENRICHMENT',//,' NUMBER 005600
      C               CELL TYPE IN FRACT         IN FRACTION        CELLS 005700
      CIN GRADIENT')                                                    005800
        DO 105  I=1, NCYTOS                                             005900
```

```
      IF (Y(J).EQ.0.0)  GO TO 90                                          006000
      ENRICH(J,I) = AA(J,I) / Y(J)                                        006100
      GO TO 95                                                            006200
90    ENRICH (J,I) = 0.0                                                  006300
95    PTCELL = SPCELS(J,I) /  TSUB(J)                                     006400
      WRITE (6,100) I,RHO(I),AA(J,I),SPCELS(J,I),PTCELL,ENRICH(J,I)       006500
100   FORMAT(1H0,1I4,8X,1F6.4,10X,1F6.4,16X,1F10.0,13X,1F10.6,12X,1F10.   006600
     C4)                                                                  006700
105  CONTINUE                                                             006800
      STOP                                                                006900
       END                                                                007000
```

Glossary of Terms

AVRHO — The density increment per pump counting unint (PUMPCN). This is calculated by the program.

CCAD — Coulter counts after dilution. These numbers are found experimentally by the user and keyed in.

CCNOBK — Coulter counts with no background. The program calculates this by subtracting the average background from the CCAD for each fraction.

CELTYP — This array is the number of cells of a specific cell type per fraction. The array columns are the fractions and the rows are the cell types. For example:

	Fraction 1	Fraction 2	Fraction 3
Blasts	3	8	0
Erythrocytes	15	29	205

CSPEED — Centrifuge speed used during the run. This is keyed on the second card.

CTIME — Time of centrifugations.

DAT — Date of experiment.

DRHO — $\Delta\rho$, the density increment per fraction.

F — Milliliter per pump count.

FRHO — The function $F(\rho)$.

IDA — Initial diluent added.

NC — Number of cards of data for each cytogram.

NO — Number of fractions used in the experiment.

NORUNS — Number of experiments to be processed at one time.

NT, NTI, NTIT, NTITL, and NTITLE — Cell names read in as five literals together so that a name up to 20 characters long can be read in. Each data card has one cell name (left-justified) such as ERYTHROCYTES. If the user wants an alphabetical list at the end the data must be entered in alphabetical

	order. Note that the order in which the names are read *must* be the same as that in which the data set CELTYP is entered.
NTYP	The number of cell types.
PTCELL	Percent of a particular cell type of the total cells.
PUMPCN	Individual pump counts for each fraction.
REF	Notebook reference.

ACKNOWLEDGMENTS

I wish to thank my students, R. L. Warters, M. A. Hirsch, W. C. Kneece, R. A. Thomas, J. T. Thornthwaite, T. A. Yopp, and L. A. Dunlap; my colleagues, S. B. Smith, W. Cieplinski, H. Lipner, and B. F. Cameron; my electrical engineers, N. Lefkove and K. Leeburn; and my programmer, S. B. Leif, for providing the data for this manuscript. Also, I wish to thank Mrs. D. H. K. Hindman for her excellent editorial assistance, Mrs. Paulette Smariga for her assistance in describing the preparation of BSA and saline solutions, and Messrs. G. Ondricek and C. Railey for the graphics. This work was supported by NIH grants CA 13441, GM 18671, American Cancer Society Grant CH 46, Damon Runyon and Walter Winchell Grant DRG-1232, and General Research Support Grant to the PCRI #5S01-RR05690. The following figures are reprinted with the kind permission of the publishers: Figures 1 and 2, *Journal of Cellular Physiology;* Figs. 22, 28, 32, 34, 36, and 37, *Journal of Histochemistry and Cytochemistry;* Figs. 35, 38, and 39 and Tables 7 and 8, *Clinical Chemistry;* Fig. 27, *Journal of Immunology;* and Figs. 3, 15–19, *Analytical Biochemistry.*

REFERENCES

Anderson, N. G., 1955, Brei fractionation, *Science* **121**:775.

Anderson, N. G., 1956, Cells and tissues, in *Physical Techniques in Biological Research* (G. Oster and A. W. Pollister, eds.), Vol. 111, pp. 299, Academic Press, New York.

Barrett, D. L., and King, E. B., 1976, Comparison of cellular recovery rates and morphologic detail obtained using membrane filter and cytocentrifuge techniques, *Acta Cytol.* **20**:174.

Brakke, M. J., 1955, Zone electrophoresis of dyes, proteins and viruses in density-gradient columns of sucrose solutions, *Arch. Biochem. Biophys.* **55**:175.

Cieplinski, W., 1972, Studies of histone V (F2c) of chicken blood and erythropoietic system, Ph.D. thesis, Johns Hopkins University.

Coulter, W. H., and Hogg, W. R., 1970, Signal modulated apparatus for generating and detecting resistive and reactive changes in a modulated current passed for particle classification and analysis. US Pat 3,502,974. (Issued 1970.)

de Duve, C., Berthet, J., and Beaufay, H., 1959, *Prof. Biophys. Biochem.* **9**:326.

Dunlap, L. A., Warters, R. L., and Leif, R. C., 1975, Centrifugal cytology III. The utilization of centrifugal cytology for the preparation of fixed, stained dispersions of cells separated by BSA buoyant density centrifugation, *J. Histochem. Cytochem.* **23**:369.

Fox, T. O., and Pardee, A. B., 1970, Animal cells: Noncorrelation of length of G1 phase with size after mitosis, *Science* **167**:80.

Fox, G. D., Joyce, J. E., and Leif, R. C., 1968 US pat 3,377,021 (to International Equipment Corp.). (Issued 1968).

Goldman, M. A., and Leif, R. C., 1973, Centrifugal cytology II. Preliminary results on a wet chemical method for rendering scanning electron microscopy samples conductive and observations on the surface morphology of human erythrocytes and Ehrlich ascites cells, *Proc. Natl. Acad. Sci. USA* **70**:3599.

Hearst, J. E., and Vinograd, J., 1961a, *Proc. Natl. Acad. Sci. USA* **47**:999.

Hearst, J. E., and Vinograd, J., 1961b, The net hydration of DNA, *Proc. Natl. Acad. Sci. USA* **47**:825.

Hearst, J. E., and Vinograd, J., 1961c, The net hydration of T-4 bacteriophage DNA and the effect of hydration on buoyant behavior in a density gradient at equilibrium in the ultracentrifuge, *Proc. Natl. Acad. Sci. USA* **47**:1005.

Hirsch, M. A., H. Lipner, and R. C. Leif, 1979, The dissociation and separation of bovine adenohypophysial cells, *J. Cell. Physiol.* (submitted)

Ingram, M., and Minter, F. M., 1969, Semiautomatic preparation of coverglass blood smears using a centrifugal device, *Am. J. Clin. Path.* **51**:214.

Jansson, S. E., Kock, B., and Wegelius, O., 1967, Separation of mast cells from the peritoneal fluid of the rat with a GE nucleopore filter, *Experientia* **23**:407.

Kneece, Jr., W. C., and Leif, R. C., 1971, The effect of pH, potassium, sodium, bicarbonate, and chloride ions and glucose on the buoyant density distribution of human erythrocytes in bovine serum albumin gradients, *J. Cell. Physiol.* **78**:357.

Kolin, A., and Luner, S. J., 1969, Continuous electrophoresis in fluid endless belts, *Anal. Biochem.* **30**:111.

Kratky, O., Leopold, H., and Stabinger, H., 1973, The determination of the partial specific volume of proteins by the mechanical oscillator technique, *Methods Enzymol.* **27**:98.

Krishan, A., 1975, Rapid flow cytofluorometric analysis of mammalian cell cycle by propidium iodide staining, *J. Cell. Biol.* **66**:188.

Legge, D. G., and Shortman, K., 1968, The effect of pH on the volume, density and shape of erythrocytes and thymic lymphocytes, *Brit. J. Haematol.* **14**:323.

Leif, R. C., 1964, The distribution of buoyant density of human erythrocytes in bovine albumin solutions, Ph.D. Thesis, California Institute of Technology.

Leif, R. C., 1968a, Density gradient system I. The formation and fractionation of density gradients, *Anal. Biochem.* **25**:271.

Leif, R. C., 1968b, Density gradient system II. A 50 channel programmable undulating diaphragm peristaltic pump, *Anal. Biochem.* **25**:283.

Leif, R. C., 1970a, The buoyant density separation of cells, in *Automated Cell Identification and Sorting* (G. L. Wied and G. F. Bahr, eds.), pp. 21–96, Academic Press, New York.

Leif, R. C., 1970b, A proposal for an automated multiparameter analyzer for cells (AMAC), in *Automated Cell Identification and Sorting* (G. L. Wied and G. F. Bahr, eds.), pp. 131–159, Academic Press, New York.

Leif, R. C., and Thomas, R. A., 1973, Electronic cell volume analysis by use of the AMAC I transducer. *Clin. Chem.* **19**:853.

Leif, R. C., and Vinograd, J., 1964, The distribution of buoyant density of human erythrocytes in bovine albumin solutions, *Proc. Natl. Acad. Sci. USA* **51**:520.

Leif, R. C., Easter, H. N., Jr., Warters, R. L., Thomas, R. A., Dunlap, L. A., and Austin, M. R., 1971, Centrifugal cytology I. A quantitative technique for the preparation of glutaraldehyde-fixed cells for the light and scanning electron microscope, *J. Histochem. Cytochem.* **19**:203.

Leif, R. C., Kneece, W. C., Jr., Warters, R. L., Grinvalsky, H., and Thomas, R. A., 1972, Density gradient system III. Elimination of hydrodynamic, wall and swirling artifacts in preformed isopycnic gradient centrifugation, *Anal. Biochem.* **45**:357.

Leif, R. C., Gall, S., Dunlap, L. A., Railey, C., Leif, S. B., and Zucker, R. M., 1975a, Centrifugal cytology IV. The preparation of fixed stained dispersions of gynecological cells, *Acta Cytol.* **19**:159.

Leif, R. C., Hudson, J., Irvin, II, G., Cayer, M., and Thornthwaite, J. T., 1975b, The identification by plaque cytogram assays and BSA density distribution of immunocompetent cells, in *Critical Factors in Cancer Immunology* (J. Schultz and R. C. Leif, eds.), pp. 103–158, Academic Press, New York.

Leif, R. C., Smith, S., Warters, R. L., Dunlap, L. A., and Leif, S. B., 1975c, Buoyant density separation of cells. I. The buoyant density distribution of guinea pig bone marrow cells, *J. Histochem. Cytochem.* **23**:378.

Leif, R. C., Ingram, D., Clay, C., Bobbitt, D., Gaddis, R., Leif, S. B., and Nordqvist, S., 1977a, Optimization of the binding of dissociated exfoliated cervico-vaginal cells to glass microscope slides, *J. Histochem. Cytochem.* **25**:538.

Leif, R. C., Nordqvist, C., Clay, C., Cayer, M., Ingram, D., Cameron, B. F., Bobbitt, D., Gaddis, R., Leif, S. B., and Cabanas, A., 1977b, A procedure for dissociating Ayre scrape samples, *J. Histochem. Cytochem.* **25**:525.

Leif, R. C., Thomas, R. A., Yopp, T. A., Watson, B. D., Guarino, V. R., Hindman, D. H. K., Lefkove, N., and Vallarino, L. M. 1977c, Development of instrumentation and fluorochromes for automated multiparameter analysis of cells, *Clin. Chem.* **23**:1492.

Megla, G. K., 1973, The PARC automatic white blood cell analyzer. *Acta Cytol.* **17**:3.

Millipore Corp., 1966, *Techniques for Exfoliative Cytology,* Bedford, Mass.

Morgan, J. F., Morton, H. J., and Parker, R. C., 1950, Nutrition of animal cells in tissue culture; initial studies on synthetic medium, *Proc. Soc. Exp. Biol. Med.* **73**:1.

Oberjat, T., Zucker, R. M., and Cassen, B., 1970, Rapid and reliable differential counts on dilute leukocyte suspensions, *J. Lab. Clin. Med.* **76**:518.

Parker, R. C., Castor, L. N., and McCullock, E. A., 1957, Altered cell strains in continuous culture: A general survey, *Spec. Pub. NY Acad. Sci.* **5**:303.

Polliack, A., Lampen, N., Clarkson, B. C., and DeHarven, E., 1973, Identification of human B and T lymphocytes by scanning electron microscopy, *J. Exp. Med.* **138**:607.

Preston, K., and Norgren, P. E., 1971, A method of preparing blood smears, US Patent 3,577,267. (Issued 1971.)

Pretlow, T. G., II, Weir, E. E., and Zettergren, J. G., 1975, Problems connected with the separation of different kinds of cells. *Int. Rev. Exp. Path.* **14**:92–204.

Seal, S. H., 1956, A method for concentrating cancer cells suspended in large quantities of fluid, *Cancer* **9**:866.

Shortman, K., 1968, The separation of different cell classes from lymphoid organs. II. The purification and analysis of lymphocyte populations by equilibrium density gradient centrifugation. *Aust. J. Exp. Biol. Med. Sci.* **46**:375.

Shortman, K., 1969a, Equilibrium density gradient separation analysis of lymphocyte populations, in *Modern Separation Methods of Macromolecules and Particles* (T. Gerritsen, ed.), Vol. 2, pp. 167–181, Wiley, New York.

Shortman, K., 1969b, The separation of lymphocyte populations on glass bead columns, in *Modern Separation Methods of Macromolecules and Particles* (T. Gerritsen, ed.), Vol. 2, pp. 91–103, Wiley, New York.

Shortman, K., Haskill, J. S., Szenberg, A., and Legge, D. G., 1967, Density distribution analysis of lymphocyte populations, *Nature* **216**:1227.

Thomas, R. A., Cameron, B. F., and Leif, R. C., 1974, Computer based electronic cell volume analysis with the AMAC II, *J. Histochem. Cytochem.* **22**:626.

Thomas, R. A., Yopp, T. A., Watson, B. D., Hindman, D. H. K., Cameron, B. F., Leif, S. B., Leif, R. C., Roque, L., and Britt, W., 1977, Combined optical and electronic analysis of cells with the AMAC transducers, *J. Histochem. Cytochem.* **25**:827.

Thornthwaite, J. T., 1974, The buoyant density distribution and plaque cytogram assay for immunocompetent cells, Master's thesis, Florida State University.

Thornthwaite, J. T., 1977, Characterization of cells involved in cell-mediated immunity, Ph.D. thesis, Florida State University.

Thornthwaite, J. T., and Leif, R. C., 1974, Plaque Cytogram assay I. Light and scanning electron microscopy of immunocompetent cells, *J. Immunol.* **113**:1897.

Thornthwaite, J. T., and Leif, R. C., 1975, Plaque Cytogram assay II. Correlation between morphology and density of antibody-producing cells, *J. Immunol.* **114**:1023.

Thornthwaite, J. T., Thornthwaite, B. N., Cayer, M. L., Hart, M. A., and Leif, R. C., 1975, A new method for preparing cells for critical point drying, in *Scanning Electron Microscopy* (O. Johari and I. Corwin, eds.), pp. 381–402, IIT Research Institute, Chicago.

Thornthwaite, J. T., Cayer, M. L., Cameron, B. F., Leif, S. B., and Leif, R. C., 1976, A technique for combined light and scanning electron microscopy of cells, in *Scanning Electron Microscopy* (O. Johari and I. Corwin, eds.), pp. 127–130, IIT Research Institute, Chicago.

Thornthwaite, J. T., Thomas, R. A., Leif, S. B., Yopp, T. A., Cameron, B. F., and Leif, R. C., 1978, The use of electronic cell volume analysis with the AMAC II to determine the optimum glutaraldehyde fixative concentration for nucleated mammalian cells, in *Scanning Electron Microscopy,* Vol. 2 (R. P. Becker and O. Johari, eds.), pp. 1123–1130, Scanning Electron Microscopy, Inc., AMF O'Hare, Illinois.

Van Dilla, M. A., Fulwyler, M. J., and Boone, I. V., 1967, Volume distribution and separation of normal human leukocytes, *Proc. Soc. Exp. Biol. Med.* **125**:367.

Vinograd, J., and Hearst, J. E., 1962, Equilibrium sedimentation of macromolecules and viruses in a density gradient. *Fortschr. Chem. Org. Naturst.* **20**:373.

Warters, R. A., 1972, Utilization of BSA buoyant density centrifugation for the enrichment of heteroagglutinates of chicken erythrocytes and Ehrlich ascites tumor cells, M.S. thesis, Florida State University.

Watson, P., 1966, A slide centrifuge: An apparatus for concentrating cells in suspension onto a microscope slide, *J. Lab. Clin. Med.* **68**:494.

Williams, N., and Shortman, K., 1972, The separation of different cell classes from lymphoid organs. The effect of pH on the buoyant density of lymphocytes and erythrocytes, *Aust. J. Biol. Med. Sci.* **50**:133.

Wintrobe, M. M., 1974, *Clinical Hematology,* 7th ed., Lea & Febiger, Philadelphia.

Wolley, R. C., Dembitzer, H. M., Herz, F., Schrieber, K., and Koss, L. G., 1976, The use of a slide spinner in the analysis of cell dispersion, *J. Histochem. Cytochem.* **24**:11.

Zucker, R. M., 1970, Fetal erythroid cell development: Density gradients and size distributions, *J. Cell. Physiol.* **75**:241.

5

Physical Separation and Characterization of Reticulocytes and Other Cell Fractions from Rat Bone Marrow, and the 1*g* Mini-Staflo

HOWARD C. MEL AND NARLA MOHANDAS

I. INTRODUCTION

Objectives of cell separation experiments can be either *analytical* or *preparative* in nature. The techniques for accomplishing such separations can be directed toward either a high-versatility, research capability or toward more focused, restricted research goals. Previous stable-flow free boundary (Staflo) methods, principally sedimentation and electrophoresis, were developed to meet both of the above kinds of cell separation needs (Mel, 1960, 1964, 1970; Tippetts *et al.,* 1967). Furthermore, previous Staflo apparatuses were conceived and developed for the widest possible range of applications regardless of the complexity or sophistication of constructions and operation. In other words, if it appeared that a given feature *might* be important or useful, it was included.

The present work represents essentially an opposite approach, more or less responding to the question: what is the simplest Staflo sedimentation apparatus that can be rapidly designed and constructed to permit satisfac-

HOWARD C. MEL • Institut de Pathologie Cellulaire, Hôpital Bicètre, Le Kremlin Bicètre, France, and Division of Medical Physics and Donner Laboratory, Lawrence Berkeley Laboratory, University of California, Berkeley, California and NARLA MOHANDAS • Institut de Pathologie Cellulaire, Hôpital Bicètre, Le Kremlin Bicètre, France, and Departments of Laboratory Medicine and Medicine, Cancer Research Institute, University of California, San Francisco, California.

tory preparative separations of selected fractions of hematopoietic cells? In particular, we were interested in reticulocyte fractions from rat bone marrow, to determine certain of their physical properties and to relate these more generally to cellular aspects of erythropoietic control. Secondary objectives, if found not be adverse to the first, would be to obtain preparative quantities of at least one granulocytic fraction (for deformability measurements) and also to obtain additional analytical information about cell population distributions within the bone marrow. A particular interest in the latter was to be able to learn more about the distribution of "rare subpopulations," that is, occasionally occurring cells of one type in populations of predominantly another type.

The simple apparatus that resulted was the 1*g* mini-Staflo. As indicated below, it was possible to achieve stable operation almost immediately, to develop successful reticulocyte-enrichment procedures, and at the same time to largely attain the ancillary preparative and analytical objectives indicated above. This approach should be equally applicable to any other limited-objective cell separation problem of scope comparable to the present work.

II. THE 1*g* MINI-STAFLO

The heart of any Staflo apparatus is the flow cell. The present flow cell contains an open, rectangular (cross-section) migration chamber, depicted schematically in Fig. 1, fed from the right at four vertically arrayed inlet entry levels, with three horizontally spaced inlets for each level. The

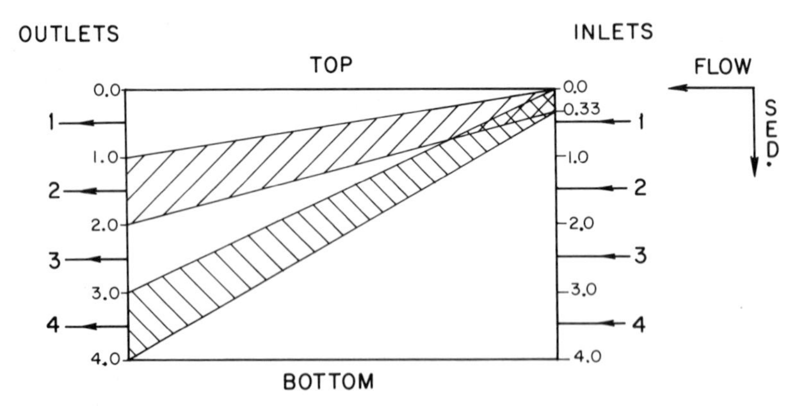

FIGURE 1. Theoretical two-component Staflo sedimentation profile in the central migration chamber of the flow cell.

central migration chamber is milled out of a larger slab of 0.5-cm lucite to have the interior dimensions: 15 cm (horizontal length) × 2.8 cm (horizontal width) × 0.5 cm (height). It is enclosed and sealed with solid lucite top and bottom pieces (not indicated in Fig. 1), all held together by screw clamps. The inlets themselves consist of four vertical columns by three horizontal rows (or twelve total) of hypodermic needles (22-gauge, cut 2.5 cm long), press-fit into holes drilled straight through the ends of the central migration chamber. Each needle is in turn force-fed through polyethylene tubing connected to a single syringe comprising part of a mechanically driven multisyringe pump. The twelve-channel outlet is identical in configuration. Each outlet delivers its exiting liquid via an 18-cm-long (0.9 mm i.d.) polyethylene tubing to the bottom of a corresponding collection container—a 20-ml plastic syringe barrel supported by its (closed) tip, as part of the 3 × 4 horizontally arranged collection system. Once the air has been purged from the system and all tips of outlet tubing are under the surface of liquid in the collection containers, this configuration assures the self-balancing hydrostatic–hydrodynamic feedback primarily responsible for the essential flow stability of the multilayer flow system (Mel, 1964).

The *sample feed* process is managed in a slightly different manner, using a special sample syringe consisting of two plastic syringe barrels fastened end to end (a "sample" barrel and a "drive" barrel), and containing a common double-ended piston of half the total barrel length. When the piston moves from one end of the double barrel to the other it empties one of the barrels and fills the other. In this way the sample syringe assembly can be mounted much closer to the flow cell inlet than can the much larger multichannel pump (i.e. within a few centimeters). This, therefore, reduces the travel of the sample suspension prior to entering the flow cell. Additional means were adopted to keep the sample cells well suspended and flowing smoothly into the flow cell. These were (1) a Teflon-coated magnetic stirring bar rotated slowly inside the sample barrel by an externally rotating magnet, and (2) a smaller-diameter (P.E. 20, i.d. = 0.38 mm) tubing connection from the outlet of the sample barrel, extending *through* the inside of the sample inlet needle, No. 1-middle inlet. (For a given volume flow rate per inlet channel, the linear flow rate is inversely proportional to the area of the inlet tubing.) The drive barrel is itself driven hydraulically through connecting tubing from a corresponding drive syringe on the multisyringe pump, and is thus constrained to drive sample into the flow cell at the same volume flow rate as for all the other pump syringes.

For all the experiments reported here a five-inlet-layer configuration was employed despite the four-layer vertical array depicted in Fig. 1. This resulted from use of the "thin sample technique" previously reported (Tippetts *et al.*, 1967) whereby the three horizontal inlets in a given vertical level can generate two or even three vertically stacked layers, simply by feeding solutions of slightly differing densities into each (or combinations) of them. Specifically, we fed the sample suspension solely into inlet No. 1-middle; a slightly denser solution was fed into inlets No. 1-front and No. 1-back; these coalesced into a single layer beneath the sample. The complete arrangement of flowing layers was then:

Layer 1a:	⅓ layer in (vertical) thickness, at the top
Layer 1b:	⅔ layer in thickness, directly beneath 1a
Layers 2,3,4:	full layer thicknesses (1.25 mm), in successive downward positions

The geometry and dimensions of the migration chamber were arrived at in consideration of the particular objectives of the cell separation experiments to be performed:

1. *Only a small number of fractions required;* thus, a 4-vertical-inlet/outlet system would be sufficient as compared with the usual 12- or 16-inlet/outlet system (Mel *et al.*, 1965; Mel, 1970). (This should not lead to a significant reduction of separation capability for the low-sedimenting, nonnucleated, hematopoietic cells of prime interest.)
2. *Comparable resolution desired for the low-sedimenting fractions;* thus the 0.125-cm (vertical) layer thickness of the previous apparatus could be and was retained.
3. *Increased preparative capacity desired without sacrifice of compact size;* most previous migration chambers had the interior dimensions of 30-cm length, 0.7 cm (horizontal) width, and 0.125-cm vertical layer thickness, leading to a layer volume of 2.625 ml. The present layer dimensions of 15 cm × 2.8 cm × 0.125 cm generate a layer volume twice as large, 5.25 ml. Consequently the average residence times and sedimentation times are twice as great, for any given syringe pump volume feed rate, using a same- or more-compact-sized flow cell. (Note: for technical definitions of these and other separation parameters see section III.)

From the standpoint of fabrication, two substantial simplifications were found possible. First, a leak-proof seal was achieved between the flat-surface top and bottom pieces and the central migration chamber (of Fig. 1) using only a thin paraffin sheet gasket in place of the more elaborate machined tongue-and-groove construction of previous models (Mel, 1964, 1970). Second, the precision-machining of the inlet/outlet end portions of previous Staflos was eliminated in favor of simple straight-through drilled holes, sized to receive the lead-in needles. While this design might be expected to reduce somewhat the margin for range of operating conditions (e.g., with respect to flow rate) prior to onset of fluid turbulance, this was found not to be a problem for the present experiments.

In sum, compared with previous models, the present limited-objective 1*g* mini-Staflo cell achieved the following: (1) approximately equal resolution, for a smaller total number of fluid layers and total fractions, thus reducing the number of gradient solutions to prepare and collected fractions to handle, (2) double the fluid capacity, in an overall more compact apparatus (flow cell), and (3) considerable simplification of fabrication without significant loss of flow and separation control.

The complete arrangement of all the elements of the Staflo apparatus is shown in Fig. 2a. These elements include the following.

A. Multichannel Variable-Speed Pump

An available 12-channel forward and reversing motor-driven multisyringe pump with simple mechanical-clutch speed control was employed, but any type of smooth-flow, multichannel, variable-speed pump could have been used. (Since only 5 different inlet solutions were employed in the present work, a 5-channel pump would have been adequate, with choice of appropriate smaller-sized syringes for layers No. 1a and No. 1b to maintain the proper layer dimensions as discussed above.) For the present flow cell and bone marrow experiments, the 40-min average residence time corresponded to 2.63 ml/h/inlet. For general use, pumping rates should be such as to provide average residence times (fluid transit times) in the range of from a few minutes to 90–120 minutes. (For rapid set-up, cleaning by flushing, etc., a rapid-flow-rate setting is also useful.)

The individual pump syringes are connected via disposable 3-way valves alternatively to a set of filling solution flasks (gradient reservoirs) or to the flow cell inlets. The 12 valves are ganged mechanically by sprocket chain so as to operate simultaneously by rotating a single lever. Each pumping syringe communicates directly with a counterpart flow cell inlet, except for the "sample driving syringe" which communicates indirectly, as described above.

B. The Flow Cell

The flow cell consists of a central, open-rectangular migration chamber surrounded (and closed) by solid top and bottom blocks of lucite (details given above); the flow cell is supported by a clamp stand, which can tilt upward or downward and thus facilitate initial purging of air, cleaning, etc.

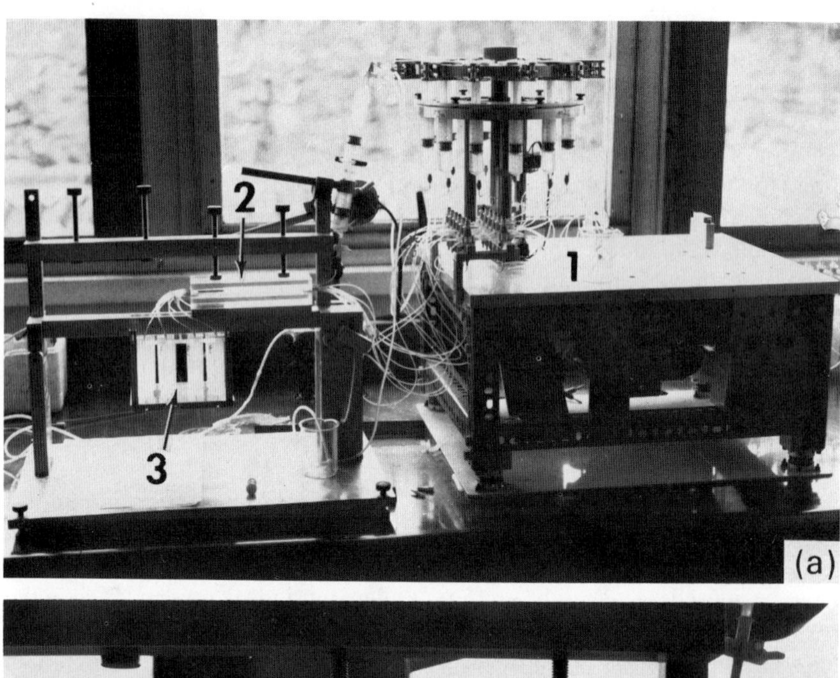

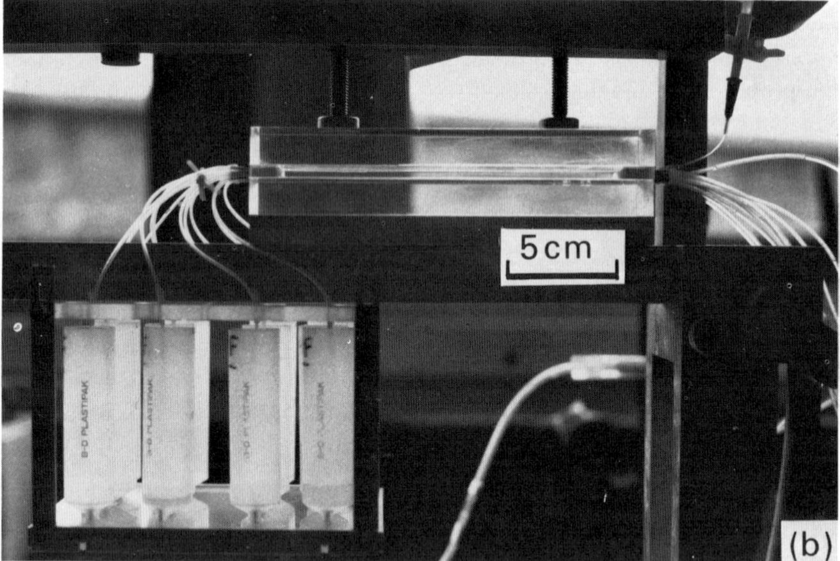

FIGURE 2. Photographs of 1*g* mini-Staflo. (a) Overview, including pump (1); flow cell (2); collection system (3). (b) Close-up of flow cell and collection system. Flow cell has internal (migration chamber) dimensions of 0.50 cm (height) × 2.8 cm (width) × 15.0 cm (length), with three horizontal × four vertical inlet–outlet arrays.

C. The Collection System

The 12-collector array of closed syringe barrels can be momentarily lowered during an experiment, elevator fashion, and another fresh array substituted, without disturbing the migration/collection pattern (additional details above). Typically this maneuver is performed some time after the initial steady-state flow configuration has been established at the start of definitive collection of separated fractions. Small, equal volumes of gradient must be present in each collection container at the time of changeover (about 1 ml), sufficient to cover the tips of the outlet tubing and thus insure continuation of the multisiphon "negative feedback" stabilization (Mel, 1964). (Air entering a single-outlet tubing can break the siphon, allowing the whole flow cell to rapidly empty out.) The 12-outlet tubings are held in a 3 × 4 geometrical arrangement matching the positions of the collection containers by being led through appropriately spaced holes in a lucite top guide-plate (best seen in Fig. 2b).

Figure 2b provides a close up view of the flow cell, clamp stand, and collection system. The bottom of the sample syringe assembly is seen at the upper right; just below it to the right are the other entering inlet tubings. The clamp stand is oversized for present purposes but used because it was available.

III. MODEL EXPERIMENTAL STUDIES AND THEORY

A. Sedimentation

The basic theoretical expression for 1g rigid particle sedimentation in a viscous medium is:

$$S = (1/g)v = (2r^2/9\eta)(\rho_{\text{part}} - \rho_{\text{med}})$$

where S is sedimentation rate; v is sedimentation velocity; r is spherical equivalent radius, η is the suspension viscosity, ρ_{part} and ρ_{med} are the density of particle and medium, respectively. The derivation of this expression is well known and will not be repeated here (e.g., see Mel and Ross, 1975). Suffice it to say that, though cells are in fact neither rigid nor spherical, and their densities are not well defined, this expression has been found to be surprisingly useful in ordering and quantitating cell sedimentation processes, despite an earlier belief that living cells were somehow anomalous in this regard (Mel, 1963).

B. Separation Criteria

In judging the needs for a cell separation experiment, in designing an experiment (selecting the parameters such as cell concentrations, duration of fraction collection, etc.), in assessing the results of a given experiment, in comparing objectively the results of different experiments and different experimental methods—for all of these purposes, it is important to have an agreed-upon set of theoretical separation concepts. We summarize below a set of four such criteria (definitions) from a recent publication (Mel and Ross, 1975), adding a fifth one dealing with resolution.

1. *Sample rate:* The total number of cells processed per unit time.
2. *Capacity:* The volume of medium (including sample suspension) handled per unit time.
3. *Recovery:* The percentage of cells from the starting sample recovered in any or all subfractions of interest.
4. *Enrichment:* The ratio of the "concentration" of a specified cell type in a given subfraction to that in the starting sample.
   a. Absolute enrichment: concentrations expressed in cells/cm^3.
   b. Relative enrichment: concentrations expressed in percentages of total cells or of a given cell type.
5. *Resolution* (of cell population A)*: The relative purity of population A compared with any other cell population B in a given fraction.

This is a minimal definition of resolution, not informative as to either the basis for the separation or the difficulty of the separation, or, hence, of the quality of the separation achieved. It does permit "cell population" to be defined either "biologically" (e.g., by morphological name, or by function), or physically, according to a measurable cell physical property such as size or sedimentation rate, or by both means simultaneously. We could thus speak of 90% resolution of erythrocytes from nonerythrocytes, or of erythrocytes in the size range $90 \pm 10\ \mu m^3$, from all other cells. For many cell separation purposes, more detailed, quantitative definitions are useful, further specifying resolution in terms of a measurable cell property (e.g., size, sedimentation rate), and expressing it relative to a particular population parameter (e.g., mode, mean, median). We thus define (as examples):

Resolution of A and B at the 15%-of-modal-size level: the percentage of cells A in a fraction, compared with A + B, where the modal size for B cells differs by 15% from that for A;

*The resolution of an *experiment* or even of a *method* is sometimes taken, in an imprecise sense, as the "best" resolution achieved (or theoretically achievable) for a component in a fraction.

Resolution of A and B at the 10%-of-mean-sedimentation-rate level: the percentage of cells A, compared with A + B, where the mean sedimentation rate for B cells differs by 10% from that for A;

most generally:

Resolution of A and B at the x% of (mode, mean, or median) of property p level: the percentage of cells A in a fraction, compared with A + B, where the (mode, mean, or median) of property p for cells B differs from that for cells A by x%.

Note that these definitions are chosen to reflect the intuitive notion that *high* resolution of A is expressed by a *large* percentage value for A cells. Note further that, as pointed out previously (Mel and Ross, 1975), certain of the criteria operate in a mutually contradictory fashion, so trade-offs must be involved in optimizing experimental design. Thus, factors increasing capacity or sample rate would typically lead to reductions in enrichment or resolution.

C. Theoretical Model Studies

We can now use these concepts in the analysis of two theoretical model studies. Figure 1 depicts an idealized, theoretical Staflo sedimentation–migration profile for two discrete component populations. Assuming the sample to contain three times as many bottom fraction cells (component B) as top fraction cells (component T), and otherwise accepting the diagram at face value, the five kinds of separation criteria would be as follows:

1. *Sample rate* (cells/h): cell sample concentration (cells/cm^3) × sample inlet feed rate, Q_s (cm^3/h) (Since the sample enters through only one-third of the layer volume, the *sample* inlet flow rate Q_s would be one-third of an entire *layer* inlet feed rate, Q_l.)
2. *Capacity* (cm^3/h): $= 4 \times Q_l$
3. *Recovery* in fraction 2: 25% of total cells (100% of T cells)
in fraction 4: 75% of total cells (100% of B cells)
overall: 100%
4. *Absolute Enrichment:* 0.33, for both T and B components. (This "dilution" arises from all of each component ending up in three times its initial volume.)

   Relative Enrichment: for component T in fraction 2: 100/25.0 = 4.0
for component B in fraction 2: 0/75.0 = 0.0
for component B in fraction 4: 100/75.0 = 1.33
of component T relative to B, in fraction 2: $4.0/0 = \infty$

5. *Resolution:* of T in fraction 2, or of B in fraction 4: 100%; of T and B in fraction 2, at the 250%-of-mean-sedimentation-velocity level: 100% (This represents the resolution actually observed as the experiment of Fig. 1 was run, where the mean sedimentation velocity of fractions 2 and 4 are seen to be $1.5 - 0.167 = 1.33$, and $3.5 - 0.167 = 3.33$, respectively, in units of layers sedimented per unit residence time. If the sedimentation velocity of component B had been only 2.33 (in the same units) B would still have migrated downward and completely out of outlet layer No. 2 (into No. 3 rather than No. 4). In this case, 100% resolution of T and B would have been achieved at the 75%-of-mean-sedimentation-velocity level.)

By inspection of Fig. 1, it is evident that the "discrete" components T and B are themselves each "populations" in the sense of sedimentation velocity, since each of their "bandwidths" increases from 0.33 layer at the inlet to 1.0 at the outlet. Thus, their respective sedimentation velocities (in units of outlet layers per unit residence time) can be characterized more precisely

$$\text{for } T\text{: } 1.33 \pm 0.33$$
$$\text{for } B\text{: } 3.33 \pm 0.33$$

Sedimentation velocity v, expressed in these general units, can be easily converted into more conventional units, for example:

$$v_{\text{av}}(\text{mm/h}) = v_{\text{av}}(\text{layers/throughput}) \times \frac{d(\text{mm/layer})}{\tau_{\text{av}}(\text{h/throughput})} \tag{2}$$

There is also the relation:

$$\tau_{\text{av}}(\text{h}) = \frac{V(\text{cm}^3/\text{layer})}{Q_l\ (\text{cm}^3/\text{h} \cdot \text{layer})} \tag{3}$$

so that equation (2) can also be written as:

$$v_{\text{av}}(\text{mm/h}) = v_{\text{av}}(\text{layers/throughput}) \times \frac{d \cdot Q_l}{V} \tag{4}$$

Using the particular dimensions of the $1g$ mini-Staflo ($d = 1.25$ mm/layer; $V = 5.25$ cm^3/layer) we can write the equations in more specific form, e.g., for equation (2):

$$v_{\text{av}}(\text{mm/h}) = \frac{1.25}{\tau_{\text{av}}(\text{h/throughput})} \times v_{\text{av}}(\text{layers/throughput}) \tag{5}$$

Finally, we note the refinement that can be made by considering the previously described three-dimensional flow properties for the Staflo, wherein the *minimum* residence time, that for the *central* (or *middle*) outlets, τ_{min}, is ⅔ as great as the τ_{av} for the whole layer, or for the whole flow cell, (Tippetts *et al.,* 1967). Thus the sedimentation velocity for the central collected fractions would be:

$$v_{cen}(\text{mm/h}) = \frac{1.25}{\tau_{min}(\text{h/throughput})} \times v(\text{layers/min throughput}) \quad (6)$$

or

$$v_{cen} = \frac{1.875}{\tau_{av}} \times v(\text{layers/av. throughput}) \quad (7)$$

Since the minimum residence times are quite uniform for all material in the central fractions, highest-resolution separations are generally available from these fractions (Tippetts *et al.,* 1967), e.g., those pictured in Fig. 4a. For the slowest sedimenting fractions, it is the highest front–back fractions that will have the best resolution since they combine the shortest sedimentation distance with the longest effective residence time. This will be seen for our marrow sedimentation results, for fraction(s) 2FB.

Results for a different assumed starting sample—a sample uniformly distributed according to sedimentation velocity—are given in Fig. 3 and Table 1. For lack of additional information, the ‘‘cell populations’’ are here defined solely in terms of their (ranges of) sedimentation velocities, in units of outlet layers per residence time. [Since these are calculated directly from the vertical geometrical relationships between the starting sample (⅓ layer initial thickness) and the outlet fractions, these values, for fractions 2 and 4, are the same as for the previous example.] Because of the finite initial sample thickness, there will necessarily be some overlap between adjacent collected fractions. That is, some of the slowest sedimenting material (starting at the bottom of the sample layer) which is mostly confined to layer 1 will be able to reach and exit by layer 2, and some of the faster material (from the top of the sample layer) which normally reaches layer 2, will be retained in layer 1. The compositions of each of the collected fractions, according to sedimentation velocity distribution (using the data of Table 1 and reconciling the sum of the collected fractions to the uniform starting sample distribution), are depicted in Fig. 3. Using equation (5), the generalized sedimentation velocity data of Table 1 can be converted into specific sedimentation velocity data applicable to any given experimental conditions. For example, using τ_{av} = 40 min (0.667 h), we calculate the sedimentation velocities of fraction 1 to fraction 4 cells to be in the range of 0.79 to 6.24 mm/h, as tabulated in the last column of Table 2. These values can in turn be normalized, using equation (1), into the sedimentation *rate*

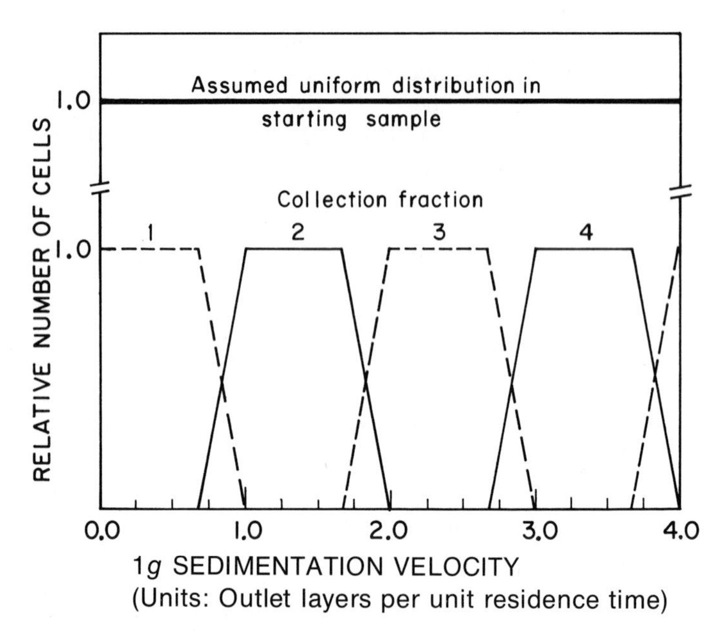

FIGURE 3. Idealized distributions of particle sedimentation velocities in Staflo collection fractions. The initial starting sample (one-third layer thick, at the top) is assumed to be uniformly distributed in sedimentation velocities.

TABLE 1
Compositions of Collection Fractions[a]

Fraction number	Sedimentation velocity			Percent overlap with adjacent fractions
	Minimum	Maximum	Mean	
1	0.00	1.0	0.42	4.2
2	0.67	2.0	1.33	8.4
3	1.67	3.0	2.33	8.4
4	2.67	4.0	3.33	8.4

[a]For theoretical Staflo sedimentation experiment of Fig. 3, in terms of $1g$ sedimentation velocities (expressed in terms of outlet layers sedimented per unit residence time).

data, tabulated in the first column of Table 2. These latter are convenient starting points for more quantitative analysis of the cell sedimentation process in terms of actual (effective) sizes and densities. As we shall see later, the bone marrow separation experiment provides a good example of the interplay of cell size and density in $1g$ sedimentation experiments.

TABLE 2
Mean Sedimentation Velocities and Rates[a]

Fraction	Mean sedimentation parameter: Sedimentation rate, $S = (1/g) \times v$ [10^{-7} s (or megasvedbergs)]	Mean sedimentation parameter: Sedimentation velocity, v (mm/h)
1	0.22	0.79
2	0.69	2.43
3	1.24	4.37
4	1.77	6.24

[a] For the theoretical sedimentation results of Table 1, assuming an average steady state residence time of 2400 s (40 min).

The numerical values of the theoretical percentages of overlap of adjacent fractions in this same hypothetical experiment are given in the final column of Table 1. The differences in these values from 100%—95.8%, 91.6%, 91.6%, and 91.6% for fractions 1, 2, 3, and 4, respectively—represent the percentages of *nonoverlap,* or of relative purity. They therefore satisfy the general definition for the resolution of each of the fractions. Though fractions 2, 3, and 4 all show the same degree of relative purity, the more detailed definition indicates resolution between adjacent fractions to be increasing with downward progressing fractions; that is, the 91.6% resolution holds at decreasing percentage differences of sedimentation rate (i.e., at the 68–75%-, 45%-, and 30%-of-mean-sedimentation-velocity level, for fractions 2, 3, and 4, respectively).

D. Experimental Particle Separation

Results for an actual model particle Staflo sedimentation separation experiment are given in Fig. 4 (5–22 μm diameter styrene divinylbenzene latex spheres; Mel, 1970). The particle sizes in Fig. 4b are means and ranges, determined by microscopic counts of several hundred particles in each fraction, using a calibrated reticle eyepiece. The upper and lower size limits calculated from assuming ideal Stokes law sedimentation behavior are given as the upper and lower solid lines in Fig. 4b; these by comparison with the actual data indicate that the sedimentation process was in fact close to ideal. [The size values for these particles and their densities (~1.055 g/ml) are comparable to those for hematopoietic cells.] A typical calculation for resolution of two adjacent fractions, 10_{cen} (13.2 μm) and 11_{cen} (14.7 μm), indicate for fraction 11_{cen} approximately 100% resolution at

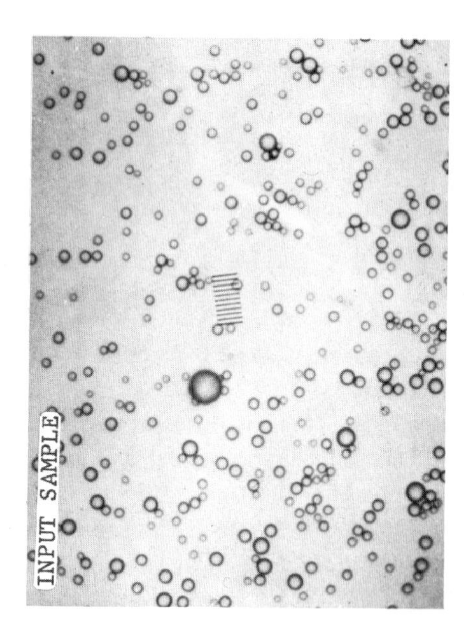
INPUT SAMPLE

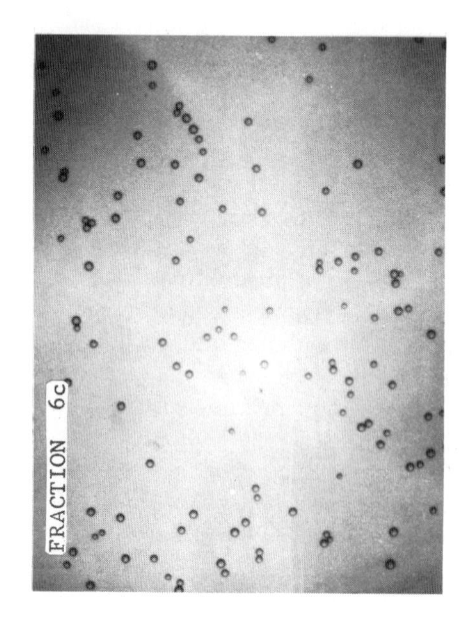
FRACTION 6c

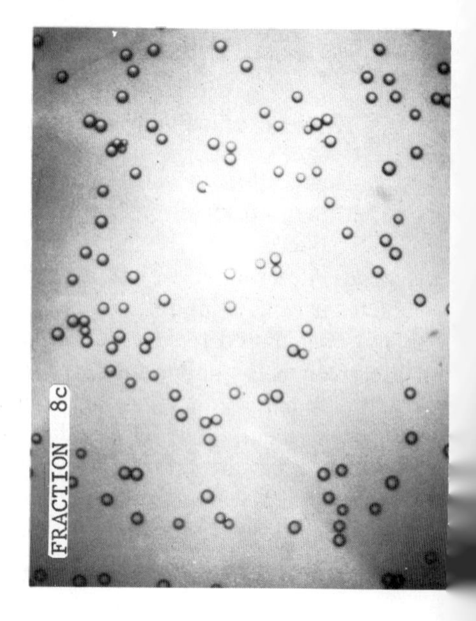
FRACTION 8c

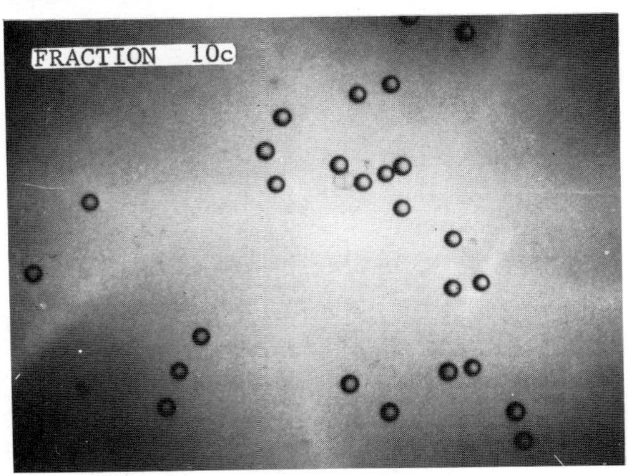

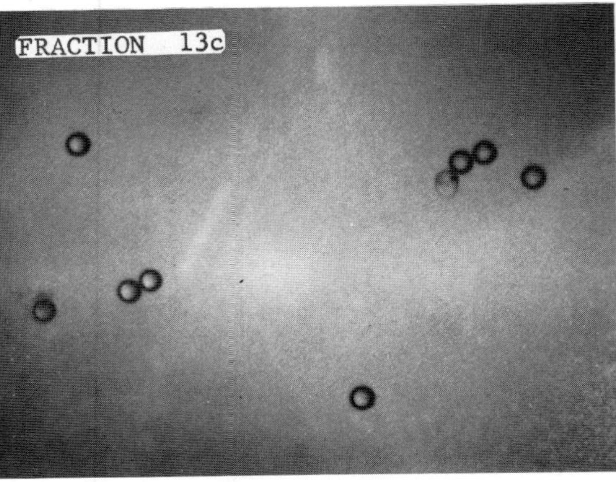

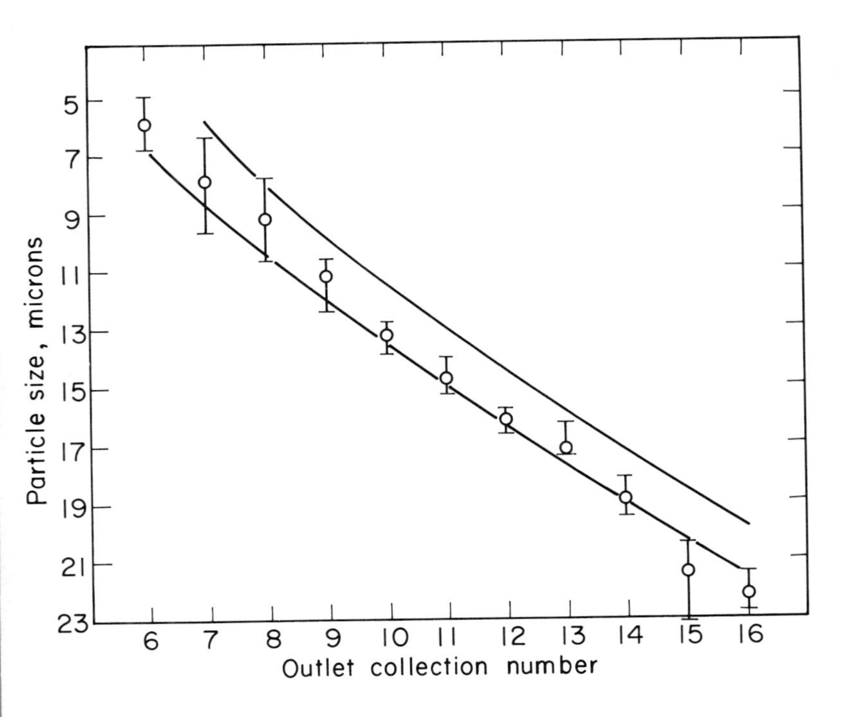

FIGURE 4. Model particle sedimentation: preparative and analytical separation for a styrene divinylbenzene latex particle suspension of diameters 5 to 22 μm. (a)Opposite page and left: Photographs of starting sample and selected collection fractions. (b)Directly above: Comparison of compositions of collection fractions, in terms of particle sizes, for limiting Stokes law behavior, using experimental data from fields such as shown in the photographs.

the 11%-of-mean-size level. (This experiment was actually carried out with a 3-horizontal × 16-vertical inlet–outlet Staflo apparatus with the same 1.25-mm layer thickness used for the 1*g* mini-Staflo, using a 28-min average residence time.)

IV. RAT BONE MARROW CELL SEPARATION

Bone marrow (and other hematopoietic tissue) displays an extraordinary cellular heterogeneity. As noted in the introduction, the conception of 1*g* mini-Staflo was motivated, in large part, by the need to preparatively fractionate rat bone marrow cells and to obtain cell subpopulations at specified or restricted stages of hematopoietic development for further study, especially enriched populations of reticulocytes and granulocytes. The biological results of this work are presented herein both for their own intrinsic interest and also to illustrate the application of the 1*g* mini-Staflo to this type of problem.

In designing these experiments the basic preparative requirement, of obtaining sufficient numbers of cells in the fractions in a reasonable time for the subsequent counting, sizing, and microscopic–cytological and deformability studies, was very much in mind. In addition it was necessary to preserve full cellular viability (not just dye exclusion capability) in order to study and quantitate the subtle movements of reticulocytes during their development and maturation. These two goals were met.

A. Cell Suspensions and Fractionation Conditions

Female Wistar rats weighing 150–220 g were used throughout this study. The marrow was removed as cylindrical blocks from the central shaft region of both femurs and was dissociated by aspiration and flushing twice through a 5/8 in. 25-gauge needle. Suspensions were then filtered through three thicknesses of 100-μm stainless steel mesh. The samples were resuspended as a single-cell suspension in phosphate-buffered saline (pH 7.4) containing 5% fetal calf serum (PBS-FCS) and 0.2% Dextran 40, at a concentration of about 20–30 × 10^6 cells/ml.

The gradient solutions consisted of the following: layer 1a—cell suspension in 0.2% Dextran 40 in PBS-FCS (cells omitted for pre-steady-state set-up); layers 1b, 2, 3, and 4—1.0%, 1.2%, 1.4%, and 1.6% Dextran in PBS-FCS, respectively. To set up the gradients in the flow cell, 7.0 ml (each) of gradient solutions (without sample) were pumped through the channel at a fast flow rate to flush out the saline solution used during assembly and for removal of air bubbles, followed by 5.25 ml each of the gradient solutions at the slow speed of the experiment (0.13 ml/min · layer, corresponding to a 40-min average residence time) to smoothly establish the layered gradients. The cell sample suspension was then switched into layer 1a (at the top of the migration chamber). Following a pre-steady-state period of one or two additional residence times, a fresh collection system was switched in place for definitive collection of fractions. In all the reticulocyte enrichment experiments, the 40-min average residence time was used and 8 to 12 ml of each of the twelve fractions were collected over a 3-to-5-hour period. Experiments were run at room temperature.

B. Compositions of Cell Fractions

The composition and material balance for separated fractions from a typical separation experiment are shown in Table 3. The starting bone marrow suspension contained 30% nonnucleated cells while the separated fractions 2FB, 2M, 3M, and 4M contained 81.6%, 67.5%, 12%, and 1.7% of nonnucleated cells, respectively. More than 65% of the nonnucleated cells in fractions 2FB and 2M were reticulocytes. Analogous to the significant enrichment and resolution of nonnucleated cells in fractions 2FB and 2M was the enrichment of nucleated cells in fraction 4M—98.3% nucleated objects, 92.3% intact nucleated cells. In a separate experiment conducted under comparable conditions, focusing attention on the compositions of nucleated cells, the ratios of granulocyte percentages to total nucleated percentages in the fractions were as follows: 2FB, 0.0/8.2; 2M, 0.0/17.2; 3M, 44.0/20.8: 4M, 77.6/12.0. Thus, for fraction 4M the resolution of granulocytes was 87%, relative to nucleated cells.

With respect to the total distribution of the starting sample in different fractions, 12.5% was collected in fraction 2FB, 14.8% in fraction 2M, 8.7%

TABLE 3
Compositions and Material Balance for Separated Fractions[a]

Fraction	Nonnucleated cells, %	Mature RBC, %	Reticulocytes, %	Total nucleated, %	Small dark (naked nuclei), %	Other nucleated cells, %	Total cells (10^6/ml)
Sample	30.0	10.0	20.0	70.1	14.3	55.8	27.3
2FB	81.6	28.3	53.3	18.4	14.2	4.2	3.41
2M	67.5	19.8	47.7	32.5	14.8	17.8	4.05
3M	12.0	3.5	8.5	88.0	10.5	77.5	2.38
4M	1.7	0.0	1.7	98.3	6.0	92.3	2.06

[a] From a typical normal rat bone marrow experiment (12/17/77). Percentages are based on total cells in each fraction.

in 3M, and 7.5% in 4M. About 50% of the cells in the starting sample settled to the bottom of the flow cell, having sedimentation velocities (either singly, or in pairs or clusters) greater than the maximum value designed to be collected in this series of experiments (1.77 megasvedbergs). The results in Table 3 indicate that the fractionation conditions chosen were in fact close to optimal for the stated objectives of reticulocyte and granulocyte preparative enrichment.

Ranges of compositions for nine separate, repeat fractionation experiments on normal rat bone marrow are given in Fig. 5. The results in Fig. 5a show the separation procedure to be reproducible, with consistent enrichments being obtained for nonnucleated cells in fractions 2FB and 2M, and for nucleated cells in 4M. For these same nine experiments the percentages of reticulocytes, based on total cells in each fraction, are given in Fig. 5b. Fractions 2FB and 2M contained on the average about 50% reticulocytes compared with the starting sample which contained on the average 20%.

C. Cytology of Cell Fractions

Figure 6 shows the photomicrographs of May-Grünwald, Giemsa-stained smears of the starting sample and fractions 2FB and 4M. The great variability in cell types and size in the starting sample is clearly seen in Fig. 6a. Figure 6b shows that nonnucleated cells comprised the vast majority of cells in fraction 2FB, and their apparent sizes are seen on the smears to be quite uniform. Immature granulocytes constituted greater than 80% of the cells in fraction 4M (Fig. 6c). A very small percentage of nonnucleated red cells including reticulocytes was consistently seen in this fraction, and occasional nucleated cells were consistently found in fractions 2FB and 2M. The possible significance of these small subpopulations with sedimentation velocities very different from their norms is considered in the discussion section (V).

In addition to the stained smears, we also made observations on the unfixed living cells from different fractions, and on this basis were able to define two classes of reticulocytes, R1 and R2 (Mel *et al.*, 1977). Motile, multilobular reticulocytes (R1) were found only in the marrow, being virtually absent in the circulating blood of normal (unstimulated) rats. Asymmetric "deep-dish" shaped, nonmotile reticulocytes (R2) made up about 70% of the normal rat marrow reticulocytes, and approximately 100% of the circulating reticulocytes. The differing percentages of reticulocytes in different fractions allowed us to establish that these two forms of reticulocytes, R1 and R2, accounted for all the reticulocytes as defined by the conventional staining methods (Mel *et al.*, 1977).

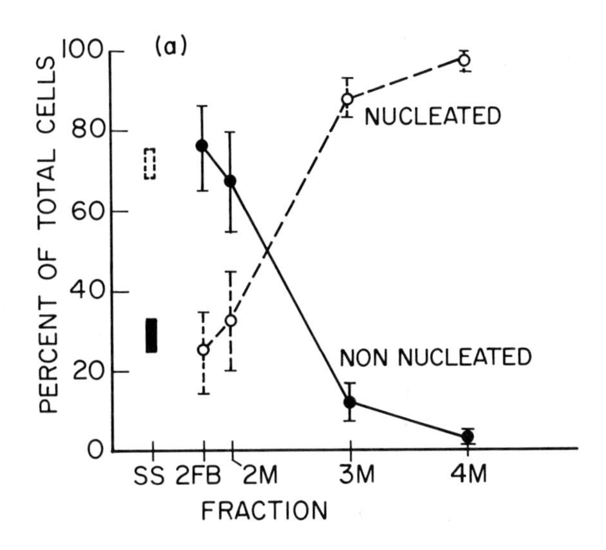

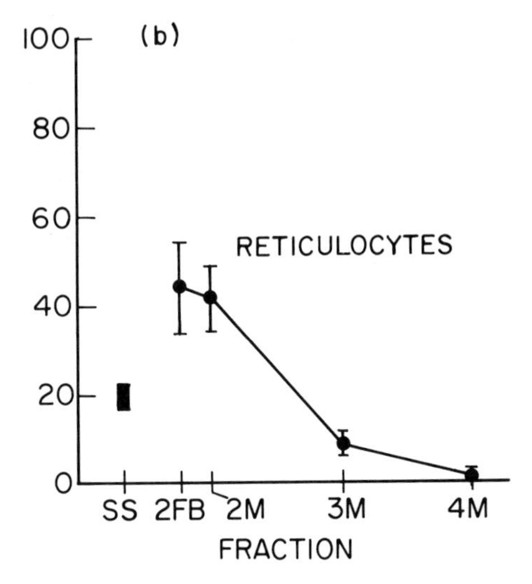

FIGURE 5. Ranges of compositions of fractionated normal bone marrow samples in nine repeat experiments: (a) nonnucleated vs. nucleated cells; (b) reticulocytes (based on total cells).

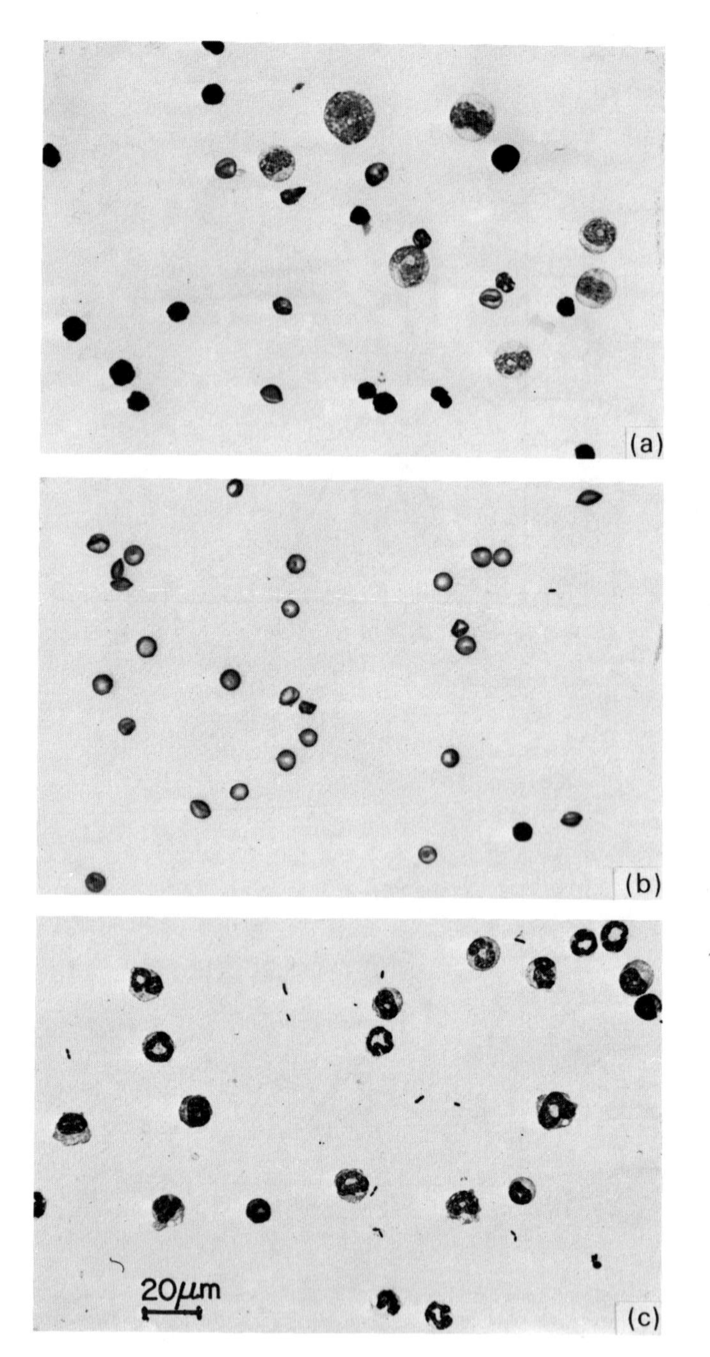

FIGURE 6. Photographs of bone marrow cell fractions: (a) starting sample; (b) fraction 2FB; (c) fraction 4M.

D. Sizing of Cell Fractions

The results of sizing using the "Cytograf" (BioPhysics Systems Inc., courtesy of SEMSA, Paris) for the starting sample and several different cell fractions are shown in Fig. 7. The size distribution of the starting sample is seen to be broad, with two apparent peaks. In contrast, the size distribution of cells in fraction 2FB is narrow and the peak channel corresponds to the first peak of the starting sample. Very few large-sized cells are present in this fraction, a result confirmed by the cytological observations. The size distribution of fraction 3M is very similar to that of the starting sample, with two apparent peaks, although slightly shifted from the corresponding ones in the starting sample. Given the compositional data of Table 3, the right-shift of the first peak is undoubtedly significant; this peak must correspond largely to the nucleated cells in the marrow that have slightly larger sedimentation velocities than the nonnucleated cells in fraction 2FB (the percentage of nonnucleated cells in 3M is on the average less than 15%).

A significant percentage of the cells in fraction 4M is found in a single peak that apparently corresponds to the second peak in the starting sample. This peak likely represents the size distribution of immature marrow granulocytes. However, a small percentage of cells with smaller size is also present in 4M. This must represent a smaller-sized but higher-density subpopulation of nucleated cells in the marrow having the same sedimentation velocity as the immature granulocytes. (The model particle studies of section III.D indicate that where particle densities are uniform, size distributions following Staflo sedimentation are also uniform.)

A comparison of the size distributions of fractions 2FB and 4M demonstrates the significant separation obtained, based on 1*g* sedimentation velocity, using the simple 1*g* mini-Staflo. The cells in fraction 2FB are seen to be 100% resolved from the large-sized cells in 4M. Fraction 4M does have some smaller-sized (and presumably higher-density) cells that overlap with cell sizes of fraction 2FB (though their sedimentation rates will overlap little, as indicated in section III.C).

E. Deformability Measurements

The deformabilities of enriched cell fractions of reticulocytes and granulocytes were measured by ektacytometry (Bessis and Mohandas, 1975). In this technique, the deformability of cells is determined by monitoring shear-stress-induced cell deformation in a couette viscometer, using laser diffractometry. The diffraction patterns of different cell fractions photographed at an applied shear stress of 100 dynes/cm^2 are shown in Fig. 8. It can be seen from this figure that biconcave red cells at zero stress give

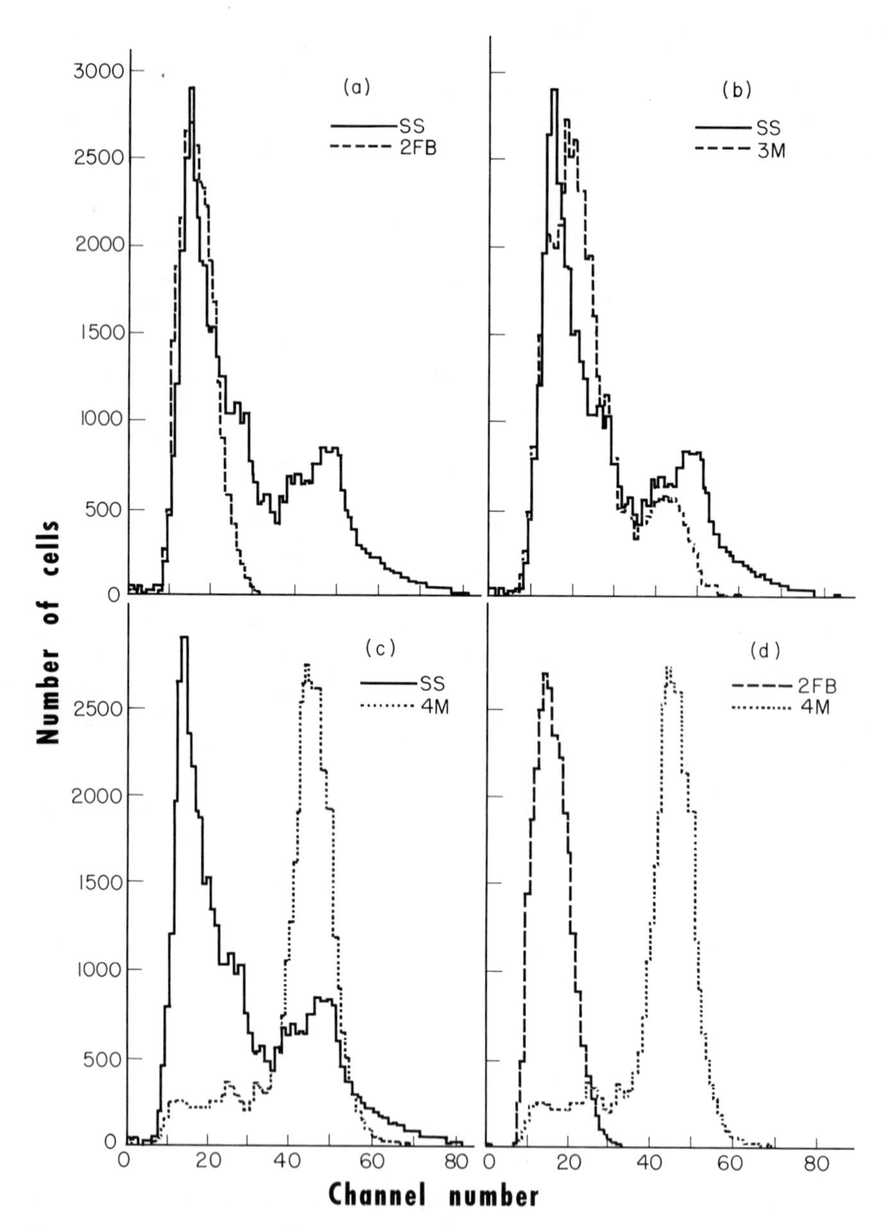

FIGURE 7. "Cytograf" sizing of bone marrow cell fractions. Each ordinate represents the number of cells per channel, each abscissa the channel number (relative cell size). Comparison of different fractions: (a) starting sample (SS) vs. fraction 2FB; (b) SS vs. 3M; (c) SS vs. 4M; (d) 2FB vs. 4M.

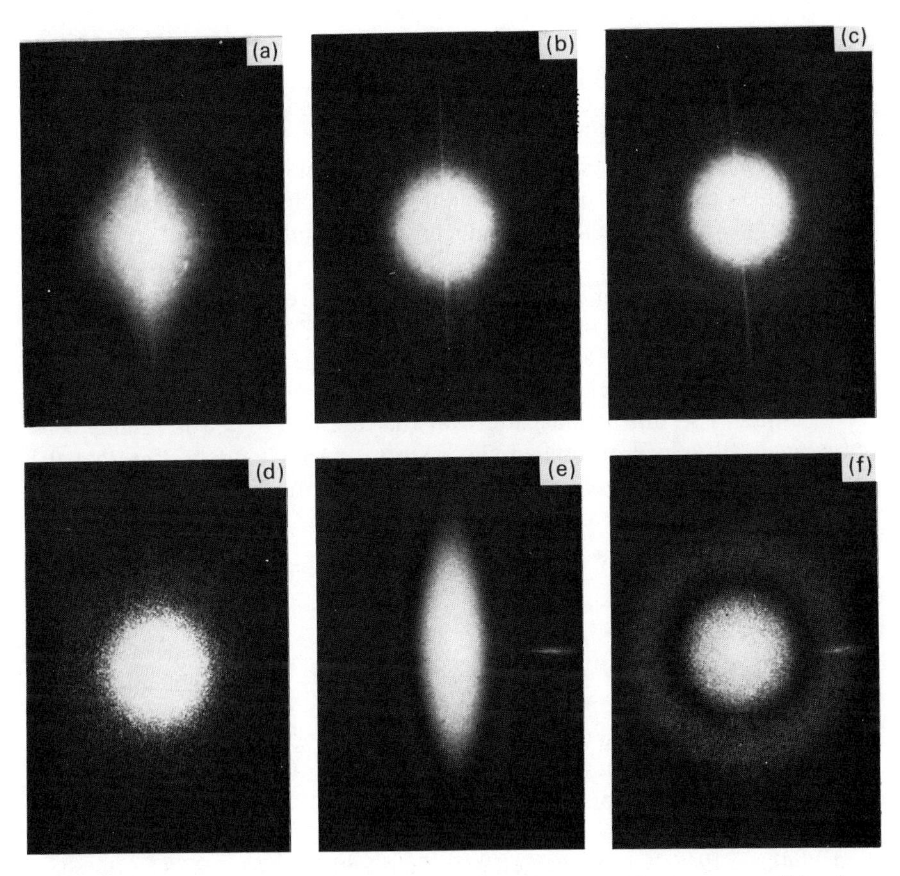

FIGURE 8. Cell deformability. Ektacytometer patterns of different bone marrow cell fractions photographed under an applied sheer stress of 100 dynes/cm^2(a–e), or 0 dynes/cm^2(f): (a) fraction 2M; (b) fraction 3M; (c) fraction 4M; (d) starting sample (SS); (e,f) blood.

a circular diffraction pattern (8f); the diameter of the diffraction rings is inversely proportional to the cell size (Bessis and Mohandas, 1975). When the red cells are deformed by the fluid shear stress of 100 dynes/cm^2 the discocytes are deformed into ellipsoids with a major axis dimension of 1.6 times that of the diameter of the discocyte, and the diffraction pattern is correspondingly elliptical (8e).

When both deformable and undeformable populations of cells are present in a sample, the resulting diffraction pattern at 100 dynes/cm^2 is a composite of an ellipse superimposed on a circle as seen in Fig. 8a for cell fraction 2M. From the intensity of the image in the circular and elliptical portions of the diffraction pattern it can be estimated that less than 30% of the cells in this fraction are deformable. As cell fraction 2M is composed 70% of nonnucleated cells, this suggests that no less than 40% of the nonnucleated cells in this fraction are undeformable or have significantly reduced deformability. Since the mature nonnucleated red cells are fully deformable, this leads us to conclude that the immature bone marrow reticulocytes have significantly reduced deformability. In fact, these data lend important support to hypotheses concerning the role of deformability in regulating maturation and release of red cells from the marrow into the circulation (Leblond *et al.*, 1971; Mel *et al.*, 1977).

The relative purity and size uniformity for the immature granulocytes of fraction 4M permitted the first deformability measurements on such a cell sample. The diffraction pattern of this fraction (8c) was found to be circular at all values of applied shear stress, strongly suggesting that the immature granulocytes of the marrow are undeformable under these conditions of measurement.

V. DISCUSSION

The cell separation methods most comparable to 1*g* Staflo sedimentation which have been applied to the hematopoietic system are the other hydrodynamically based ones. These include isopycnic gradient centrifugation (Evans *et al.*, 1974; Splinter and Reiss, 1974; Leif *et al.*, 1975), zonal centrifugation (Anderson, 1968, Boone *et al.*, 1968; Egan and Garrett, 1974), and the Staput system, for static sedimentation at unit gravity (Miller and Phillips, 1969; Glass *et al.*, 1975; Tulp and Bent, 1975). The detailed descriptions and the theoretical basis of these methods have been extensively reviewed (Pretlow *et al.*, 1975; Mel and Ross, 1975) and will also be found elsewhere in this volume. Ideally, the results from such different experimentation should be compared according to the separation criteria presented in section III or according to some other such set of criteria. Since no consensus has yet emerged on this matter, and since cell separations are carried out for widely differing purposes and their results reported in widely varying forms in varying degrees of completeness, such comparisons have not generally been possible. With the increased quantitative attention being paid to this subject, it is to be hoped that this situation will be ameliorated in the future, particularly for the benefit of the novice interested in a separation task but faced with a bewildering set of options as to how best to proceed.

To put the biological results of this paper into such a context, we calculate from Table 3 and from section IV.B the following: *sample rate:*

1.4 to 2.2 × 10^4 cells/s; total *capacity:* 8.75 × 10^{-3} ml/s; *recovery:* 50 to 60% (of cells processed); *absolute enrichment:* nonnucleated cells (2FB) 0.34, reticulocytes (2FB) 0.33, granulocytes (4M) 0.22, *relative enrichment:* nonnucleated cells (2FB) 2.72, reticulocytes (2FB) 2.67, granulocytes (4M) 2.87, granulocytes relative to nonnucleated cells (4M) 45.6, nonnucleated cells compared to granulocytes (2FB) ∞; *resolution:* nonnucleated cells (2FB) 81.6%, granulocytes relative to nucleated cells (4M) 87%. (For other data on hematopoietic cell fractionation by Staflo methods see Mel, 1963, 1970; Mel *et al.,* 1965.)

Partial comparisons can be made with results from two of the above-cited authors. From the Leif *et al.* (1975) buoyant density work (using BSA gradients): *relative enrichment:* nonnucleated cells, 2.11; granulocytes, 3.09; nonnucleated cells compared to granulocytes (fraction 1.0236), 48.9; granulocytes compared to nonnucleated cells (fraction 1.0646), 4.17; *resolution:* nonnucleated cells, 53.8%; granulocytes, 53.8%. Evans *et al.* (1974) removed the nonnucleated cells by lysis, so comparisons can be made for their Ficoll gradient results only for nucleated cells. For these they achieved, *resolution:* granulocytes, 85%.

The biological results presented here along with the above analysis, lead to two simple conclusions: (1) the hematopoietic cell separations achieved were able to satisfy the several goals set at the outset of this work; and (2) the simplified 1*g* mini-Staflo appears to serve at least as well as (if not better than) other available tools for these purposes.

The results cited and compared above, and indeed most cell separation results, are quite naturally slanted toward the major components in a mixture. Another level of interest, mentioned in section IV, is that of "rare subpopulations." Examples are the small numbers of reticulocytes in our fraction 4M, and the very infrequent intact nucleated cells in our fractions 2FB. These subpopulations are consistently found; they are physically very different from the majority of cells sharing the same Greek-based names (and the same sedimentation rates); they are easy to detect, in a great excess of very different-appearing cell types; and they may well have considerable significance beyond their small numbers, as clues for understanding mechanisms of normal and pathological hematopoiesis.

A final word should be added about the overall approach to any cell separation task. The planning and design of an optimal experiment is altogether a complex process, in some ways still as much an art form as a science. In any case it is a multidimensional trade-off of many different kinds of elements. If an apparatus is to be purchased or fabricated, factors such as initial cost, complexity of operation, expense and difficulty of maintenance, cost of gradient materials, etc., must be factored in, as well as the scientific criteria discussed in this paper. One different class of separation method may be cited as an illustration—cell sorting methods (e.g., see Steinkamp *et al.,* 1974). Such methods are inherently capable of extremely high resolution and offer great potential versatility. The price for these advantages is often minimal sample rate and capacity, and greater difficulty of keeping the cells alive. The practical matters of cost and complexity must also be seriously considered. Finally, along with all other cell separation methods they have their own particular set of scientific limitations (e.g., they do not appear readily adapted to separations according to sedimentation rate or surface charge density).

Whether the advantages of any given separation method outweigh the disadvantages is a question that cannot be answered *in abstracto,* but only in response to clearly delineated needs for a well defined problem. Given the enormous variety of cells and cell properties, of biological problems that can benefit from separations, and of differently perceived needs for solving these problems, a wide variety of methods and approaches will no doubt continue to be of use in the elusive search for the ultimate optimum.

VI. SUMMARY AND CONCLUSIONS

A simplified 1*g* mini-Staflo is described, which was designed and constructed for limited-objective preparative and analytical studies on bone marrow cells, but which would also be applicable to other separations of comparable scope. For the present experiments the cell separations, carried out by continuous-flow 1*g*-rate sedimentation, are seen to be based primarily on differences in cell size, though contributions from density differences are not negligible.

A set of theoretical separation criteria is described which enables quantitative analysis and meaningful comparison of different experiments and of different methods. These are illustrated by application to model theoretical and experimental particle separations, and to the hematopoietic cell separation results. In most separation experiments described in the literature, insufficient information is provided to evaluate some or most of these parameters: sample rate, capacity, recovery, enrichment, and resolution. It is hoped that the concepts presented here (or a similar set of agreed-upon parameters) may become widely utilized in the future to bring more systematization and order to this kind of work.

The bone marrow fractionation results reported gave rise to sufficient quantities of enriched viable reticulocytes and granulocytes to conduct size, deformability, and live-cell cytology studies on the fractions. This work permitted defining two new classes of reticulocytes and obtaining evidence that reticulocyte deformability serves as an important control variable for release of marrow reticulocytes into the circulation. In addition, the first Ektacytometer measurements were carried out on fractions of immature marrow granulocytes, indicating these cells to be undeformable. Analysis of these marrow separation results indicates the 1g mini-Staflo to be an excellent method (from the standpoint of resolution, enrichment, and other preparative separation parameters) in comparison with other single-step hydrodynamically based methods.

ACKNOWLEDGMENTS

We thank B. Cavadini and Stéphanie Mel de Fontenay for their excellent technical assistance. This work was supported by INSERM, France (Unité 48, Institut de Pathologie Cellulaire), U.S. Energy Research and Development Administration, and USPHS Grant HL 07100.

REFERENCES

Anderson, N. G., 1968, Preparative particle separation in density gradients, *Q. Rev. Biophys.* **1**:217.

Bessis, M., and Mohandas, N., 1975, A diffractometric method for the measurement of cellular deformability, *Blood Cells* **1**:307.

Boone, C. W., Harell, G. S., and Bond, H. E., 1968, The resolution of mixtures of viable mammalian cells into homogeneous fractions by zonal centrifugation, *J. Cell Biol.* **36**:369.

Egan, P. M., and Garrett, J. V., 1974, Separation of abnormal cells in the peripheral blood by means of the zonal centrifuge, *J. Clin. Pathol.* **27**:741.

Evans, W. H., Wolf, M. M., and Chabnev, B. A., 1974, Concentration of immature and mature granulocytes from normal human bone marrow, *Proc. Soc. Exp. Biol. Med.* **146**:526.

Glass, J., Lavidor, L. M., and Robinson, S. H., 1975, Use of cell separation and short-term culture techniques to study erythroid cell development, *Blood* **46**:705.

Leblond, P. F., LaCelle, P. L., and Weed, R. I., 1971, Cellular deformability: A possible determinant of the normal release of maturing erythrocytes from the bone marrow, *Blood* **37**:40.

Leif, R. C., Smith, S. B., Warters, R. L., Dunlap, L. A., and Lief, S. B., 1975, Buoyant density separation of cells. I. The buoyant density distribution of guinea pig bone marrow cells, *J. Histochem. Cytochem.* **23**:378.

Mel, H. C., 1960, Electrophoretic interaction studies by the stable flow free boundary method, *Science* **132**:1255.

Mel, H. C., 1963, Sedimentation properties of nucleated and non-nucleated cells in normal rat bone marrow, *Nature* **200**:423.

Mel, H. C., 1964, Stable-flow free boundary (STAFLO) migration and fractionation of cell mixtures. I. Apparatus and hydrodynamic feedback principles, *J. Theoret. Biol.* **6**:159.

Mel, H. C., 1970, Stable-flow free boundary cell fractionation as an approach to the study of hematopoietic disorders, in *Proceedings 8th Annual Hanford Biology Symposium 1968* (W. J. Clarke *et al.*, eds.), pp. 665–686, Oak Ridge, Tennessee.

Mel, H. C., and Ross, D. W., 1975, Biophysics of cell separations, *Q. Rev. Biophys.* **8**:421.

Mel, H. C., Mitchell, L. T., and Thorell, B., 1965, Continuous free-flow fractionation of cellular constituents in rat bone marrow, *Blood* **25**:63.

Mel, H. C., Prenant, M., and Mohandas, N., 1977, Reticulocyte motility and form. Studies on maturation and classification, *Blood* **49**:1001.

Miller, R. G., and Phillips, R. A., 1969, Separation of cells by velocity sedimentation, *J. Cell. Physiol.* **73**:191.

Pretlow, T. G., Weir, E. E., and Zettergren, J. G., 1975, Problems connected with the separation of different kinds of cells, in *International Review of Experimental Pathology* (G. W. Richter and M. A. Epstein, eds.), pp. 91–204, Academic Press, New York.

Splinter, Th. A. W., and Reiss, M., 1974, Separation of lymphoid-line cells according to volume and density, *Exp. Cell Res.* **89**:343.

Steinkamp, J. A., Romero, A., Horan, P. K., and Crissman, H. A., 1974, Multiparameter analysis and sorting of mammalian cells, *Exp. Cell Res.* **84**:15.

Tippetts, R. D., Mel, H. C., and Nichols, A. V., 1967, Stable-flow free-boundary (STAFLO) electrophoresis: Three-dimensional fluid flow properties and applications to lipoprotein studies, in *Chemical Engineering in Medicine and Biology* (D. Hershey, ed.), pp. 505–540, Plenum Press, New York.

Tulp, A., and Bont, W. S., 1975, An improved method for the separation of cells by sedimentation at unit gravity, *Anal. Biochem.* **67**:11.

Index